Endocrine Tumor Syndromes and Their Genetics

Frontiers of Hormone Research

Vol. 41

Series Editor

Ashley B. Grossman Oxford

Endocrine Tumor Syndromes and Their Genetics

Volume Editor

Constantine A. Stratakis Bethesda, Md.

18 figures, 8 in color, and 24 tables, 2013

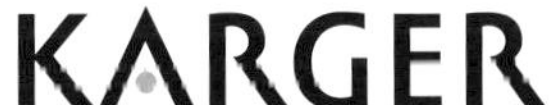

Basel · Freiburg · Paris · London · New York · New Delhi · Bangkok · Beijing · Tokyo · Kuala Lumpur · Singapore · Sydney

Constantine A. Stratakis, MD, D(med)Sci
Bethesda, Md.

Library of Congress Cataloging-in-Publication Data

Endocrine tumor syndromes and their genetics / volume editor, Constantine A. Stratakis.
p. ; cm. -- (Frontiers of hormone research, ISSN 0301-3073 ; v. 41)
Includes bibliographical references and index.
ISBN 978-3-318-02330-5 (hard cover : alk. paper) -- ISBN 978-3-318-02331-2 (e-ISBN)
I. Stratakis, Constantine A. II. Series: Frontiers of hormone research ; v. 41. 0301-3073
[DNLM: 1. Endocrine Gland Neoplasms--genetics. 2. Multiple Endocrine Neoplasia--genetics. 3. Neurofibromatosis 1--genetics. 4. Peutz-Jeghers Syndrome--genetics. 5. von Hippel-Lindau Disease--genetics. W1 FR946F v.41 2013 / WK 140]

616.99'44042--dc23

2013000040

Bibliographic Indices. This publication is listed in bibliographic services, including Current Contents® and PubMed/MEDLINE.

www.karger.com
Printed in Switzerland on acid-free and non-aging paper (ISO 9706) by Reinhardt Druck, Basel
ISSN 0301–3073
e-ISSN 1662–3762
ISBN 978–3–318–02330–5
e-ISBN 978–3–318–02331–2

Contents

Foreword

With the sequencing of the human genome in 2000, it was anticipated that most human disease would come into focus and that our increased understanding of molecular biology would initiate a whole range of new effective therapies. That this has not, for the most part, come about has led to a reconsideration as to the relevance of DNA technology to modern medicine. It is evident that the task of comprehending and treating human disease remains complex and difficult. However, there is one area in which our increased molecular knowledge has led to a considerable increase in our understanding of disease, and that is in endocrine oncology. We now realize that many 'sporadic' endocrine tumours arise on a background of germline mutations, even in the apparent absence of other syndromic features. This is particularly the case for phaeochromocytomas and paragangliomas, where as many as 30% of patients presenting with these tumours may have a 'genetic syndrome'. These are exciting times, and I am delighted that Constantine Stratakis has undertaken to review the current 'state of the art'. As a major contributor to this area, he has been able to bring together a stellar group of contributors to summarise our current knowledge. While the impact of our understanding of these germline syndromes on somatic tumour aberrations is less than might have been anticipated, these new findings have provided insights into novel signalling pathways which cannot but enhance our understanding of tumorigenesis in general.

From a personal point of view, I am really happy to have initiated this volume, which is the last in the series where I have been Editor-in-Chief. It has been a real pleasure having the freedom to choose the most engaging and fast-moving areas of modern endocrinology for the 'Frontiers' series, and I sincerely thank my talented clinical and scientific volume editors over the years who have made this series so successful. I am also very grateful to Thomas Nold (Karger Publishers) who has assisted me over much of this time, and has frequently but gently prodded me in the right direction in the most diplomatic manner. I am delighted that Prof. Ezio Ghigo is to take over the series, and I leave in his safe and experienced hands a series which I am sure will continue to flourish.

Ashley B. Grossman, Oxford

Preface

What Is New in the Genetics of Endocrine Tumors? From Classic Multiple Neoplasia Syndromes to Various Germline or Somatic Mutations in Sporadic Tumors

Contemporary genome-sequencing studies indicate that each human carries as many as 100 loss-of-function mutations with more than 20 genes completely inactivated [1]. In a recent Editorial, I stated that 'a patient can have as many genetic variants as he damn pleases' [2]. Hence, the subtitle of this note, which serves as an introduction to a wonderful collection of articles, written by leaders in the field, as updates on the genetics of endocrine tumors: 'From classic multiple neoplasia syndromes to various germline or somatic mutations in sporadic tumors'. The order of the reports in the book follows the theme of the subtitle [3–13] that is also the theme of this introductory note.

In other words, the description of the classic multiple endocrine neoplasia (MEN) syndromes, MEN1, MEN2, von Hippel-Lindau disease (VHLD) and Carney complex (CNC) [3–6], and their molecular elucidation led to the description of new associations: MEN 4, the paraganglioma syndromes, and Carney triad, the newest form of MEN to be described [7–9]. The description of these latter associations became possible after the germline genetic defects were identified in the former, because it became clear that a number of patients with pituitary tumors, pheochromocytomas, paragangliomas and other adrenal tumors did not have MEN1, MEN2, VHLD or CNC. In turn, the newly described associations allowed for the investigation of cohorts of patients with sporadic or inherited endocrine tumors, many of them with mutations in genes that were not previously suspected to be involved in endocrine tumors, such as, for example, the gene coding for the aryl hydrocarbon receptor interacting protein or AIP or cyclin-dependent kinases and their inhibitors. Today, a number of previously thought sporadic endocrine tumors are found to be predisposed to germline defects, some of these being simple genetic variants that do not always cause disease. This is well described in the chapters on pituitary, thyroid and parathyroid tumors in this book [10–12]. Finally, the careful investigations of cohorts of patients with genetic conditions that we knew them to be at the periphery of endocrinology, such as Peutz-Jeghers syndrome, neurofibromatosis or tuberous sclerosis, led to the description of a variety of endocrine tumors [13] and pointed to the respective molecular pathways and their potential involvement in endocrine tumorigenesis.

A book cannot capture everything that is going on in a field and, in our days, it is quickly relatively outdated. But a book like this should aspire to reflect the theme of the moment, represent the most significant advances of the field at present, and provide a useful compendium for at least the near future. I do believe the chapters in these series reflect well the changing world of modern genetics in endocrine tumors and its impact on clinical practice beyond the obvious implications for our understanding of endocrine tumor formation, molecular biology of cancer, in general, and the potential therapeutic implications.

It is indeed a new world out there for the practicing clinician. Every time we see a patient with the admittedly rare endocrine tumor, we now have to think somewhat differently from the past. We have to be knowledgeable about the associations described in this book (and suspicious of many new ones that have yet to be described) and be able to incorporate systems biology information into our daily clinical practice. When I proposed paraphrasing Hickam's dictum, 'a patient can have as many genetic variants as he damn pleases', I did not say that all sequence defects that are identified today by modern sequencing methods cause various diseases; the truth is far more complicated [2]. The evidence is that there is some redundancy, safety loops, and a tremendously complex molecular balance in human biology. But variants are there, in our genomes, and they do influence biology and how we respond to the environment; clinicians have to incorporate modern genetics in their daily practice. Likewise, educators and researchers have to introduce molecular pathways and their genetic variability in their teachings and understanding, respectively, of classic physiology and pathophysiology.

I thank Karger Publishers for asking me to edit this book; all staff members were wonderful to work with. A huge thank you goes to all our authors who provided timely their work product; our audience, I hope, will agree with me on the outstanding quality of all submissions. Finally, there was no research funding that was used for this editorial text and the opinions and statements made above are not those of the agencies or other organizations that have funded my official duties as a National Institutes of Health Senior Investigator.

Constantine A. Stratakis
North Bethesda, Md., USA

References

1 MacArthur DG, Balasubramanian S, Frankish A, Huang N, Morris J, Walter K, Jostins L, Habegger L, Pickrell JK, Montgomery SB, Albers CA, Zhang ZD, Conrad DF, Lunter G, Zheng H, Ayub Q, DePristo MA, Banks E, Hu M, Handsaker RE, Rosenfeld JA, Fromer M, Jin M, Mu XJ, Khurana E, Ye K, Kay M, Saunders GI, Suner MM, Hunt T, Barnes IH, Amid C, Carvalho-Silva DR, Bignell AH, Snow C, Yngvadottir B, Bumpstead S, Cooper DN, Xue Y, Romero IG; 1000 Genomes Project Consortium, Wang J, Li Y, Gibbs RA, McCarroll SA, Dermitzakis ET, Pritchard JK, Barrett JC, Harrow J, Hurles ME, Gerstein MB, Tyler-Smith C: A systematic survey of loss-of-function variants in human protein-coding genes. Science 2012;335:823–828.

2 Stratakis CA: Patients can have as many gene variants as they damn well please': why contemporary genetics presents us daily with a version of Hickam's dictum. J Clin Endocrinol Metab 2012; 97:E802–E804.

3 Agarwal SK: Multiple Endocrine Neoplasia Type 1; in Stratakis CA (ed): Endocrine Tumor Syndromes and Their Genetics. Front Horm Res. Basel, Karger, 2013, vol 41, pp 1–15.

4 Lodish M: Multiple Endocrine Neoplasia Type 2; in Stratakis CA (ed): Endocrine Tumor Syndromes and Their Genetics. Front Horm Res. Basel, Karger, 2013, vol 41, pp 16–29.

5 Chou A, Toon C, Pickett J, Gill AJ: von Hippel-Lindau Syndrome; in Stratakis CA (ed): Endocrine Tumor Syndromes and Their Genetics. Front Horm Res. Basel, Karger, 2013, vol 41, pp 30–49.

6 Espiard S, Bertherat J: Carney Complex; in Stratakis CA (ed): Endocrine Tumor Syndromes and Their Genetics. Front Horm Res. Basel, Karger, 2013, vol 41, pp 50–62.

7 Lee M, Pellegata NS: Multiple Endocrine Neoplasia Type 4; in Stratakis CA (ed): Endocrine Tumor Syndromes and Their Genetics. Front Horm Res. Basel, Karger, 2013, vol 41, pp 63–78.

8 Dahia PLM: Novel Hereditary Forms of Pheochromocytomas and Paragangliomas; in Stratakis CA (ed): Endocrine Tumor Syndromes and Their Genetics. Front Horm Res. Basel, Karger, 2013, vol 41, pp 79–91.

9 Carney JA: Carney Triad; in Stratakis CA (ed): Endocrine Tumor Syndromes and Their Genetics. Front Horm Res. Basel, Karger, 2013, vol 41, pp 92–110.

10 Gadelha MR, Trivellin G, Hernández-Ramírez LC, Korbonits M: Genetics of Pituitary Adenomas; in Stratakis CA (ed): Endocrine Tumor Syndromes and Their Genetics. Front Horm Res. Basel, Karger, 2013, vol 41, pp 111–140.

11 Bauer AJ: Clinical Behavior and Genetics of Nonsyndromic, Familial Nonmedullary Thyroid Cancer; in Stratakis CA (ed): Endocrine Tumor Syndromes and Their Genetics. Front Horm Res. Basel, Karger, 2013, vol 41, pp 141–148.

12 Hendy GN, Cole DEC: Genetic Defects Associated with Familial and Sporadic Hyperparathyroidism; in Stratakis CA (ed): Endocrine Tumor Syndromes and Their Genetics. Front Horm Res. Basel, Karger, 2013, vol 41, pp 149–165.

13 Kalkan E, Waguespack SG: Endocrine Tumors Associated with Neurofibromatosis Type 1, Peutz-Jeghers Syndrome and Other Familial Neoplasia Syndromes; in Stratakis CA (ed): Endocrine Tumor Syndromes and Their Genetics. Front Horm Res. Basel, Karger, 2013, vol 41, pp 166–181.

Stratakis CA (ed): Endocrine Tumor Syndromes and Their Genetics.
Front Horm Res. Basel, Karger, 2013, vol 41, pp 1–15 (DOI: 10.1159/000345666)

Multiple Endocrine Neoplasia Type 1

Sunita K. Agarwal

Metabolic Diseases Branch, National Institute of Diabetes and Digestive and Kidney Diseases, NIH, Bethesda, Md., USA

Abstract

Multiple endocrine neoplasia type 1 (MEN1) is an autosomal-dominant tumor syndrome characterized by the occurrence of tumors in multiple endocrine tissues and nonendocrine tissues. The three main endocrine tissues most frequently affected by tumors are parathyroid (95%), enteropancreatic neuroendocrine (50%) and anterior pituitary (40%). Tumors are caused by a heterozygous germline-inactivating mutation in the *MEN1* gene (1st hit) followed by somatic inactivating mutation or loss of the normal copy of the gene (2nd hit), leading to complete loss of function of the encoded protein menin. Most of the disease features and tumors are recapitulated in mouse models with heterozygous germline loss of the *Men1* gene. Also, tissue-specific tumors are observed in mouse models with homozygous somatic loss of the *Men1* gene specifically in MEN1-associated endocrine tissues. Hence, mouse models could serve as possible surrogates for studying MEN1 and related states. To gain insights into MEN1 pathophysiology, menin-interacting partners and pathways have been identified to investigate its tumor suppressor and other functions. Also, the 3D crystal structure of menin has been deciphered which could be useful to reveal the relevance of *MEN1* gene mutations and menin's interactions. This chapter covers clinical, genetic and basic findings about the MEN1 syndrome, *MEN1* gene and its product protein menin.

Multiple endocrine neoplasia type 1 (MEN1) is an autosomal-dominant tumor syndrome with no gender bias and with an approximate prevalence of 1 in 30,000 individuals. The disease, first described in two families in 1954, manifests as multiple hormone-secreting tumors, hormone nonsecreting tumors and nonendocrine tumors [1–3]. The disease manifests in adults around 40–50 years of age; however, early onset of the disease has been observed in a few children before the age 10 years [3]. Germline heterozygous mutation in the *MEN1* tumor suppressor gene encoding menin, located on chromosome 11q13, predisposes to the development of tumors. This chapter covers the clinical, genetic and basic findings about the MEN1 syndrome, *MEN1* gene and its protein product menin.

Table 1. Tumors associated with the MEN1 syndrome

Tumors	% penetrance (at age 40)
Endocrine (hormone-secreting or NF)	
Parathyroid	90
Entero-pancreatic neuroendocrine	
Gastrinoma*	40
Insulinoma	10
NF*, PPoma*	20
Glucagonoma*, VIPoma*, Somatostatinoma*, etc.	2
Anterior pituitary	
Prolactinoma	20
GH + prolactin secreting	5
GH secreting	5
NF	5
ACTH-secreting	2
Adrenal	
Cortex NF	25
Medulla	1
Foregut carcinoid	
Gastric ECLoma NF	10
Thymic carcinoid* NF	4
Bronchial carcinoid* NF	2
Nonendocrine	
Facial angiofibroma	85
Truncal collagenoma	70
Lipoma	30
Meningioma	5
Barrett's esophagus	5
Leiomyoma	
Uterus (in female)	30
Esophagus	5
Ependymoma	1

NF = Nonfunctioning; GH = growth hormone; PPoma = tumor secreting pancreatic polypeptide; VIPoma = tumor secreting vasoactive intestinal polypeptide; ECLoma = tumor of enterochromaffin-like cells; ACTH = adrenocorticotropic hormone.
* Tumor type with malignant potential for 25% or more cases.
Modified from Agarwal et al. [18].

Clinical Characteristics of MEN1

MEN1 is characterized by the occurrence of tumors in multiple endocrine tissues and in nonendocrine tissues (table 1). The three main endocrine tissues most frequently affected by tumors in MEN1 are parathyroid (95%), enteropancreatic neuroendocrine (50%) and anterior pituitary (40%). Typical MEN1 is defined as tumor in two of the three main endocrine tissues, which in familial MEN1, includes at least one relative with tumor in one of the three main endocrine tissues [3]. In addition, an MEN1 patient could present with many other hormone-secreting, hormone nonsecreting and nonendocrine tumors: adrenal cortical tumor, foregut carcinoid (bronchial, thymic or of the gastric enterochromaffin-like cells), facial angiofibroma, truncal collagenoma, lipoma, meningioma, Barrett's esophagus, leiomyoma (uterine in females, or in the esophagus), and ependymoma [3]. Approximately 25% of MEN1 patients die from cancer due to malignant gastrinoma (enteropancreatic neuroendocrine tumor) or foregut carcinoid tumor [3].

Primary hyperparathyroidism from parathyroid hormone-secreting multiple parathyroid adenomas is usually the first clinical manifestation observed in MEN1 patients typically between 20 and 25 years of age [3]. In a few patients, the first clinical manifestation has been observed as tumors of the enteropancreatic neuroendocrine tissues (multiple gastrinoma) or anterior pituitary (prolactinoma) [3]. Eventually the patients develop various combinations of the 20 or more tumor types associated with the MEN1 syndrome (table 1). MEN1-associated endocrine tumors are named after the hormones that these tissues produce because majority of these tumors secrete excessive amounts of hormone. Some endocrine tumors can be hormone non-secreting, therefore, clinically nonfunctioning (NF). The frequently observed skin lesions, facial angiofibroma (85%), truncal collagenoma (70%), and lipoma (30%) have been considered to be helpful for presymptomatic diagnosis prior to the appearance of the hormone-secreting tumors [3]. The earliest manifestation of MEN1 has been reported in two cases of insulinoma at age 6 years, and one case with pituitary macro-adenoma secreting prolactin and growth hormone at age 5 years or earlier [3]. Hence, routine periodic monitoring for tumors in asymptomatic MEN1 at-risk individuals by biochemical tests (for substances secreted by the hormone-secreting tumors) and imaging tests has been recommended beginning in early childhood at age 5 years [3].

Genetics of MEN1

Genetic linkage studies in kindreds, and loss-of-heterozygosity (LOH) studies in tumors established linkage of the MEN1 syndrome to chromosome 11q13 in 1988 [4]. Subsequently, in 1997, the *MEN1* gene was identified by a positional cloning approach [5, 6]. The 9-kb *MEN1* gene contains 10 exons transcribed into a 2.8-kb mRNA which encodes a 610 amino acid protein named menin (NCBI Reference Sequence: NM_130799.2, human menin isoform-2). Screening of the coding region and splice junctions has identified a heterozygous germline mutation of the *MEN1* gene in 70% of typical MEN1 index cases (familial or sporadic). No germline promoter mutations have been reported, and large deletions have been reported as rare in the *MEN1* gene [7]. Germline-inactivating mutation (1st hit) predisposes to the development of tumors in adults; tumors arise after loss of the remaining normal copy of the *MEN1* gene (2nd hit), classifying the *MEN1* gene as a tumor suppressor gene. More than 95% of tumors from MEN1 patients show LOH at chromosome 11q13 [7].

MEN1 gene mutation analysis has helped to identify the cause of various sporadically occurring tumors of the same types that are observed in the MEN1 syndrome. Somatic LOH at chromosome 11q13 is observed in 5–50% of such noninherited commonly occurring sporadic tumors [7]. Somatic *MEN1* gene mutation analysis has revealed that a fraction of these tumor types possess inactivating mutation in the *MEN1* gene: parathyroid adenoma (18%), gastrinoma (38%), insulinoma (14%), VIPoma (57%), nonfunctioning pancreatic tumor (16%), glucagonoma (60%), adrenocortical tumor (2%), bronchial carcinoid (35%), anterior pituitary tumor (3.5%), angiofibroma (10%) and lipoma (28%) [7].

Mutations in the *MEN1* gene are dispersed over the entire coding region with no significant hot spots, and no significant genotype/phenotype correlation with the tumor spectrum or with the clinical characteristics. More than 1,000 mutations have been reported which comprise: frame-shift deletions or insertions (40%), nonsense (20%), missense (25%), splice-site alterations (8%), in-frame deletions or insertions (6%), and large deletions (1%) [Agarwal and Marx, unpubl., 7]. Thus, 70–75% of the *MEN1* gene mutations are inactivating causing premature protein truncation, while many mutations (such as rare missense in nonfamilial cases) can be classified as mutations of unknown clinical significance due to lack of available assays that could provide evidence for an adverse physiological consequence of such mutations.

Identification of the genetic cause of the disease has become useful for the diagnosis of at-risk carriers affected by MEN1, and to rule out the disease in unaffected relatives of mutation-positive individuals. Although finding a pathologic *MEN1* gene mutation predicts the MEN1 syndrome, absence of mutation in a patient with MEN1 tumors does not exclude the possibility that the individual is affected with MEN1 [3].

Patients with incomplete MEN1 characteristics have been described as MEN1-like, where tumor occurs in as few as one of the three main MEN1-associated endocrine tissues [8]. In the 30% of MEN1 index cases without a germline *MEN1* gene mutation or in those cases that are MEN1-like but without an identified *MEN1* gene mutation, mutations could occur in regions not interrogated by typical screening methods, or mutations could occur in other genes. Candidate gene mutation analysis or whole genome/exome sequencing approaches could help identify the causative genes. The *p27* gene encoding one of the cyclin-dependent kinase inhibitors (CDKI) is one such candidate gene. Homozygous germline-inactivating mutation of the *p27* gene was found in a laboratory rat strain with a tumor spectrum similar to MEN1 and MEN2 with an additional feature of cataract (a syndrome named MENX) [for details about MEN2, see chapter by Lodish and for MENX, see chapter by Chou et al., this vol.]. Subsequently, the heterozygous germline p27 gene mutation has been reported in a few human MEN1-like cases. The CDKI genes consist of two families with total 7 members, the INK4 family (*p15*, *p16*, *p18* and *p19*) and the Cip/Kip family (*p21*, *p27* and *p57*), that negatively regulate progression through the cell cycle by inhibiting specific cyclin-CDK complexes. Possible rare heterozygous germline mutations have been observed in four CDKI genes (*p15*, *p18*, *p21* and *p27*) in index cases with MEN1 or MEN1-like disease [9]. In the OMIM database, MEN syndrome with the *p27* gene mutation was named MEN4 [see chapter by Chou et al., this vol., for details about MEN4]. No obvious genotype/phenotype correlation has emerged from the analysis of the few CDKI gene mutations reported in MEN1 and MEN1-like index cases. Interestingly, a mouse model with combined knockout of the *p18* and *p27* genes has shown features similar to MEN1 and MEN2A underscoring the importance of finding rare germline mutations in CDKI genes in human MEN1 and related states [10].

Mouse Models of MEN1

To study the consequence of *MEN1* gene loss, conventional and conditional knockout mouse models have been generated. Mice with germline homozygous loss of the *Men1* gene (*Men1–/–*) die in utero between embryonic days 10.5 and 14.5 [11]. Approximately 30–40% of the embryos show delayed development with craniofacial abnormalities, defective neural tube closure, heart hypertrophy, abnormal liver organization, hemorrhages, and edemas [11]. Mice with germline heterozygous loss of the *Men1* gene (*Men1+/–*) have been generated in four different laboratories (in Australia, France, UK and USA). These mice gestate normally, but are tumor prone. After 9–16 months, they develop endocrine tumors similar to those in the human MEN1 syndrome: parathyroid tumors, pancreatic islet tumors (mainly insulinoma; also, glucagonoma, glucagon + insulin mixed-hormone tumors, or gastrinoma), anterior pituitary tumors (mainly prolactinoma; also, GH-secreting somatotropinoma), adrenal cortical tumors, thyroid tumors, gonadal tumors (Leydig cells in male, or ovarian stroma in female), mammary gland tumors, and lipomas [11]. Tumors in conventional *Men1+/–* mice exhibit loss of the wild-type *Men1* allele (LOH), thus supporting a tumor suppressor role of the *Men1* gene in these tissues [11].

Conditional homozygous knockouts of the *Men1* gene in various MEN1-associated target tissues in mice have been generated using floxed *Men1* alleles and Cre-recombinase under the control of different tissue-specific promoters: parathyroid hormone promoter (PTH-Cre, for parathyroid cells), rat insulin promoter (Rip-Cre, for islet β-cells), glucagon promoter (GLU-Cre, for islet α-cells), and Pdx1 promoter (Pdx1-Cre for whole pancreas, exocrine and endocrine). After 9 months, mice with parathyroid-specific *Men1* gene knockout develop parathyroid hyperplasia and hypercalcemia [11]. Pancreatic islet β-cell-specific *Men1* gene knockout mice develop insulinomas (adenoma or carcinoma) at an earlier age (6 months) than the conventional *Men1+/–* mice [11]. Also, pancreatic α-cell-specific *Men1* gene knockout mice after 12 months show mostly insulinomas rather than the expected glucagonomas – a phenotype attributed to trans-differentiation of α-cells into β-cells, or the possible involvement of paracrine signals that induce β-cell proliferation [11, 12]. Despite loss of the *Men1* gene in the whole pancreas, Pdx1-Cre-driven *Men1* gene knockout mice develop tumors only in the endocrine pancreatic β-cells (insulinomas) after 10–12 months [11]. These observations highlight the importance of menin as a tumor suppressor in the parathyroid cells, and pancreatic β-cells. Although loss of menin expression occurs early in embryogenesis in the conditional knockout mice, delayed tumor formation implicates other hits for tumor formation.

Another mouse model with liver-specific homozygous *Men1* gene knockout develops normally, and lacks tumors in the liver, suggesting that *Men1* gene loss in the liver (a non-MEN1 target tissue) is tolerated and a tissue-specific action of menin is required for tumor suppression in MEN1-associated target tissues [11].

Some tumor types are specific to MEN1 in mouse, e.g. bilateral pheochromocytoma, and gonadal tumors are not observed in human MEN1 patients. Also, islet tumors in the conventional and conditional *Men1* gene knockout mouse models begin with polyclonal hyperplasia, a precursor stage observed in mice but not in humans. Pancreatic tissue from these mice could serve as a unique approach to study tumor progression and to identify other possible hits after *Men1* gene loss that play a role in tumorigenesis.

A MEN1 mouse model (germline *Men1*+/–) has been used to study the efficacy of anti-angiogenesis treatment (anti-VEGF-A monoclonal antibody, mAb G6–31) [13]. This treatment inhibited pituitary tumor growth in situ and in transplants, and lowered the elevated serum prolactin level. Also, similar efficacy was observed against pancreatic islet tumors [13]. Hence, mouse models could serve as possible surrogates for studying MEN1 and related states.

Menin-Null Cell Lines

To gain molecular insights about MEN1, a critical resource is the availability of cell lines from the tumor types associated with the disease. Cell lines from human or mouse MEN1-associated endocrine tissues with biallelic inactivation of the *MEN1* gene have not yet been established. Menin-null mouse embryonic stem cells (ESCs) and menin-null immortalized mouse embryonic fibroblasts (MEFs) have been derived using embryos from the mouse models of MEN1 [14–16]. A menin-null Leydig cell tumor cell line (LCT10) has been derived from a male *Men1*+/– mouse with Leydig cell tumor (testicular interstitial cell tumor, a tumor type not found in human MEN1 cases) [17]. Reconstituted expression of menin in the menin-null MEFs or in the LCT10 cell line delays progression through the cell cycle and reduces their proliferation rate, in agreement with the tumor suppressor function of menin [16, 17]. MEFs have been used extensively for the functional analysis of menin.

Wild-type and menin-null ESCs have been used for in vitro differentiation into pancreatic islet-like endocrine cells to generate homogeneous populations of cells to serve as an alternative source of menin-null endocrine cells [18]. Such cells have been used for genomewide studies to compare wild-type and menin-null cells for gene expression changes and other assays [18]. Thus, mouse ESCs could be used for generating other MEN1-associated endocrine cell types by in vitro differentiation protocols to aid in the analysis of endocrine-specific tumor suppressor functions of menin.

Menin Expression and Function

Menin is a ubiquitously expressed 67-kDa predominantly nuclear protein highly conserved in animal species (with no known homologs in yeast and nematodes). Localization to the nucleus is mediated by the two nuclear localization signals (NLS), NLS1 (amino acid residues 479–497) and NLS2 (amino acid residues 588–608), and a third accessory NLS, NLSa (amino acid residues 546–572) [7]. Most of the nonsense and frame-shift mutations in the *MEN1* gene predict premature protein truncation and thus loss of NLS, preventing the normal localization of menin in the nucleus.

Menin is reported to undergo phosphorylation at 6 different amino acid residues – Ser394, Thr397, Thr399, Ser487, Ser543, and Ser583 – constitutively (Ser543), or in response to DNA damage (Ser394 and Ser487) or upon loss of phosphorylation at Ser394 (Thr397 and Thr399) [19]. The importance of menin phosphorylation in tumorigenesis remains to be determined.

The primary amino acid sequence of menin is conserved but does not show any obvious homologous domains or motifs that would allow prediction about its biological function. Menin has not been shown to possess any enzymatic activity. Therefore, to uncover the physiologic processes perturbed upon loss of menin that lead to tumor formation, many proteins that interact directly or form a complex with menin have been identified. Work from many laboratories, using various protein/protein interaction methods, has reported approximately 40 different proteins that could partner with menin implicating a role for menin in the pathways and processes regulated by these interacting partners (table 2). Menin partners include DNA-binding transcription factors, chromatin modifying proteins and complexes, transcription initiation or elongation proteins, DNA-repair proteins associated with response to DNA damage, a protein responsible for mutant-protein degradation, signaling mediators in the cytoplasm, and cytoplasmic proteins associated with the cytoskeleton, cell division, adhesion or motility. Through interaction with transcription factors or chromatin-modifying protein complexes, menin acts as a transcriptional regulator either as a repressor or activator of transcription. This chapter will focus on some aspects of the interaction of menin with the transcription factor JUND, and with the chromatin-modifying mixed lineage leukemia (MLL) complex.

Table 2. Proteins reported to partner with menin

Functional categories and protein partners
Transcription
Transcription factors
JUND
c-MYB
NFκB – p50, p52, p65
PEM
RUNX2 (BMP2 signaling)
SMADs – SMAD1, SAMD3, SMAD5 (TGFβ signaling)
TCF3/TCF4/β-catenin (Wnt signaling)
VDR, RAR, PPARγ, ERα (nuclear hormone receptors)
Chromatin modification
HDACs/mSIN3A
LEDGF
MLL1/MLL2 (H3K4me3)
(ASH2L/hDPY30/HCF-2/MLL/RBBP5/RPB2/WDR5 complex)
Transcription initiation or elongation
RNAPII isoforms (pSer5 and pSer2)
SKIP/c-MYC (HIV-1 Tat:P-TEFb transcription)
DNA repair
ASK
CHES1
FANCD2
RPA2
Mutant-protein degradation
CHIP
Signaling mediators in the cytoplasm
AKT1
FOXO1
NM23β
Cytoskeleton/cell division/adhesion/motility
GFAP
IQGAP1
NMMHC-IIA
Vimentin

Readers may refer to other articles and reviews that cover more protein partners mentioned in table 2.

Menin Interaction with JUND

A conventional yeast two-hybrid library screening with menin identified JUND as a menin-interacting partner in two different laboratories [20, 21]. Menin interacts directly with JUND, a member of the activator protein-1 (AP1) transcription factor family that consists of JUN (JUNB, c-JUN, and JUND) and FOS (c-FOS, FRA-1 and FRA-2) proteins [20, 21]. JUN and FOS are cellular homologs of viral oncogenes that bind to specific DNA sequences, the TPA-responsive element (TRE), to activate transcription. The activity of the AP1 complex consisting of JUN/JUN homodimers or JUN/FOS heterodimers has been linked to cancer and neoplastic transformation. However, no mutations in the *JUN* or *FOS* genes have been identified so far. Through their target genes, AP1 proteins have been reported to regulate processes such as cell proliferation, differentiation, apoptosis, angiogenesis, cell motility and invasiveness.

Menin specifically interacts with JUND in multiple protein/protein interaction assays, and does not interact directly with other AP1 family members [20, 21]. In reporter assays, menin represses transcription activated by JUND [20, 21]. Although menin does not interact physically with c-JUN, in reporter assays menin enhances transcription activated by c-JUN [20]. The transcriptional activation domains of the JUN transcription factors are located at their N-terminus and the DNA binding and dimerization region (bZIP domain) is located at their C-terminus. The menin-interacting region is located at the N-terminus of JUND [20, 21]. Synthetic mutations in JUND that disrupt menin interaction have been isolated by reverse yeast two-hybrid screening, which mapped the menin-interacting region in JUND to the PGAP motif (corresponding to amino acid residues 33–36 in human JUND, or 41–44 in mouse JunD) [22]. JUND can suppress growth of normal MEFs; however, JUND is unable to suppress growth of menin-null MEFs [23]. Furthermore, experiments conducted in JUND-null MEFs have shown that a JUND mutant that lacks menin-binding (mouse JUND-G42E, corresponding to human JUND amino acid residue G34) converts the growth-suppressing JUND into a growth-promoting factor [23]. JUND-null MEFs stably expressing this menin-interaction-deficient JUND mutant form tumors in nude mice highlighting the oncogenic property of this mutant [Agarwal and Marx, unpubl.]. Disease-associated missense mutations in menin located at amino acid residues 139–242 impair binding to JUND [20]. These observations strongly suggest that the menin/JUND partnering plays an important role in tumor suppression. Target genes and pathways regulated by this partnering of menin remain to be determined.

In contrast to mice with homozygous knockout of *c-Jun* and *JunB* genes, inactivation of the *JunD* gene in mice does not lead to embryonic lethality perhaps due to genetic redundancy from the other members of the AP1 family as shown by knockin mouse models where JunB and JunD could substitute for c-Jun in embryonic development [24]. Homozygous *JunD* gene knockout mice although viable and healthy, exhibit: postnatal growth retardation, age-dependent defective spermatogenesis, enhanced cardiomyocyte apoptosis and fibrosis, chronic kidney disease, and increased bone formation [24, 25]. Transgenic mice broadly expressing JunD (controlled by the ubiquitin promoter) are viable and normal, but show reduced proliferation of lymphoid cells [26]. Whether these phenotypes, or the phenotypes described above in the mouse models of MEN1, are modified upon loss or gain of menin/JUN partnering is not known.

Genetic studies in the fruit fly, *Drosophila*, support the function of menin to modulate JUN activity. The *Drosophila melanogaster* menin (Mnn1) shows 47% amino acid identity with human menin. Unlike the early embryonic lethality of the *Men1–/–* mice described above, homozygous *mnn1*-null flies are viable and fertile [27]. Interestingly, flies with localized overexpression of Mnn1 show defects in thoracic closure (cleft thorax), a phenotype similar to insufficient activity of DJun (only a single *Jun* gene is present in *Drosophila*, i.e. the *DJun* gene) [27]. Mnn1 does not interact with DJun in biochemical assays; however, genetic experiments in flies have shown that overexpression of Mnn1 in a heterozygous DJun background or together with over-expression of a dominant negative DJun caused a more severe thoracic cleft phenotype [27]. These observations indicate that this complex interaction of menin with JUN proteins is evolutionarily conserved, and important for normal development.

Menin Interaction with the MLL Complex

Menin is an integral component of two similar MLL complexes, containing either MLL1 or MLL2. Mass spectrophotometric analysis of anti-menin immunoprecipitates of HeLa or HEK293T cells identified a protein complex containing RPB2 (large subunit of RNA Pol II), MLL2, Menin, ASH2L, RBBP5, WDR5, and hDPY30 [28]. Mass spectrophotometric analysis of anti-MLL1 immunoprecipitates of K562 erythroleukemia cells identified a protein complex containing MLL1 (MLL^N and MLL^C), HCF-2, Menin, ASH2L1, ASH2, RBBP5 and WDR5 [29].

These menin-MLL complexes have an enzymatic activity (histone methyltransferase, HMTase) catalyzing a specific covalent histone modification, trimethylated histone H3 on lysine 4 (H3K4me3) [28, 29]. H3K4me3 is associated with activation of gene transcription. In these complexes, menin interacts directly with MLL, the human homolog of *Drosophila* trithorax [30]. Several disease-associated menin missense mutants are impaired for MLL interaction, and highly reduced HMTase activity is observed in anti-menin immunoprecipitates from cells expressing the same menin missense mutants [28]. These findings highlight the functional significance of menin/MLL partnering showing that H3K4me3 would be lost on specific genes in the absence of menin resulting in repression of gene transcription.

The importance of the menin/MLL partnering and menin-dependent H3K4me3 in MEN1-associated tumorigenesis has been studied in a mouse model with tissue-specific combined loss of menin and the H3K4me2/H3K4me3 demethylase Rbp2 in pancreatic β-cells [31]. Loss of Rbp2 H3K4 demethylase activity would allow H3K4me3 on specific genes even in the absence of menin-MLL complex activity, and rescue tumor formation driven by menin loss. *Rbp2* gene loss substantially decreased tumor burden and enhanced median survival age from 45 weeks (*Men1* gene knockout in β-cells) to 69 weeks (combined knockout of *Men1* and *Rbp2* genes in β-cells) [31]. This rescue of tumorigenesis from inhibition of RBP2 (and its histone demethylase activity) reveals RBP2 as a potential cancer therapeutic target for further studies.

Translocations involving the MLL gene are a common cause of acute lymphoid and myeloid leukemias (the so-called mixed lineage leukemia). During normal hematopoiesis, MLL regulates the expression of specific *HOX* genes. Leukemic MLL translocations upregulate the expression of HOXA7, HOXA9 or the HOX cofactor MEIS1, which block hematopoietic differentiation thereby promoting leukemogenesis [29]. Furthermore, menin serves as an adaptor to link MLL with LEDGF (lens epithelium-derived growth factor), another chromatin-associated protein, on specific *HOX* genes [30]. Some menin missense mutants show impaired LEDGF interaction, while retaining interaction with MLL, but they are deficient in MLL/menin-associated HMTase activity [30]. Work done in different laboratories has shown that interaction with menin is critical for the oncogenic function of MLL fusion proteins. In contrast to its tumor suppressor function in MEN1, menin acts as an oncogenic co-factor of MLL in leukemia.

Studies exploring the association of menin in the chromatin-modifying MLL-complex have led to the identification of H3K4me3-dependent menin-regulated genes such as the *HOX* genes, the CDKI genes *p18* and *p27*, and genes at the imprinted *MEG3* locus [18, 32–34]. The *HOX* gene family consists of 39 genes located in 4 clusters on different chromosomes. They are highly conserved transcription factors that regulate the development of the embryonic body plan during embryogenesis. Dysregulated expression of *HOX* genes has been noted in leukemia and in solid tumors including in sporadic and MEN1-associated parathyroid tumors [35]. Reduced expression of CDKI genes *p18* and *p27* that negatively regulate progression through the cell cycle has been observed in islet tumors from the mouse models of MEN1 [32]. The *MEG3* locus contains co-ordinately regulated imprinted genes, and downregulation of these genes have been observed in sporadic pituitary tumors [36]. These investigations have provided valuable insights into the functional role of the menin/MlLL complex partnering.

3D Crystal Structure of Menin

For many years, efforts to decipher the crystal structure of menin were unsuccessful in several laboratories perhaps due to disordered internal fragments that could hinder protein crystallization. After the deletion of such unstructured regions, two different laboratories (both from the University of Michigan) have since successfully obtained menin crystals [37, 38]. They determined the crystal structure of *Nematostella* menin (the starlet sea anemone) and human menin using X-ray diffraction at resolutions of 1.95 and 2.5 Å, respectively. Based on the prediction of disordered regions, deletion of an unstructured loop (amino acid residues 426–442) and truncation of the C-terminus (amino acid residues 487–539) in *Nematostella* menin and deletion of a single internal unstructured loop (amino acid residues 460–519) in human menin yielded protein that crystallized easily [37, 38]. The structures of human and *Nematostella* menin are very similar (PBD ID: human, 3U84; *Nematostella*, 3RE2). The 3D shape of menin is described as a curved left 'hand' with a pocket formed by its 'thumb' and 'palm'. The basic structure reveals four domains in menin: an N-terminal domain consisting of a long β-hairpin, a transglutaminase-like domain that forms the 'thumb', a helical 'palm' domain of eight α helices that contain three tetratricopeptide (TRP) motifs, and a carboxy-terminal 'fingers' domain that has no homology with any known motifs [37, 38]. The transglutaminase-like domain in menin is predicted to lack enzymatic activity [37, 38]. Given the number of proteins that have been reported to partner with menin, the presence of TRP motifs is of interest because TRP is a structural motif known to serve as a scaffold for protein-protein interactions and the assembly of multiprotein complexes [37, 38]. Although menin participates in transcriptional regulation, no DNA-binding interface has been located in the 3D structure of menin to indicate direct binding of menin to DNA.

Disease-related mutations, missense (n = 60) and in-frame deletions (n = 10) are localized in all the different domains in the 3D structure of menin, changing buried residues, thus predicting destabilization of the menin structure and loss of protein function [37, 38]. Several menin missense mutant proteins have been shown to express poorly in cells because they are targeted to the proteasome and rapidly degraded [39]. Mapping of *MEN1* gene mutations to the menin structure could be informative for exploring the consequence of mutations of unknown clinical significance, and to distinguish pathologic and benign mutations.

The crystal structure of human menin individually with its partners JUND or MLL1, or together with MLL1 and LEDGF reveal that binding of JUND and MLL1 to menin is mutually exclusive [38]. These structures show that menin contains a deep pocket (in the 'palm' domain) that binds short peptides of JUND (amino acid residues 27–47) or MLL1 (amino acid residues 6–25) [38]. In the menin-MLL1-LEDGF complex, menin could bind to MLL1 through the peptide pocket while LEDGF was located at a distinct surface formed by the interaction of menin and MLL1 [38]. Structural features of menin with other partners remain to be determined.

Conclusions

Clinical, genetic and basic findings about MEN1, the *MEN1* gene and menin have advanced the understanding of this disease. Identification of a germline *MEN1* gene mutation in at-risk individuals allows early monitoring for tumors. Mouse models and protein interaction studies have helped explore the critical biological function(s) of menin. These studies have revealed candidate protein partners and menin-dependent target genes that should be studied further to understand the exact mechanisms of action of menin in normal physiology and actions potentially perturbed during tumor formation. The 3D crystal structure of menin will facilitate such investigations. Applications of this knowledge will help develop new diagnostic methods and treatment options for MEN1 and related states, and for similar sporadic tumors.

Acknowledgments

This work was supported by the Intramural Research Program of the NIH, National Institute of Diabetes and Digestive and Kidney Diseases (Project No. 1ZIADK075035-03).

References

1 Moldawer MP, Nardi GL, Raker JW: Concomitance of multiple adenomas of the parathyroids and pancreatic islets with tumor of the pituitary: a syndrome with a familial incidence. Am J Med Sci 1954;228:190–206.

2 Wermer P: Genetic aspects of adenomatosis of endocrine glands. Am J Med 1954;16:363–371.

3 Brandi ML, Gagel RF, Angeli A, et al: Guidelines for diagnosis and therapy of MEN type 1 and type 2. J Clin Endocrinol Metab 2001;86:5658–5671.

4 Larsson C, Skogseid B, Oberg K, Nakamura Y, Nordenskjold M: Multiple endocrine neoplasia type 1 gene maps to chromosome 11 and is lost in insulinoma. Nature 1988;332:85–87.

5 Chandrasekharappa SC, Guru SC, Manickam P, et al: Positional cloning of the gene for multiple endocrine neoplasia-type 1. Science 1997;276:404–407.

6 Lemmens I, Van de Ven WJ, Kas K, et al: Identification of the multiple endocrine neoplasia type 1 (MEN1) gene. The European consortium on MEN1. Hum Mol Genet 1997;6:1177–1183.

7 Thakker RV: Multiple endocrine neoplasia type 1 (MEN1). Best Pract Res Clin Endocrinol Metab 2010;24:355–370.

8 Agarwal SK, Ozawa A, Mateo CM, Marx SJ: The MEN1 gene and pituitary tumours. Horm Res 2009;71(suppl 2):131–138.

9 Agarwal SK, Mateo CM, Marx SJ: Rare germline mutations in cyclin-dependent kinase inhibitor genes in multiple endocrine neoplasia type 1 and related states. J Clin Endocrinol Metab 2009;94: 1826–1834.

10 Franklin DS, Godfrey VL, Lee H, Kovalev GI, Schoonhoven R, Chen-Kiang S, Su L, Xiong Y: CDK inhibitors p18(Ink4c) and p27(Kip1) mediate two separate pathways to collaboratively suppress pituitary tumorigenesis. Genes Dev 1998;12:2899–2911.

11 Piret SE, Thakker RV: Mouse models for inherited endocrine and metabolic disorders. J Endocrinol 2011;211:211–230.

12 Lu J, Herrera PL, Carreira C, Bonnavion R, Seigne C, Calender A, Bertolino P, Zhang CX: Alpha cell-specific MEN1 ablation triggers the transdifferentiation of glucagon-expressing cells and insulinoma development. Gastroenterology 2010;138: 1954–1965.

13 Korsisaari N, Ross J, Wu X, Kowanetz M, Pal N, Hall L, Eastham-Anderson J, Forrest WF, Van Bruggen N, Peale FV, Ferrara N: Blocking vascular endothelial growth factor-a inhibits the growth of pituitary adenomas and lowers serum prolactin level in a mouse model of multiple endocrine neoplasia type 1. Clin Cancer Res 2008;14: 249–258.

14 Novotny E, Compton S, Liu PP, Collins FS, Chandrasekharappa SC: In vitro hematopoietic differentiation of mouse embryonic stem cells requires the tumor suppressor menin and is mediated by Hoxa9. Mech Dev 2009;126:517–522.

15 Ji Y, Prasad NB, Novotny EA, Kaur S, Elkahloun A, Chen Y, Zhang RZ, Chu ML, Agarwal SK, Marx SJ, Collins FS, Chandrasekharappa SC: Mouse embryo fibroblasts lacking the tumor suppressor menin show altered expression of extracellular matrix protein genes. Mol Cancer Res 2007;5:1041–1051.
16 Schnepp RW, Mao H, Sykes SM, Zong WX, Silva A, La P, Hua X: Menin induces apoptosis in murine embryonic fibroblasts. J Biol Chem 2004;279: 10685–10691.
17 Hussein N, Casse H, Fontaniere S, Morera AM, Asensio MJ, Bakeli S, Lu JL, Coste I, Di Clemente N, Bertolino P, Zhang CX: Reconstituted expression of menin in MEN1-deficient mouse Leydig tumour cells induces cell cycle arrest and apoptosis. Eur J Cancer 2007;43:402–414.
18 Agarwal SK, Jothi R: Genome-wide characterization of menin-dependent h3k4me3 reveals a specific role for menin in the regulation of genes implicated in MEN1-like tumors. PLoS One 2012; 7:e37952.
19 Francis J, Lin W, Rozenblatt-Rosen O, Meyerson M: The menin tumor suppressor protein is phosphorylated in response to DNA damage. PLoS One 2011; 6:e16119.
20 Agarwal SK, Guru SC, Heppner C, Erdos MR, Collins RM, Park SY, Saggar S, Chandrasekharappa SC, Collins FS, Spiegel AM, Marx SJ, Burns AL: Menin interacts with the AP1 transcription factor JUND and represses JUND-activated transcription. Cell 1999;96:143–152.
21 Gobl AE, Berg M, Lopez-Egido JR, Oberg K, Skogseid B, Westin G: Menin represses JUND-activated transcription by a histone deacetylase-dependent mechanism. Biochim Biophys Acta 1999;1447:51–56.
22 Knapp JI, Heppner C, Hickman AB, Burns AL, Chandrasekharappa SC, Collins FS, Marx SJ, Spiegel AM, Agarwal SK: Identification and characterization of JUND missense mutants that lack menin binding. Oncogene 2000;19:4706–4712.
23 Agarwal SK, Novotny EA, Crabtree JS, Weitzman JB, Yaniv M, Burns AL, Chandrasekharappa SC, Collins FS, Spiegel AM, Marx SJ: Transcription factor JUND, deprived of menin, switches from growth suppressor to growth promoter. Proc Natl Acad Sci USA 2003;100:10770–10775.
24 Meixner A, Karreth F, Kenner L, Penninger JM, Wagner EF: JUN and JUND-dependent functions in cell proliferation and stress response. Cell Death Differ 2010;17:1409–1419.
25 Thepot D, Weitzman JB, Barra J, Segretain D, Stinnakre MG, Babinet C, Yaniv M: Targeted disruption of the murine JUND gene results in multiple defects in male reproductive function. Development 2000;127:143–153.
26 Meixner A, Karreth F, Kenner L, Wagner EF: JUND regulates lymphocyte proliferation and T helper cell cytokine expression. Embo J 2004;23:1325–1335.
27 Cerrato A, Parisi M, Santa Anna S, Missirlis F, Guru S, Agarwal S, Sturgill D, Talbot T, Spiegel A, Collins F, Chandrasekharappa S, Marx S, Oliver B: Genetic interactions between *Drosophila melanogaster* menin and Jun/Fos. Dev Biol 2006;298:59–70.
28 Hughes CM, Rozenblatt-Rosen O, Milne TA, Copeland TD, Levine SS, Lee JC, Hayes DN, Shanmugam KS, Bhattacharjee A, Biondi CA, Kay GF, Hayward NK, Hess JL, Meyerson M: Menin associates with a trithorax family histone methyltransferase complex and with the hoxc8 locus. Mol Cell 2004;13: 587–597.
29 Yokoyama A, Wang Z, Wysocka J, Sanyal M, Aufiero DJ, Kitabayashi I, Herr W, Cleary ML: Leukemia proto-oncoprotein MLL forms a SET1-like histone methyltransferase complex with menin to regulate Hox gene expression. Mol Cell Biol 2004; 24:5639–5649.
30 Yokoyama A, Cleary ML: Menin critically links MLL proteins with LEDGF on cancer-associated target genes. Cancer Cell 2008;14:36–46.
31 Lin W, Cao J, Liu J, et al: Loss of the retinoblastoma binding protein 2 (RBP2) histone demethylase suppresses tumorigenesis in mice lacking RB1 or MEN1. Proc Natl Acad Sci USA 2011;108:13379–13386.
32 Karnik SK, Hughes CM, Gu X, Rozenblatt-Rosen O, McLean GW, Xiong Y, Meyerson M, Kim SK: Menin regulates pancreatic islet growth by promoting histone methylation and expression of genes encoding p27Kip1 and p18INK4c. Proc Natl Acad Sci USA 2005;102:14659–14664.
33 Scacheri PC, Davis S, Odom DT, Crawford GE, Perkins S, Halawi MJ, Agarwal SK, Marx SJ, Spiegel AM, Meltzer PS, Collins FS: Genome-wide analysis of menin binding provides insights into MEN1 tumorigenesis. PLoS Genet 2006;2:e51.
34 Wang P, Lin C, Smith ER, Guo H, Sanderson BW, Wu M, Gogol M, Alexander T, Seidel C, Wiedemann LM, Ge K, Krumlauf R, Shilatifard A: Global analysis of H3K4 methylation defines MLL family member targets and points to a role for MLL1-mediated H3K4 methylation in the regulation of transcriptional initiation by RNA polymerase II. Mol Cell Biol 2009;29:6074–6085.
35 Shen HC, Rosen JE, Yang LM, Savage SA, Burns AL, Mateo CM, Agarwal SK, Chandrasekharappa SC, Spiegel AM, Collins FS, Marx SJ, Libutti SK: Parathyroid tumor development involves deregulation of homeobox genes. Endocr Relat Cancer 2008;15: 267–275.

36 Zhou Y, Zhang X, Klibanski A: MEG3 noncoding RNA: a tumor suppressor. J Mol Endocrinol 2012; 48:R45–R53.
37 Murai MJ, Chruszcz M, Reddy G, Grembecka J, Cierpicki T: Crystal structure of menin reveals binding site for mixed lineage leukemia (MLL) protein. J Biol Chem 2011;286:31742–31748.
38 Huang J, Gurung B, Wan B, Matkar S, Veniaminova NA, Wan K, Merchant JL, Hua X, Lei M: The same pocket in menin binds both MLL and JUND but has opposite effects on transcription. Nature 2012;482: 542–546.
39 Canaff L, Vanbellinghen JF, Kanazawa I, Kwak H, Garfield N, Vautour L, Hendy GN: Menin missense mutants encoded by the MEN1 gene that are targeted to the proteasome: restoration of expression and activity by chip SIRNA. J Clin Endocrinol Metab 2012;97:E282–E291.

Sunita K. Agarwal, PhD
National Institutes of Health, NIDDK, Metabolic Diseases Branch
Bldg 10, Room 8C-101
9000 Rockville Pike
Bethesda, MD 20892 (USA)
E-Mail SunitaA@mail.nih.gov

Stratakis CA (ed): Endocrine Tumor Syndromes and Their Genetics.
Front Horm Res. Basel, Karger, 2013, vol 41, pp 16–29 (DOI: 10.1159/000345667)

Multiple Endocrine Neoplasia Type 2

Maya Lodish

Section on Endocrinology and Genetics, Eunice Kennedy Shriver National Institute of Child Health and Human Development, National Institutes of Health, Bethesda, Md., USA

Abstract

Multiple endocrine neoplasia type 2 (MEN2) is an autosomal-dominant cancer syndrome characterized by variable penetrance of medullary thyroid carcinoma(MTC), pheochromocytoma (PHEO), and primary hyperparathyroidism (PHPT). MEN2 consists of two clinical subtypes, MEN2A and MEN2B. Familial medullary thyroid cancer is now viewed as a phenotypic variant of MEN2A with decreased penetrance for PHEO and PHPT rather than a distinct entity. All subtypes are caused by gain-of-function mutations of the RET proto-oncogene. Genotype-phenotype correlations exist that help predict the presence of other associated endocrine neoplasms as well as the timing of thyroid cancer development. Recognition of the clinical entity in individuals and families at risk of harboring a germline *RET* mutation is crucial for the management and prevention of associated malignancies. Recent guidelines released by the American Thyroid Association regarding the management of MTC will be summarized in this chapter.

Overview

Multiple endocrine neoplasia type 2 (MEN2) occurs in 1:200,000 live births, and is an autosomal-dominant syndrome characterized by predisposition to neuroendocrine tumors [1]. The first clinical subtype of MEN2, MEN2A, is characterized by medullary thyroid cancer (MTC), pheochromocytoma (PHEO), and primary hyperparathyroidism (PHPT). MEN2A accounts for 70–80% of individuals with MEN2. MTC is frequently the first neoplastic manifestation in MEN2A patients, with thyroid cancer occurring as early as in the first 5 years of life. MTC is a calcitonin-producing tumor that arises from the parafollicular C cells of the thyroid gland, which are derived from the embryonic neural crest. Two rare variants of MEN2A have been identified, one with Hirschsprung's disease and the other with cutaneous lichen amyloidosis [2, 3]. In families without an established diagnosis of MEN2A, patients typically present with a neck mass between the ages of 15 and 20 years. The risk of developing MTC in MEN2A is between 70 and 95%, while approximately 50% of individuals with MEN2A develop PHEO and 10–30% develop primary PHPT [4, 5].

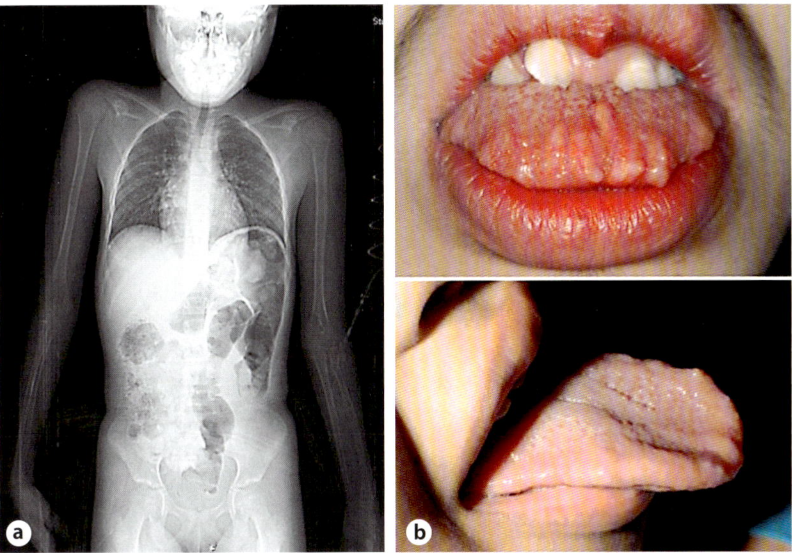

Fig. 1. a Computed tomography scout film showing dilated bowel due to ganglioneuromatosis of the gastrointestinal tract in MEN2B. **b** Mucosal neuromas on the anterior surface of the tongue in MEN2B.

The second inherited subtype of MEN2, MEN2B, accounts for only 5% of MEN2. MEN2B is characterized by MTC in all affected individuals, in addition to variable presentation of PHEO, a Marfanoid body habitus, mucosal and eyelid neuromas, and ganglioneuromatosis of the gastrointestinal tract (fig. 1). Patients with MEN2B do not develop PHPT. Distinct early clinical manifestations in MEN2B include inability to shed tears and gastrointestinal symptoms including abdominal distension, megacolon, diarrhea or constipation [6, 7]. MTC in MEN2B is characterized by a clinically aggressive course; affected individuals who do not undergo prophylactic thyroidectomy in infancy are likely to develop metastatic MTC. Prior to the recommendation for prophylactic thyroidectomy, the mean age of death in MEN2B was 21 years [1]. Approximately 50% of individuals with MEN2B develop PHEOs, which are often bilateral.

Familial MTC (FMTC) was previously categorized as a separate, third subtype of MEN2A. Now, however, FMTC is viewed as a phenotypic variant of MEN2A with decreased penetrance for PHEO and primary PHPT rather than a distinct entity [8]. FMTC accounts for 10–20% of MEN2 cases; only the thyroid gland is affected in these patients by definition. In general, FMTC patients present later with MTC than those with MEN2A or MEN2B, usually between 20 and 40 years of age.

MTC is the most common cause of death in patients with MEN2A, MEN2B and FMTC [9]. Carriers of all variants of inherited MTC have a high penetrance for developing thyroid cancer: 90% of carriers of such predisposition eventually are diag-

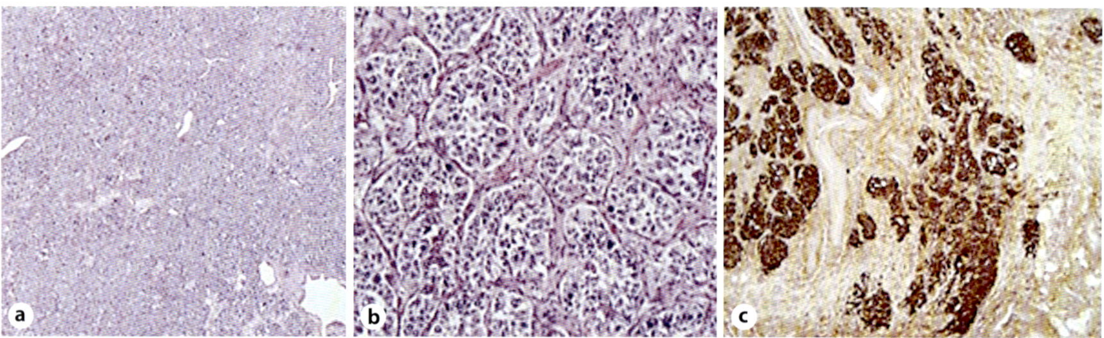

Fig. 2. a Low power view of medullary carcinoma of the thyroid comprised of nests of spindle-shaped cells containing amyloid. **b** High-power detail. **c** Calcitonin immunohistochemical staining of MTC.

nosed with MTC and present with a palpable thyroid nodule or elevation of calcitonin levels [10]. The most frequent systemic manifestation of MTC is diarrhea, which is associated with elevated plasma calcitonin and poor prognosis. On histopathology, MTC is a malignant tumor originating from the calcitonin-producing (C cells) of the thyroid gland (fig. 2a, b). C cell hyperplasia is a precursor to MTC, in which clusters of C cells extend beyond the basement membrane. Positive immunohistochemical staining with calcitonin antibodies is also found in MTC (fig. 2c).

History

MEN2A was originally described by Sipple [11], who in 1961 published the case of a man who died of intracranial hemorrhage and autopsy findings were consistent with PHEO, MTC, and parathyroid hyperplasia. The following year, Cushman [12] put forth a link between these endocrine tumors, which led to the classification of MEN2 as a unique entity. Linkage analysis in families with MEN2 led to the discovery of the *RET* proto-oncogene in chromosome 10 as the causative gene in this syndrome in 1993 [13–15]. MEN2 is the first inherited neoplasia syndrome in which a clear genotype-phenotype association was made, notably between the *RET* genotype and the MEN2 phenotype [5].

In 1966 the constellation of findings associated with MEN2B including thick lips, tongue lesions, MTC and PHEO was described in a patient and his family members by Williams and Pollock [16]. Nearly 30 years later in 1994, distinct activating mutations in the *RET* proto-oncogene were found to cause MEN2B [17, 18]. Following these discoveries, it became possible to identify relatives of patients with these syndromes who have inherited a mutated *RET* allele and in whom MTC is almost certain to develop. Because MTC is not curable once it metastasizes beyond the thyroid, it is now recommended that all patients with MTC and especially young members of kindreds with MEN2A and MEN2B have genetic screening performed to determine if they are carriers of a *RET* mutation [19].

Structure and Function of *RET*

The *RET* proto-oncogene is located on chromosome 10q11.2 and includes 21 exons. *RET* (REarranged during Transfection) was first identified by Takahashi et al. [20] in 1985. *RET* encodes a receptor tyrosine kinase with key roles in cell growth, differentiation, and survival. Receptor dimerization leads to autophosphorylation of intracellular tyrosine residues, which subsequently activate downstream pathways of signal transduction [21]. The role of the *RET* oncogene in the development of MTC has been well characterized. Activating *RET* germline mutations have been identified as the primary cause of all the hereditary MTC syndromes: approximately a quarter to a third of all sporadic MTC cases and up to 98% of MEN2 cases have a germline *RET* mutation leading to constitutive activation of the *RET* receptor; somatic *RET* mutations account for another quarter to half of all sporadic MTCs [5].

The specific site of the particular mutated residue within the RET protein has been correlated to phenotypic differences among patients with inherited MTC [22]. For example, patients with MEN2A characteristically have missense mutations in exon 10 (codons 609, 610, 611, 618 and 620) and exon 11 (codon 634) [19]. These mutations affect one of the six cysteine residues present in the *RET* extracellular domain [23]. Mutations in these cysteine residues lead to receptor homodimerization via the formation of disulfide bonds, rendering the receptor activated regardless of the presence of ligand. The natural history of MTC in MEN2A is highly variable between different *RET* mutations and even among members of the same family. In the case of MEN2B, more than 95% of patients have a mutation at exon 16 (codon 918), in the tyrosine kinase domain of the protein. This mutation renders the receptor activated in its monomeric state, and leads to increased phosphorylation of intracellular tyrosine residues [24]. Patients with FMTC harbor mutations in exons 10, 11, 13 (codon 768) and 14 (codons 804 and 806) [19].

RET Gene and Practice Recommendations

MEN2 is a well-defined hereditary cancer syndrome in which genetic testing is considered part of the standard management for relatives who are at-risk. Therefore, *RET* molecular genetic testing should be offered to at-risk family members. The risk to family members of having a *RET* mutation differs according to the subtype of MEN2. In MEN2A, the majority (95%) of individuals have inherited the mutation from a parent, while the remaining 5% have a de novo germline mutation [25]. In contrast, in MEN2B, the overall rate of de novo mutations in MEN2B appears to be 50% but for certain mutations (i.e. the 918 codon) the rate may be substantially higher [26]. As is the case with autosomal-dominant disorders, each child of an individual with MEN2 has a 50% chance of inheriting the *RET* mutation. Early detection of at-risk children leads to prophylactic thyroidectomy in a timely fashion, potentially averting the risk of metastatic MTC.

Current practice recommends performing prophylactic thyroidectomy prior to the development of MTC in at-risk patients [9]. In fact, total thyroidectomy is indicated in patients with inherited *RET* mutations, regardless of the plasma calcitonin level. Specific genotype-phenotype correlations have been established that associate the clinical aggressiveness of MTC with the mutated codon of the RET protein, as outlined in table 1 [19]. Therefore, the timing and extent of prophylactic surgery is dictated by germline analysis of mutations. The dilemma arises in terms of balancing the risk of surgical morbidity from performing the thyroidectomy at an early age with doing the surgery prior to the development of metastatic MTC. In 1999, the 7th International Workshop on MEN published a consensus statement that was the first to classify *RET* mutations into risk levels. They correlated patient genotypes with clinical aggressiveness of hereditary MTC, and created guidelines for the timing of prophylactic thyroidectomy: the patients at highest risk include those with MEN2B and *RET* mutations in codons 883 or 918 [5, 19]. The guidelines call for prophylactic thyroidectomy in these patients within the first year of life. Patients with MEN2A or FMTC who have mutations in codons 611, 618, 620, and 634 are at high risk and thyroidectomy should be undertaken prior to the age of 5 years, whereas the timing of surgery of patients with other mutations can be individualized; such a decision, however, should never be left for later than childhood [5, 9, 19]. In 2009, the American Thyroid Association (ATA) published updated recommendations for clinical and genetic diagnostic testing and treatment options for MTC, in which the age at which prophylactic thyroidectomy is performed can be guided by the codon position of the *RET* mutation [8]. The risks of aggressive MTC based on genotype are defined in the ATA guidelines. For example, level D is associated with the highest risk of developing aggressive MTC. These risk levels are then used to guide the timing of prophylactic thyroidectomy as outlined in table 2. For those patients identified by screening to have inherited a mutated *RET* allele who go on to have prophylactic thyroidectomy, 5- and 10-year survival rates approach 100% [9, 27, 28]. In patients with sporadic MTC, however, genetic screening has rarely been applied; these patients often present with metastatic disease [27, 28].

For individuals with a *RET* mutation who have not had a thyroidectomy, annual biochemical screening with calcitonin is recommended, followed by thyroidectomy if results are elevated. Calcitonin is secreted by the C cells of the thyroid and is used as a marker of disease in MTC. Historically, stimulated calcitonin testing was performed by measurement of calcitonin following intravenous administration of the

Table 1. Genotype-phenotype correlations and risk levels for aggressive medullary thyroid cancer

Mutation	Exon	ATA risk level*	MEN2 phenotype	Penetrance	
				PHPT	PHEO
G321R	5	A	FMTC/MEN2A	–	–
531/9 bp duplication	8	A	FMTC/MEN2A	–	–
532 duplication	8	A	FMTC	–	–
C515S	8	A	FMTC/MEN2A	–	–
G533C	8	A	FMTC/MEN2A	–	R
R600Q	10	A	FMTC/MEN2A	–	–
K603E	10	A	FMTC/MEN2A	–	–
Y606C	10	A	FMTC	–	–
C609F/R/G/S/Y	10	B	FMTC/MEN2A, HSCR	MI	R
C611R/G/F/S/W/Y	10	B	FMTC/MEN2A, HSCR	MI	R
C618R/G/F/S/Y	10	B	FMTC/MEN2A, HSCR	MI	MI
C620R/G/F/S/W/Y	10	B	FMTC/MEN2A, HSCR	MI	MI
C630R/F/S/Y	11	B	FMTC/MEN2A	R	R
D631Y	11	B	FMTC	–	–
633/9 base pair duplication	11	B	FMTC/MEN2A	MI	MI
C634R	11	C	MEN2A, CLA	MI	MA
C634G/F/S/W/Y	11	C	FMTC/MEN2A, CLA	MI	MA
634/12 bp duplication	11	B	FMTC/MEN2A	MI	–
635/insertion ELCR;T636P	11	A	FMTC/MEN2A	–	–
S649L	11	A	FMTC/MEN2A	R	–
K666E	11	A	FMTC/MEN2A	–	MI
E768D	13	A	FMTC/MEN2A	R	R
N777S	13	A	FMTC/MEN2A	–	–
L790F	13	A	FMTC/MEN2A	R	R/MI
Y791F	13	A	FMTC/MEN2A	MI	MI
V804L	14	A	FMTC/MEN2A	MI	R
V804M	14	A	FMTC/MEN2A	R	R
V804M+V778I	13/14	B	FMTC/MEN2A	–	–
V804M+E805K	14	D	MEN2B	–	MA
V804M+Y806C	14	D	MEN2B	–	MA
V804MþS904C	14/15	D	MEN2B	MI	–
G819K	14	A	FMTC	–	–
R833C	14	A	FMTC	–	–
R844Q	14	A	FMTC	–	–
R866W	15	A	FMTC/MEN2A	–	–
A883F	15	D	MEN2B	–	MA
S891A	15	A	FMTC/MEN2A	R	R
R912P	16	A	FMTC/MEN2A	–	–
M918T	16	D	MEN2B	–	MA

Adapted from Kloos et al. [8]. * Risk from aggressive MTC: level D is highest risk.
MA = Majority; MI = minority; R = rare; PHPT = primary hyperparathyroidism; PHEO = pheochromocytoma; HSCR = Hirschsprung disease; CLA = cutaneous lichen amyloidosis.

Table 2. Recommended interventions based on ATA risk level of genotype

ATA risk level	Age of prophylactic thyroidectomy	Age to begin screening for PHEO	Age to begin screening for PHPT
Level D	as soon as possible within first year of life	8 years	N/A
Level C	before age 5 year	8 years	8 years
Level B	consider before 5 years, may delay if criteria met[1]	8 years for those with codon 630 mutation, 20 years for all others	8 years for those with codon 630 mutation, 20 years for all others
Level A	may delay surgery beyond age 5 year if criteria met[1]	20 years	20 years

[1] A normal annual basal ± stimulated serum calcitonin, normal annual neck ultrasound examination, and family history of less aggressive MTC.

secretagogue pentagastrin, which is not currently available in the United States and many other countries. In addition, current calcitonin assays have superior sensitivities, as low as 1–2 pg/ml. In the present time, most experts believe that there is rarely a need for stimulated calcitonin testing in the diagnosis or follow-up of MTC [8]. Guidelines call for annual serum calcitonin screening to begin for children with MEN2B at 6 months and at age 3–5 years for children with MEN2A or FMTC, and to continue as indicated post-thyroidectomy [8].

Mutations in the *RET* proto-oncogene causing MEN2 are listed in table 1. The algorithm for molecular genetic testing is presented in the most recent ATA MTC practice guidelines [8]. For all patients with isolated MTC, or with MTC along with PHPT or PHEO, initial testing should include sequencing of exons 10, 11 and 13–16 of *RET*. If this initial testing is negative, potential reflex testing should include full sequencing of the coding region. For individuals with MTC along with features suggestive of MEN2B, targeted mutation analysis or sequencing of exons 15 and 16 for M918T and A883F is warranted.

Summary of Current Optimal Therapeutic Practices for MTC

MTC is relatively unresponsive to radiation therapy and to standard chemotherapeutic regimens [27, 29]. Radiation therapy has only a palliative role in the treatment of MTC [30]. Surgery remains the only standard treatment for patients with MTC: total thyroidectomy that is performed before MTC grows or spreads beyond the gland is currently the only curative therapy. It is recommended that surgery be performed by a center with experience in MEN2. The thyroid surgeon must incorporate knowledge of the patient's genotype into the decision regarding surgical approach. In a prophy-

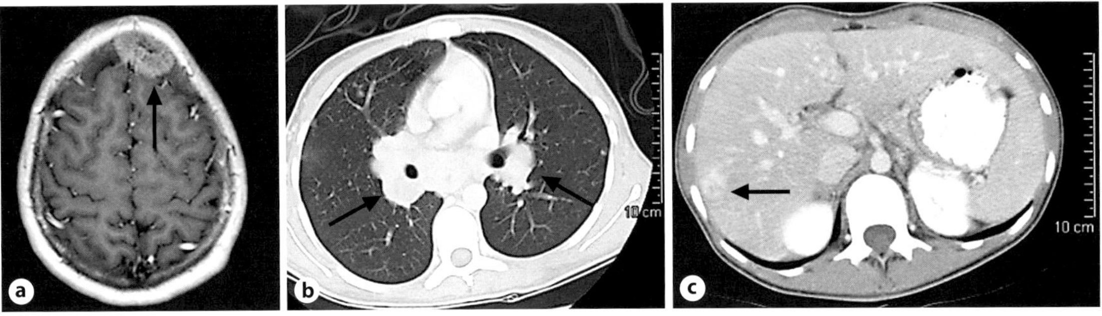

Fig. 3. Metastatic MTC to the skull (**a**), hilar lymph nodes (**b**) and liver (**c**).

lactic thyroidectomy, a total thyroidectomy should be performed and routine central compartment dissection is not warranted. However, in the setting of a clinically evident tumor, central neck dissection should be performed along with total thyroidectomy [8]. Specific recommendations regarding evaluation and management of metastatic MTC are outlined in the ATA guidelines and are beyond the scope of this chapter.

Once MTC metastasizes, it has a tendency to spread to local and regional lymph nodes (cervical and mediastinal), and more distantly to bone, lung, and liver (fig. 3) [27]. Although MTC is often widely metastatic, it tends to be a slow growing tumor. Patients with metastatic disease continue to have 5- and 10-year survival rates of 80 and 70%, respectively. Decreased survival in MTC can be correlated with the stage of diagnosis. Survival also varies by the extent of local disease, with 10-year survival rates as high as 95% for patients with disease confined to the thyroid gland, and rates as low as 40% for those with distant metastases [31].

Because approximately 50% of individuals with MTC have recurrent disease after total thyroidectomy and neck dissection, surveillance for recurrent MTC is paramount [32]. Annual serum calcitonin is indicated in all individuals with MTC who have undergone thyroidectomy, with more frequent follow-up indicated for those with residual disease [8]. Imaging indicated for localization of metastatic disease in these patients includes neck ultrasound, chest and neck computed tomography (CT), contrast-enhanced magnetic resonance imaging (MRI) of liver, bone MRI of the spine and pelvis, as well as bone scan [8].

Treatment of MTC with Tyrosine Kinase Inhibitors

The only current cure for patients with MTC is total thyroidectomy performed at an early stage, when the disease is confined to the thyroid gland. Standard chemotherapy and radiation have not been shown to be effective. Rationally designed small molecular compounds that affect tyrosine kinase-dependent oncogenic pathways, tyrosine kinase inhibitors (TKIs) have emerged recently as treatment for patients with MTC. Vandetanib is an orally available TKI that targets vascular endothelial growth factor-dependent tumor angiogenesis and epidermal growth factor receptor and *RET*-dependent tumor cell proliferation. Like other small molecule TKIs in this class of anticancer agents, vandetanib competes with ATP and blocks autophosphorylation and signal transduction. Vandetanib was approved by the Federal Drug Administration for use in patients with locally advanced or metastatic medullary thyroid cancer in April 2011. A randomized, double blind phase III trial of vandetanib in patients with advanced MTC demonstrated therapeutic efficacy [33]. Another tyrosine kinase inhibitors, sorafenib showed suggestion of clinical benefit for patients with sporadic MTC in a phase II clinical trial [34]. Sunitinib has also shown effectiveness in MTC and well-differentiated thyroid carcinoma in a phase II clinical trial [35]. The use of these agents is limited by the development of resistance; multiple drug therapy may hold promise for future studies.

Pheochromocytomas in MEN2 Syndromes

Pheochromocytomas develop in approximately 50% of patients with MEN2A or MEN2B [36]. The timing of the development of PHEO is usually after the presentation of MTC; however, it is the presenting disease in 13–30% of individuals with MEN2A [37, 38]. Nodular or diffuse hyperplasia of the adrenal medulla occurs as a precursor to the development of PHEO, and on histopathological examination, bilateral adrenal medullary disease is usually found [36]. Malignant transformation of PHEO occurs in approximately 4% of the cases [39].

Evaluation and Treatment of Pheochromocytoma

Recommendations for the management of PHEO in MEN2A syndromes have evolved from bilateral adrenalectomy, to unilateral adrenalectomy, and most recently to cortical-sparing adrenalectomy as the treatment of choice. Because of the high likelihood of the development of a contralateral PHEO, older surgical recommendations called for bilateral adrenalectomy in MEN2A and MEN2B once the diagnosis of PHEO was made, regardless of clear evidence of tumor in both glands. This approach led to the lifelong need for glucocorticoid replacement therapy and the risk of death from adrenal insufficiency. In the 1990s, recommendations advocated for the more conservative approach of single gland resection via laparoscopic adrenalectomy for unilateral disease. In their series of 23 patients with MEN2 syndromes who underwent unilateral adrenalectomy, Lairmore et al. [36] reported that 48% of the patients did not develop a PHEO in the contralateral adrenal gland during at least 10 years of follow-up. Even more recently, minimally invasive cortical-sparing adrenalectomy has been very successful in terms of both low risk of local recurrence and reducing the risk of Addisonian crisis [40, 41]. Asari et al. [41] reported outcomes in 13 patients with MEN2A and hereditary PHEO who underwent adrenal sparing surgery; only 5 of the 13 patients (38%) developed recurrence in the contralateral gland. In addition, 22% of their patients experienced Addisonian crisis, including a death, after bilateral adrenalectomy. Asari et al. [41] concluded that cortical-sparing adrenalectomy and close monitoring of the remnant may be the treatment of choice for hereditary bilateral PHEO in MEN2A, as overall recurrence is low.

Screening for Pheochromocytoma

The majority of PHEOs in MEN2A syndromes are intra-adrenal and benign; however, the potential for malignancy does exist. As is the case with the development of MTC, there is also a *RET* codon-specific, age-related risk for development of PHEO. The median age of presentation of PHEO in MEN2B is in the mid-20s [42, 43]. Machens et al. [44] investigated the timing of development of PHEO in a series of 206 *RET* mutation carriers. Based on their data, annual biochemical screening for PHEO was recommended from age 10 years in carriers of *RET* mutations in codons 918, 634 and 630, and from age 20 years in the remainder [44]. According to the 2009 ATA guidelines for the management of MTC, PHEO screening should begin by age 8 years for MEN2B and mutated *RET* codons 634 and 630; otherwise by age 20 years for other *RET* mutations [8].

Current recommendations call for biochemical screening for PHEO with measurement of plasma metanephrines or measurement of 24-hour collections for urinary catecholamines or metanephrines [45]. Epinephrine and norepinephrine are the most common metabolites found to be elevated in MEN2 [46]. If levels are elevated, adrenal imaging with CT or MRI should be performed. [^{18}F]-fluorodopamine positron emission tomography (PET) is a superior imaging modality for PHEO localization and further evaluation, with superior sensitivity as compared to ^{123}I-metaiodobenzylguanidine and ^{111}In-pentetreotide scintigraphy [47]. There is not a consensus on specific recommendations for regular adrenal imaging in the setting of normal metabolic screening for individuals with MEN2.

Patients with MEN2 should be screened for PHEO prior to any surgical procedure so that appropriate adrenergic blockade can be administered. Therefore, PHEO must be excluded or treated prior to surgery for MTC. Special care should be taken to ensure that female *RET* mutation carriers are screened for PHEO before or during early pregnancy to avoid the potential of hypertensive crisis activated by pregnancy or delivery [8]. Once identified, patients with phechromocytoma must undergo proper preoperative management with α- and β-blockade to minimalize adverse events associated with induction of anesthesia and surgery [48].

Primary Hyperparathyroidism

Between 15 and 30% of individuals with MEN2A will develop primary hyperparathyroidism (PHPT) [19, 28]. Periodic screening with albumin-corrected calcium or ionized calcium is recommended; if serum calcium is elevated along with inappropriately normal or elevated PTH, the diagnosis of PHPT is suspected. PHPT usually presents years after the diagnosis of MTC and most individuals have no symptoms associated with elevated calcium. In one study of 56 patients affected by PHPT among 249 MEN2A patients, the median age at diagnosis was 37.6 years, and PHPT was asymptomatic in 68% of the patients [49]. Another group looked at 67 patients with MEN2A and PHPT where the median age at diagnosis of PHPT was 38 years, and PHPT was asymptomatic in 84% of the patients [50]. These studies suggest that MEN2A-related PHPT is generally associated with mild, often asymptomatic hypercalcemia, although hypercalcuria and renal calculi may occur. Although some patients had recurrences 5–15 years after the first parathyroidectomy, resection of only macroscopically enlarged glands generally appears sufficient. Subtotal or total parathyroidectomy with autotransplantation is associated with a high rate of hypoparathyroidism.

Surveillance with annual serum calcium and PTH levels should begin by age 8 years in carriers of *RET* mutations in codons 630 and 634, and by age 20 years in carriers of other MEN2A *RET* mutations [8]. Treatment recommendations for PHPT associated with MEN2A vary according to the particular *RET* mutation. Resection and autotransplantation of parathyroid tissue are performed at the time of thyroidectomy when there is evidence of PHPT. The ATA MTC guidelines recommend that in individuals with a strong family history of PHPT or with *RET* mutations carrying high risk of PHPT, devascularized normal parathyroid glands should be autografted into the forearm, while those individuals with lower risk conferring mutations may have the parathyroid tissue autografted into either the forearm or the sternocleidomastoid muscle. This will help to preserve the remaining parathyroid tissue in the likely scenario of the patient requiring repeat neck operations for recurrent MTC, thus avoiding hypoparathyroidism. For MEN2A patients who have had prior thyroidectomy who later get PHPT, these individuals require preoperative localization using sestamibi and CT scans. In patients with persistent or recurrent PHPT, and in those who are suboptimal surgical candidates, medical therapy with calcimimetics may play a role. Calcimimetics reduce PTH secretion by increasing the sensitivity of parathyroid calcium-sensing receptors to extracellular calcium. Cinalcet, an oral calcimimetic, has been studied in a randomized double-blind placebo controlled study and has shown effectiveness in reducing PTH concentrations and PTH levels in patients with PHPT [51]. While cinacalcet may prove to be an attractive alternative to surgery in patients with PHPT, it is unknown if cinalcet will prove useful in patients with MEN2A-associated PHPT, and use in these patients is not documented.

Conclusion

MEN2 is an autosomal-dominant hereditary cancer syndrome caused by gain-of-function mutations in the *RET* proto-oncogene. MEN2A is defined as the presence of MTC, PHEO and PHPT. MEN2B is a multiple tumor syndrome associated with MTC, marfanoid habitus, ganglioneuromatosis of the oral mucosa and GI tract, and PHEO. Early screening of family members who may be affected by MEN2 is associated with improved prognosis. The timing of prophylactic thyroidectomy is guided by the ATA risk level of *RET* mutations. Surveillance for PHEO and PHPT is indicated in select groups of patients with specific *RET* mutations.

References

1 Moline J, Eng C: Multiple endocrine neoplasia type 2: an overview. Genet Med 2011;13:755–764.

2 Gagel RF, Levy ML, Donovan DT, Alford BR, Wheeler T, Tschen JA: Multiple endocrine neoplasia type 2a associated with cutaneous lichen amyloidosis. Ann Intern Med 1989;111:802–806.

3 Verdy M, Weber AM, Roy CC, Morin CL, Cadotte M, Brochu P: Hirschsprung's disease in a family with multiple endocrine neoplasia type 2. J Pediatr Gastroenterol Nutr 1982;1:603–607.

4 Howe JR, Norton JA, Wells SA Jr: Prevalence of pheochromocytoma and hyperparathyroidism in multiple endocrine neoplasia type 2A: results of long-term follow-up. Surgery 1993;114:1070–1077.

5 Eng C, Clayton D, Schuffenecker I, et al: The relationship between specific RET proto-oncogene mutations and disease phenotype in multiple endocrine neoplasia type 2. International RET mutation consortium analysis. JAMA 1996;276:1575–1579.

6 Wray CJ, Rich TA, Waguespack SG, Lee JE, Perrier ND, Evans DB: Failure to recognize multiple endocrine neoplasia 2B: more common than we think? Ann Surg Oncol 2008;15:293–301.

7 Brauckhoff M, Machens A, Hess S, Lorenz K, Gimm O, Brauckhoff K, Sekulla C, Dralle H: Premonitory symptoms preceding metastatic medullary thyroid cancer in MEN 2B: an exploratory analysis. Surgery 2008;144:1044–1050.

8 Kloos RT, Eng C, Evans DB, Francis GL, Gagel RF, Gharib H, Moley JF, Pacini F, Ringel MD, Schlumberger M, Wells SA Jr: Medullary thyroid cancer: management guidelines of the American Thyroid Association. Thyroid 2009;19:565–612.

9 Skinner MA, Moley JA, Dilley WG, Owzar K, Debenedetti MK, Wells SA Jr: Prophylactic thyroidectomy in multiple endocrine neoplasia type 2A. N Engl J Med 2005;353:1105–1113.

10 Ponder BA, Ponder MA, Coffey R, Pembrey ME, Gagel RF, Telenius-Berg M, Semple P, Easton DF: Risk estimation and screening in families of patients with medullary thyroid carcinoma. Lancet 1988;i:397–401.

11 Sipple JH: Association of pheochromocytoma with carcinoma of thyroid gland. Am J Med 1961;31:163.

12 Cushman P: Familial endocrine tumors – report of two unrelated kindred affected with pheochromocytomas, one also with multiple thyroid carcinomas. Am J Med 1962;32:352–360.

13 Mathew CG, Chin KS, Easton DF, et al: A linked genetic marker for multiple endocrine neoplasia type 2A on chromosome 10. Nature 1987;328:527–528.

14 Donis-Keller H, Dou S, Chi D, Carlson KM, Toshima K, Lairmore TC, Howe JR, Moley JF, Goodfellow P, Wells SA Jr: Mutations in the RET proto-oncogene are associated with MEN2A and FMTC. Hum Mol Genet 1993;2:851–856.

15 Mulligan LM, Kwok JB, Healey CS, et al: Germ-line mutations of the RET proto-oncogene in multiple endocrine neoplasia type 2A. Nature 1993;363:458–460.

16 Williams ED, Pollock DJ: Multiple mucosal neuromata with endocrine tumours – a syndrome allied to Von Recklinghausens disease. J Pathol Bacteriol 1966;91:71–80.

17 Hofstra RM, Landsvater RM, Ceccherini I, et al: A mutation in the RET proto-oncogene associated with multiple endocrine neoplasia type 2B and sporadic medullary thyroid carcinoma. Nature 1994;367:375–376.

18 Carlson KM, Dou S, Chi D, Scavarda N, Toshima K, Jackson CE, Wells SA Jr, Goodfellow PJ, Donis-Keller H: Single missense mutation in the tyrosine kinase catalytic domain of the RET proto-oncogene is associated with multiple endocrine neoplasia type 2B. Proc Natl Acad Sci USA 1994;91:1579–1583.
19 Brandi ML, Gagel RF, Angeli A, et al: Guidelines for diagnosis and therapy of MEN type 1 and type 2. J Clin Endocrinol Metab 2001;86:5658–5671.
20 Takahashi M, Ritz J, Cooper GM: Activation of a novel human transforming gene, ret, by DNA rearrangement. Cell 1985;42:581–588.
21 Arighi E, Borrello MG, Sariola H: RET tyrosine kinase signaling in development and cancer. Cytokine Growth Factor Rev 2005;16:441–467.
22 Lodish MB, Stratakis CA: RET oncogene in MEN2, MEN2B, MTC and other forms of thyroid cancer. Expert Rev Anticancer Ther 2008;8:625–632.
23 Asai N, Iwashita T, Matsuyama M, Takahashi M: Mechanism of activation of the ret proto-oncogene by multiple endocrine neoplasia 2A mutations. Mol Cell Biol 1995;15:1613–1619.
24 Santoro M, Carlomagno F, Romano A, et al: Activation of RET as a dominant transforming gene by germline mutations of MEN2A and MEN2B. Science 1995;267:381–383.
25 Schuffenecker I, Ginet N, Goldgar D, Eng C, Chambe B, Boneu A, Houdent C, Pallo D, Schlumberger M, Thivolet C, Lenoir GM: Prevalence and parental origin of de novo RET mutations in multiple endocrine neoplasia type 2A and familial medullary thyroid carcinoma. Le Groupe d'Etude des Tumeurs a Calcitonine. Am J Hum Genet 1997;60:233–237.
26 Carlson KM, Bracamontes J, Jackson CE, Clark R, Lacroix A, Wells SA Jr, Goodfellow PJ: Parent-of-origin effects in multiple endocrine neoplasia type 2B. Am J Hum Genet 1994;55:1076–1082.
27 Kebebew E, Ituarte PH, Siperstein AE, Duh QY, Clark OH: Medullary thyroid carcinoma: clinical characteristics, treatment, prognostic factors, and a comparison of staging systems. Cancer 2000;88:1139–1148.
28 Modigliani E, Cohen R, Campos JM, Conte-Devolx B, Maes B, Boneu A, Schlumberger M, Bigorgne JC, Dumontier P, Leclerc L, Corcuff B, Guilhem I: Prognostic factors for survival and for biochemical cure in medullary thyroid carcinoma: results in 899 patients. The GETC Study Group. Groupe d'etude des tumeurs a calcitonine. Clin Endocrinol (Oxf) 1998;48:265–273.
29 Quayle FJ, Moley JF: Medullary thyroid carcinoma: including MEN 2A and MEN 2B syndromes. J Surg Oncol 2005;89:122–129.
30 Brierley J, Tsang R, Simpson WJ, Gospodarowicz M, Sutcliffe S, Panzarella T: Medullary thyroid cancer: analyses of survival and prognostic factors and the role of radiation therapy in local control. Thyroid 1996;6:305–310.
31 Roman S, Lin R, Sosa JA: Prognosis of medullary thyroid carcinoma: demographic, clinical, and pathologic predictors of survival in 1252 cases. Cancer 2006;107:2134–2142.
32 Cohen MS, Moley JF: Surgical treatment of medullary thyroid carcinoma. J Intern Med 2003;253:616–626.
33 Wells SA Jr, Robinson BG, Gagel RF, Dralle H, Fagin JA, Santoro M, Baudin E, Elisei R, Jarzab B, Vasselli JR, Read J, Langmuir P, Ryan AJ, Schlumberger MJ: Vandetanib in patients with locally advanced or metastatic medullary thyroid cancer: a randomized, double-blind phase III trial. J Clin Oncol 2012;30:134–141.
34 Lam ET, Ringel MD, Kloos RT, Prior TW, Knopp MV, Liang J, Sammet S, Hall NC, Wakely PE Jr, Vasko VV, Saji M, Snyder PJ, Wei L, Arbogast D, Collamore M, Wright JJ, Moley JF, Villalona-Calero MA, Shah MH: Phase II clinical trial of sorafenib in metastatic medullary thyroid cancer. J Clin Oncol 2010;28:2323–2330.
35 Carr LL, Mankoff DA, Goulart BH, Eaton KD, Capell PT, Kell EM, Bauman JE, Martins RG: Phase II study of daily sunitinib in FDG-PET-positive, iodine-refractory differentiated thyroid cancer and metastatic medullary carcinoma of the thyroid with functional imaging correlation. Clin Cancer Res 2010;16:5260–5268.
36 Lairmore TC, Ball DW, Baylin SB, Wells SA Jr: Management of pheochromocytomas in patients with multiple endocrine neoplasia type 2 syndromes. Ann Surg 1993;217:595–601.
37 Rodriguez JM, Balsalobre M, Ponce JL, Rios A, Torregrosa NM, Tebar J, Parrilla P: Pheochromocytoma in MEN 2A syndrome. Study of 54 patients. World J Surg 2008;32:2520–2526.
38 Frank-Raue K, Rybicki LA, Erlic Z, et al: Risk profiles and penetrance estimations in multiple endocrine neoplasia type 2A caused by germline RET mutations located in exon 10. Hum Mutat 2011;32:51–58.
39 Modigliani E, Vasen HM, Raue K, et al: Pheochromocytoma in multiple endocrine neoplasia type 2: European study. The Euromen Study Group. J Intern Med 1995;238:363–367.
40 Alesina PF, Hinrichs J, Meier B, Schmid KW, Neumann HP, Walz MK: Minimally invasive cortical-sparing surgery for bilateral pheochromocytomas. Langenbecks Arch Surg 2012;397:233–238.

41 Asari R, Scheuba C, Kaczirek K, Niederle B: Estimated risk of pheochromocytoma recurrence after adrenal-sparing surgery in patients with multiple endocrine neoplasia type 2A. Arch Surg 2006;141: 1199–1205; discussion 1205.
42 O'Riordain DS, O'Brien T, Crotty TB, Gharib H, Grant CS, van Heerden JA: Multiple endocrine neoplasia type 2B: more than an endocrine disorder. Surgery 1995;118:936–942.
43 Leboulleux S, Travagli JP, Caillou B, Laplanche A, Bidart JM, Schlumberger M, Baudin E: Medullary thyroid carcinoma as part of a multiple endocrine neoplasia type 2B syndrome: influence of the stage on the clinical course. Cancer 2002;94:44–50.
44 Machens A, Brauckhoff M, Holzhausen HJ, Thanh PN, Lehnert H, Dralle H: Codon-specific development of pheochromocytoma in multiple endocrine neoplasia type 2. J Clin Endocrinol Metab 2005;90: 3999–4003.
45 Chen H, Sippel RS, O'Dorisio MS, Vinik AI, Lloyd RV, Pacak K: The North American Neuroendocrine Tumor Society consensus guideline for the diagnosis and management of neuroendocrine tumors: pheochromocytoma, paraganglioma, and medullary thyroid cancer. Pancreas 2010;39:775–783.
46 Ilias I, Pacak K: Diagnosis, localization and treatment of pheochromocytoma in MEN 2 syndrome. Endocr Regul 2009;43:89–93.
47 Ilias I, Chen CC, Carrasquillo JA, Whatley M, Ling A, Lazurova I, Adams KT, Perera S, Pacak K: Comparison of $^{6-18}$F-fluorodopamine PET with ^{123}I-metaiodobenzylguanidine and ^{111}In-pentetreotide scintigraphy in localization of nonmetastatic and metastatic pheochromocytoma. J Nucl Med 2008; 49:1613–1619.
48 Pacak K: Preoperative management of the pheochromocytoma patient. J Clin Endocrinol Metab 2007;92:4069–4079.
49 Kraimps JL, Denizot A, Carnaille B, Henry JF, Proye C, Bacourt F, Sarfati E, Dupond JL, Maes B, Travagli JP, Boneu A, Roger P, Houdent C, Barbier J, Modigliani E: Primary hyperparathyroidism in multiple endocrine neoplasia type IIa: retrospective French multicentric study. Groupe d'Etude des Tumeurs a Calcitonine (GETC, French Calcitonin Tumors Study Group), French Association of Endocrine Surgeons. World J Surg 1996;20:808–812.
50 Raue F, Kraimps JL, Dralle H, Cougard P, Proye C, Frilling A, Limbert E, Llenas LF, Niederle B: Primary hyperparathyroidism in multiple endocrine neoplasia type 2A. J Intern Med 1995;238:369–373.
51 Peacock M, Bilezikian JP, Klassen PS, Guo MD, Turner SA, Shoback D: Cinacalcet hydrochloride maintains long-term normocalcemia in patients with primary hyperparathyroidism. J Clin Endocrinol Metab 2005;90:135–141.

Maya Lodish, MD
Section on Endocrinology and Genetics, Eunice Kennedy Shriver National Institute of Child Health and Human Development, National Institutes of Health
Building 10-CRC, Room 1–3330, 10 Center Drive, MSC 1103, Bethesda, MD 20892 (USA)
E-Mail lodishma@mail.nih.gov

Stratakis CA (ed): Endocrine Tumor Syndromes and Their Genetics.
Front Horm Res. Basel, Karger, 2013, vol 41, pp 30–49 (DOI: 10.1159/000345668)

von Hippel-Lindau Syndrome

Angela Chou[a] · Christopher Toon[b–d] · Justine Pickett[b] · Anthony J. Gill[b–d]

[a]Department of Anatomical Pathology, St Vincents Hospital, Darlinghurst, N.S.W., Departments of [b]Anatomical Pathology and [c]Northern Cancer Translational Research Unit, Royal North Shore Hospital, St Leonards, N.S.W., and [d]University of Sydney, Sydney, N.S.W., Australia

Abstract

von Hippel-Lindau (VHL) disease is an autosomal-dominant familial cancer syndrome associated with mutations of the *VHL* tumor suppressor gene (3p25–26). Its estimated incidence ranges from 1 in 36,000 to 1 in 53,000 with a penetrance of up to 95% by age 60. Genotype-phenotype correlation divides VHL into two broad clinical subtypes. Type 1 VHL is predominantly associated with large deletion or truncation mutations which result in an encoded protein with very little or no activity. It is associated with retinal and CNS hemangioblastoma and renal cell carcinoma but not pheochromocytoma. Type 2 is usually associated with missense mutations encoding a protein with limited activity and includes pheochromocytoma. It is further classified into three other subtypes (2A, 2B, 2C) based on the presence of hemangioblastoma and renal cell carcinoma. Visceral cysts in the kidney, pancreas and epididymis, nonfunctioning pancreatic neuroendocrine tumors which often show distinctive clear cell cytology, endolymphatic sac tumors and head and neck paragangliomas are well recognized but less common presenting features. Surveillance of carriers can reduce the burden of disease and is best performed in specialist referral centers with due consideration given to both the complex molecular pathogenesis and psychosocial aspects of the disease.

von Hippel-Lindau (VHL) disease is a familial multisystem syndrome associated with germline mutation of the *VHL* tumor suppressor gene which spans 10 kb at chromosome 3p25 (OMIM 193300). It occurs in approximately 1 in 36,000 live births [1]. By age 60, the gene has a penetrance of 95% [1]. VHL patients are predisposed to retinal hemangioblastoma (commonly called 'retinal angioma'), central nervous system hemangioblastoma, pheochromocytoma, renal cell carcinoma, pancreatic neuroendocrine tumors, endolymphatic sac tumors and benign renal, epididymal and pancreatic cysts. Genotype-phenotype correlation divides VHL into two broad clinical subtypes based on the absence (type 1) or presence (type 2) of pheochromocytoma [2]. Type 2 VHL is further subclassified into three subtypes (2A, 2B, 2C) based on the presence or absence of hemangioblastoma and renal cell carcinoma. The management of VHL patients requires routine surveillance and a multidisciplinary approach due to multisystem involvement. Early detection and surgical intervention currently offers the best hope of diminishing the burden of disease. Despite advances in treatment and improved understanding of the underlying molecular pathogenesis, the outlook for VHL patients remains guarded, with a median survival of approximately 49 years [3]. In this review, we summarize the historical, clinical, pathological, genetic and molecular features of VHL syndrome.

Historical Perspectives

The first components of VHL syndrome began to be recognized in the late 19th century. These earliest observations of the disease have been summarized by Melmon and Rosen [4]. Briefly, in 1879 Panas and Remy illustrated a retinal hemangioblastoma but misclassified it as 'cystic detachment of the retina'. Between 1882 and 1902 Fuchs, von Dzialowski and Leplat all independently described patients with compatible ophthalmic findings but classified the lesions as 'arteriovenous aneurysms'. In 1894, Collins described the histopathology of three enucleations from a brother and sister. He concluded that the disease was hereditary and, although he used the term 'capillary nevus', his description of the retinal pathology in these cases ('made up of a plexus of numerous very thin-walled blood vessels and there are in [them] cystic spaces') indicates that the lesions he recognized were retinal hemangioblastomas. Collins did not recognize the extraocular components of the syndrome.

Initially unaware of Collins' work, in 1904 von Hippel published clinical data describing the progression of retinal disease in 2 patients. Seven years later, having become aware of Collins' work and being able to perform histological examination on a subsequently enucleated eye from one of his original patients, von Hippel described the pathological findings in terms similar to Collins as 'angiomatosis retinae'. One of von Hippel's patients subsequently died and underwent a full autopsy reported by Brandt in 1921. It was the unexpected findings in this autopsy that led to extraocular disease being recognized as part of this syndrome. Vascular tumors were found in the cerebellum, base of the brain and spinal cord. There were cysts in the kidneys, pancreas and epididymides as well as tumors in the kidneys, several ribs and a vertebra. Brandt's literature review revealed that in at least 10% of all reported cases of 'angiomatosis retinae', signs of central nervous system neoplasia were also identified. Most memorably, he highlighted a previous case report of brothers with retinal disease who had earned their living as tightrope walkers before the onset of cerebellar dysfunction!

These observations allowed Lindau to revisit the syndrome in 1926 and describe the retinal, cerebral and visceral components of the disease as one cohesive entity. Importantly he recognized that the retinal lesions and CNS lesions showed similar morphological features and identified retinal disease in two of his own cases who were thought clinically to only have cerebellar tumors. Although he was aware of the visceral components of the disease, Lindau did not emphasize them as he considered them benign and clinically insignificant. Thus, despite the fact that of the 16 new cases he reported, 8 had pancreatic cysts, 10 renal cysts and 6 renal tumors, Lindau used the term 'central nervous system angiomatosis' for this syndrome and emphasized the CNS manifestations at the expense of visceral disease.

The entity which is now known as a cerebellar hemangioblastoma came to be known as a 'Lindau tumor' while the morphologically identical lesion in the retina was known as a 'von Hippel tumour'. By the time of Melmon and Rose's review in 1964, the hereditary syndrome was known as 'Lindau disease'. This term was gradually replaced by 'von-Hippel Lindau (VHL)' disease in the 1970s.

Molecular Genetics

The *VHL* tumor suppressor gene maps to 3p25.3, spans 10 kb and contains three exons which are transcribed into two spliced mRNAs differing by the presence (isoform I) or absence (isoform II) of exon 2 [5]. No endogenous protein has been described associated with isoform II and it is likely that isoform 1 is the only form that results in functional protein. Isoform 1 results in two translation products – a 28- to 30-kDa 213 amino acid protein (pVHL30) and an 18- to 19-kDA 160 amino acid protein (pVHL19). The pVHL19 differs from pVHL30 by the absence of the first 53 amino acids. These first 53 amino acids of pVHL30 are less evolutionarily conserved than the remainder of the protein which shows strong interspecies homology [6].

Since 1993 more than 900 kindreds with *VHL* mutations have been reported (http://www.umd.be/) and germline mutations have been identified in more than 95% of non-mosaics with classical disease [6, 7]. Most patients with VHL have a strong family history, however approximately 20% of UK and USA cases appear to occur from de novo mutations [8]. Studies from China report a higher incidence of apparently de novo cases – approximately 55% [9].

The reported mutations can be divided into three distinct classes [10]. Approximately 40% are large genomic deletions (0.5–250 kb) resulting in removal of one or more exons usually due to Alu-mediated recombination [11]. Missense mutations and mutations predicted to cause a truncated protein (nonsense, frameshift insertions and deletions, splice site mutations) account for approximately equal numbers of the remainder. To date no mutations have been reported in the first 53 amino acids of pVHL30 [6].

Type 1 VHL (pheochromocytoma absent or rare) is usually associated with large (e.g. exon) deletions and truncating mutations which result in a nonfunctional protein [12]. In contrast, most type 2 families are associated with missense mutations which appear to encode a protein with some, albeit limited, activity [12]. Some mis-

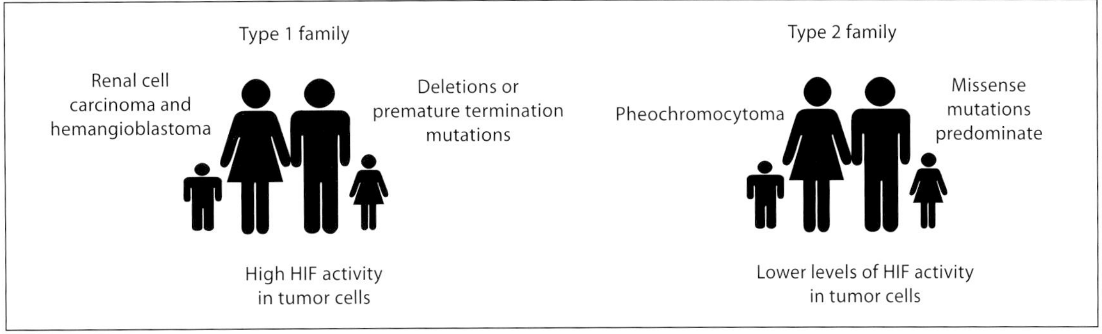

Fig. 1. Genotype-phenotype correlation in VHL syndrome families. HIF = Hypoxia inducible factor.

Table 1. VHL disease genotype-phenotype correlation

Type 1
- Usually associated with exon deletions and truncating mutations
- Susceptibility to hemangioblastoma
- No phemochromocytoma

Type 2
- Usually associated with missense mutation
- Susceptibility to pheochromocytoma
- *Type 2A:* susceptible to hemangioblastomma but rarely to renal cell carcinoma
- *Type 2B:* susceptible to hemangioblastoma and renal cell carcinoma
- *Type 2C:* susceptible only to pheochromocytoma

sense mutations which are predicted to alter pVHL protein folding and therefore cause complete disruption of the pVHL structure and function may result in a type 1 phenotype. A summary of genotype-phenotype correlation are outlined in table 1 and figure 1. Homozygous missense mutations of *VHL* may cause isolated congenital polycythemia syndromes.

VHL Protein

Both pVHL19 and pVHL30 are widely expressed in adult and fetal tissue. They appear to have a role in development by controlling transcriptional elongation during embryogenesis [13]. pVHL30 is found predominantly in the cytoplasm, with lower amounts in the nucleus or associated with cell membranes. In contrast, pVHL19 is equally distributed between the cytoplasm and nucleus and is unassociated with membranes. Despite these differences in cellular compartment locations and size, both proteins share similar biological profiles, and may be referred to collectively as pVHL.

Table 2. Clinical diagnostic criteria for VHL disease [4]

Patients without a family history of VHL
– Two or more CNS hemangioblastomas
or
– One CNS hemangioblastoma and a visceral tumor (excluding epididymal or renal cysts)
Patients with a family history of VHL disease
– One CNS hemangioblatoma
or
– Pheochromocytoma
or
– Clear cell renal carcinoma

Hypoxia inducible factors (HIF1 and HIF2) are DNA-binding transcription factors which act as master transcriptional activators for 100–200 genes that promote cellular adaptation and growth under hypoxic conditions. pVHL has been shown to form a complex with elongin B, elongin C, Cullin-2 and Rbx1 (VCB-Cul2 complex), which regulates the ubiquitin mediated proteolytic degradation of the α subunits of HIF1 and HIF2 [14–18]. Briefly, in the presence of oxygen, proline hydroxylase enzymes are able to modify the α subunits of HIF which in turn facilitates pVHL binding and ubiquitin-mediated degradation, resulting in destabilization and loss of function of the HIF heterodimer. However, in the presence of either hypoxia (in which case the α subunits of HIF are unmodified and cannot bind pVHL) or if pVHL is absent or inactive, then HIF1 and HIF2 are stabilized and act as transcription factors for the hypoxic response (fig. 2). This hypoxic response affects glucose uptake and metabolism, angiogenesis, extracellular matrix formation, chemotaxis and cell proliferation and is therefore directly implicated in the tumorigenesis of VHL neoplasms [19].

Other less well understood roles of pVHL are independent of HIF activity and include inhibition of atypical protein kinase C-mediated cellular signaling to regulate apoptosis, binding to the hydroxylated α-chain of collagen IV and interaction with fibronectin to enable intact extracellular matrix assembly, regulation of NKκB by inhibiting phosphorylation of nuclear factor-kappa B (NFκB) against Card9 and regulation of β-catenin/Wnt signaling by stabilization of Jade-1 [20, 21]. pVHL has also been found to bind clusterin (a glycoprotein involved in multiple biological processes including cell survival and apoptosis) and mediate K63-linked ubiquitination and nuclear translocation [22].

Clinical Features

VHL syndrome can be diagnosed by formal genetic testing in an at-risk individual or by clinical criteria. These clinical criteria were initially proposed by Melmon and Rosen [4] and are summarized in table 2. Briefly, the diagnosis of VHL can be made

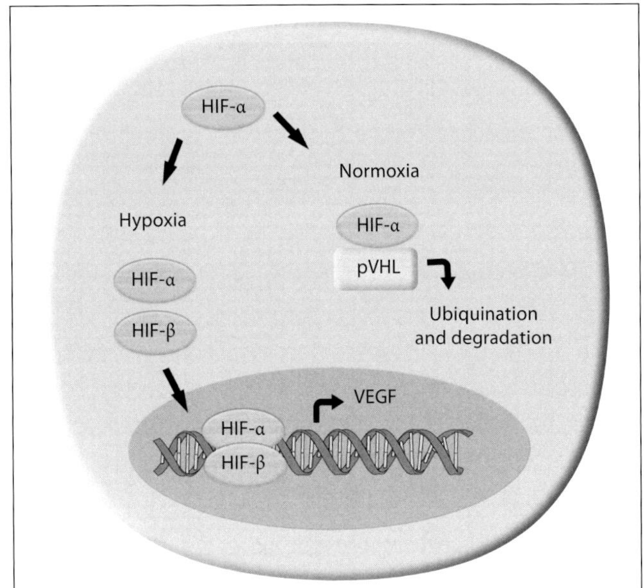

Fig. 2. HIF shuttles between the cytoplasm (where it is under negative feedback control by pVHL-mediated ubiquination and degradation) and the nucleus where it acts as a transcripter activator for many genes. In this simplified example, HIF promotes angiogenesis via activation of VEGF.

clinically if a single VHL-associated tumor (that is a hemangioblastoma, pheochromocytoma or clear cell renal carcinoma) occurs in an individual with a family history of VHL. The diagnosis can also be made clinically in the absence of a family history if a second VHL associated tumor occurs in an individual with hemangioblastoma (that is two or more hemangioblastomas or both a hemangioblastoma and a pheochromocytoma or clear cell renal carcinoma). As approximately 20% of VHL disease results from de novo mutations, the absence of a family history in no way excludes the diagnosis. VHL is thought to cause up to 33% of CNS hemangioblastomas [23], 50% of retinal hemangioblastomas [24], 1% of renal carcinoma [25], 50% of apparently isolated familial pheochromocytoma and 11% of patients with apparently sporadic pheochromocytoma [6]. Therefore, the possibility of VHL should at least be considered whenever one of these neoplasms is encountered.

The median age of first presentation is 22 years (mean of approximately 25 years) [26]. The most common lesions are in the central nervous system (retinal and cerebellar hemangioblastoma), kidney (clear cell renal cell carcinoma, renal cyst), adrenal gland/paraganglia (pheochromocytoma/paraganglioma), pancreas (neuroendocrine tumors, pancreatic cyst, serous cystadenoma) and middle ear (endolymphatic sac tumor) [27]. Other less common lesions include broad ligament cystadenomas and epididymal cystadenomas. Retinal hemangioblastoma and endolymphatic sac tumor usually present the earliest (mean 25 and 22 years, respectively) followed by pheochromocytoma (mean 24 years), cerebellar hemangioblastoma (mean 30 years), spinal hemangioblastoma (mean 33.3 years), pancreatic neuroendocrine tumor (36 years) and renal cell carcinoma (40 years) [26, 28, 29].

The frequency of each neoplasm varies depending on the clinical phenotype [27]. Overall, retinal hemangioblastoma occurs most frequently (73%) followed by cerebellar hemangioblastoma (57%), renal cell carcinoma (35%), spinal hemangioblastoma (25%), pheochromocytoma (20%) and pancreatic neuroendocrine tumor (12%) [26, 29].

Retinal and CNS Hemangioblastoma

Although they are commonly termed 'retinal angiomas', the ophthalmic lesions of VHL show identical histological features to the CNS tumors and are better classified as hemangioblastomas. They are the most common tumors of VHL syndrome and usually occur in the peripheral retina or juxtapapillary regions. About 50% of cases are multifocal and/or bilateral [30]. Diagnosis is usually made by simple dilated fundoscopy, with fluorescein angiography being used only if there is uncertainty. The cumulative risk of blindness has been estimated at 30% in patients with retinal hemangioblastomas [30]. Most small peripheral lesions can be adequately treated with laser photocoagulation while larger lesions may require cryotherapy. Lesions at the optic disc are monitored for progression before treatment due to the risk of optic nerve damage. There have been isolated case reports of response to anti-angiogenic therapy with vascular endothelial growth factor receptor inhibitors [31, 32].

CNS hemangioblastomas occur most commonly in the spinal cord, cerebellum, brainstem and rarely supratentorially [33]. These lesions demonstrate a growth pattern characterized by periods of quiescence alternating with periods of active growth [33]. Symptomatic presentation is variable and only 41% of patients will present symptomatically during long-term follow-up (mean follow-up 12.5 years) [34, 35]. Presentation depends on the exact anatomical site of the lesion and includes symptoms of increased intracranial pressure (hydrocephalus, nausea, vomiting), limb/truncal ataxia, hyperreflexia, hypesthesia, dysesthesia, bladder and bowel complaints [33]. Due to the variable growth rate of hemangioblastoma, surgical removal of a stable asymptomatic lesion is generally not indicated. Resection of symptomatic lesions using microsurgical techniques with coagulation and division of the circumferential vessels feeding the tumor is the current standard of care [36]. In the case of a cystic lesion with an intramural nodule, only the nodule is resected as the surrounding capsule is composed of reactive gliosis and not neoplastic tissue. Therefore, the cyst wall usually collapses after surgery [34].

Spinal lesions comprise nearly half of CNS hemangioblastomas. They usually occur in the cervical and thoracic spinal cord, and are commonly located at the dorsal nerve root zone. At 6-month follow-up after surgery, 96% of patients will be stable with symptomatic improvement. However, intramedullary or ventral spinal cord lesions are more likely to be associated with significant postoperative morbidities [37].

Brainstem lesions account for 10–15% of cases and usually occur at the floor of the 4th ventricle, dorsal aspect of the medulla oblongata or the cervicomedullary junction. Presenting symptoms include swallowing difficulties, headache, sensory difficulties and impaired gait. Most patients will remain functionally stable and symptom-free while 18% will show symptomatic deterioration post-surgery. Approximately 16% of these patients will show symptomatic improvement [38]. Stereotactic radiotherapy has been proposed as an alternative therapeutic option for difficult lesions; however, the effectiveness and side effect profile of the treatment requires further validation [39].

Magnetic resonance imaging (MRI) with gadolinium contrast is the imaging modality of choice for detecting hemangioblastoma. The typical radiological features include a well-demarcated contrast-enhancing lesion, usually associated with a cyst [36].

Retinal and CNS hemangioblastoma demonstrate similar gross and histological features. On gross examination, the tumors are bright red or orange/yellow. A solid component is always present, but this often co-exists with a cystic element; the classic gross appearance being that of a vascular mural nodule within a cystic cavity. Cyst formation is believed to occur as a result of peritumoral edema due to the increased vascular permeability of these neoplasms, and can account for a significant amount of the tumor's mass effect [40].

The neoplastic cells within a hemangioblastoma are the 'stromal' cells [41, 42]. These are distributed within a prominent network of small-caliber vascular channels. They have abundant clear cytoplasm, imparted by the presence of cytoplasmic vacuoles containing lipid. A degree of degenerative nuclear atypia may be present [43]. Cellular and reticular variants of both VHL-associated and sporadic hemangioblastomas have been described, with the cellular variant comprising a minority of tumors. This variant is composed of epithelioid cells forming columns and alveolar structures within a less prominent vascular network, and may be associated with a higher risk of recurrence [44].

The stromal cells of hemangioblastoma typically show positive immunohistochemical staining for S100, inhibin, vimentin and neuron-specific enolase. They are negative for cytokeratins, and for EMA [43]. The major differential diagnosis in the setting of VHL is metastatic renal cell carcinoma. This is complicated by the fact that areas of metastatic renal cell carcinoma have been described within hemangioblastomas [45]. A recent study has proposed the use of a combined panel of PAX-2 and PAX-8 (positive in renal cell carcinoma) and inhibin-A (positive in hemangioblastoma) as a sensitive and specific way of distinguishing these tumors [46].

The neoplastic stromal cells in hemangioblastoma are believed to originate from the hemangioblast; a precursor cell of mesodermal derivation which has undergone embryologic arrest. These cells have the potential for both hematopoietic and endothelial differentiation [47]. In an autopsy study performed on patients with VHL, multiple microscopic 'tumorlets' were discovered within the cerebellum and spinal nerve roots. These were composed of small undifferentiated cells showing positive immunohistochemical staining for neuron-specific enolase, with a prominent capillary network, and were interpreted as representing precursor lesions [48].

The development of hemangioblastomas in VHL correlate well with HIF dysfunction and evidence suggests that precursor lesions arise due to developmental arrest during embryogenesis. In patients with CNS hemangioblastoma, developmental arrest structures can be found in VHL patients but not in sporadic cases [49].

Clear Cell Renal Cell Carcinoma and Renal Cysts

Renal cell carcinoma is the major cause of death in VHL patients. Multiple and bilateral lesions usually occur [25]. Multiple renal cysts often occur but usually do not compromise renal function.

Routine annual imaging detects small lesions with low risk of distant metastasis. A small lesion is usually monitored until it reaches 3 cm, when nephron-sparing surgical resection can be offered [50]. Multiple renal surgeries may eventually compromise renal function and result in end stage renal failure [51]. Renal transplantation does not appear to adversely affect the underlying course of disease and VHL is not usually considered an exclusion criterion for transplant [52].

The full range of lesions may be seen in the same kidney, and can be present as microscopic foci adjacent to resected tumors [53, 54]. Simple cysts are lined by a single layer of epithelial cells. In contrast to sporadic renal cysts, the epithelial cells lining the cysts associated with VHL often demonstrate clear cytoplasm. Atypical cysts are lined by 2–3 layers of epithelial cells with clear cytoplasm. The renal cell carcinomas which arise in VHL are always of clear cell type (sometimes known as 'conventional clear cell renal carcinoma'). Clear cell renal cell carcinoma occurring in VHL is usually low grade (Fuhrman nuclear grade 1–2). It is typically circumscribed and may have a pseudocapsule. A cystic component is not uncommon, and carcinomas may be seen arising in lesions with an appearance otherwise in keeping with simple or atypical cysts.

In renal cell carcinoma, HIF dysfunction is necessary, but does not appear sufficient for tumor development. Recently, the critical role of pVHL in microtubule dynamics, in particular the maintenance and function of the primary cilium, has been elucidated [55–57]. The primary cilium is intimately involved in chemical and mechanical signal transduction, linking environmental cues to cell cycle control [58]. Thoma et al. [59] showed that pVHL is involved in cilia maintenance in kidney-derived cell lines and that renal cysts in VHL patients demonstrated reduced frequencies of primary cilia. The authors proposed that the disruption of the ciliary maintenance signaling pathways due to loss of HIF-independent pVHL function increases the vulnerability of cells to cilia loss thereby promoting the formation of cysts.

Similar defects in cilia maintenance have also been described by Montani et al. [60] who showed that in kidneys of VHL patients, shortening or loss of cilia is found in the spectrum of VHL lesions including cysts and renal cell carcinoma. Further supporting renal cysts as a precursor lesion of renal cell carcinoma in VHL patients, the *CA9* gene product was found in both these lesions in this study. In VHL, pVHL inactivation with resultant activation of HIF-dependent pathways caused activation of the *CA9* gene. The *CA9* gene product, carbonic anhydrase IX, functions to promote reversible hydration of carbon dioxide. Using immunohistochemistry, carbonic anhydrase IX can be demonstrated in VHL related renal cell carcinoma, cystic lesions and also in patchy single histologically normal tubular cells. This finding suggests that pVHL inactivation is shared by all VHL renal lesions and that renal cysts are a precursor lesion of renal cell carcinoma.

The transcription factor NF-κB has recently emerged as an important component in renal cell carcinoma tumorigenesis. Activation of NF-κB is found in VHL associated clear cell renal carcinomas, due to defective regulation by the VHL-HIF pathway. This results in a tumor cell survival advantage via enhanced resistance to apoptosis, increased angiogenesis and drug resistance [61]. In view of this, NF-κB inhibition may represent a potential therapeutic strategy [62].

Pheochromocytoma/Paraganglioma

Most of these tumors (more than 90%) occurring in association with VHL are pheochromocytomas arising within the adrenal gland [63]. Extra-adrenal paragangliomas may occur, as carotid body, vagal, or para-aortic neoplasms. The adrenal tumors may be bilateral (44%), or involve the same gland in a metachronous fashion. They have been reported to be smaller and more often nonfunctional than sporadic tumors. This may reflect a screening bias rather than a quality inherent to VHL-associated pheochromocytomas [64]. Although metastasis has been reported, the overall risk of malignancy associated with VHL disease is considerably lower than in other pheochromocytomas and has been estimated at 3% [65].

Some histologic features have been reported to occur in VHL-associated pheochromocytomas which differ from those seen when the tumors occur in other syndromes or sporadically. These include a thick vascular tumor capsule, myxoid stroma, rounded small to medium-sized tumor cells with interspersed small vascular channels, prominent amphophilic or clear cytoplasm, lack of hyaline globules, lack of nuclear atypia or mitoses, and an absence of adjacent adrenal medullary hyperplasia. While these features may be clues to the diagnosis of VHL, there is considerable overlap with sporadic tumors [66].

In contrast to renal cell carcinoma and hemangioblastoma, HIF dysfunction does not appear to be associated with the development of pheochromocytoma suggesting an alternative HIF-independent pathway to the tumorigenesis. Lee et al. [67] found in type 2 VHL, mutant pVHL affected apoptotic pathways. They postulated that inherited pheochromocytomas occur due to apoptotic escape of sympathetic neuronal progenitors during fetal development.

Pancreatic Neuroendocrine Tumor and Pancreatic Cyst

Pancreatic involvement by VHL can manifest as cystic lesions or pancreatic neuroendocrine tumors (PNET). The cystic lesions have been termed 'VHL-associated serous cystic neoplasms' and manifest as single or multiple benign cysts in 17–56% of patients [68, 69]. The most common of these lesions are unilocular cysts lined by a single layer of bland epithelium containing cytoplasmic glycogen. Multilocular lesions also occur, with an appearance very similar to sporadic microcystic or macrocystic adenomas. A notable point of difference when compared to the solitary well-defined sporadic lesion is the often ill-defined nature of many VHL-associated serous cystic neoplasms, which can involve the pancreas in a multifocal or even diffuse 'sponge-like' fashion [70, 71].

VHL-related PNETs may be multiple and are invariably nonfunctioning. Approximately 8% of the tumors will be malignant and the single best predictor of malignancy is tumor size greater than 3 cm [29, 72]. Compared to sporadic pancreatic neuroendocrine tumors, VHL tumors are more likely to show histological features associated with aggressive behavior, such as extrapancreatic extension, invasion of surrounding tissue, vascular invasion, perineural invasion and liver metastasis; Ki-67 immunohistochemistry as a marker of cell proliferation range from 1 to 25% [73]. Similar to sporadic PNET the prognosis after surgery is generally good. The mortality rate for PNET is lower than for hemangioblastoma and renal carcinoma and has been estimated to be 6% [73].

Pancreatic neuroendocrine tumors in VHL show no apparent predilection for any site within the pancreas. The tumors are circumscribed and of variable color. They may demonstrate conventional pancreatic neuroendocrine tumor histology; however, focal or diffuse clear cell areas are common and serve as a clue to the diagnosis of VHL [74]. Microadenomas (≤5 mm), some with clear cells, are usually found in the adjacent pancreas and are described in more than 70% of patients operated on for pancreatic neuroendocrine tumors [75].

The tumors show positive immunohistochemistry for synaptophysin and chromogranin. This may be helpful in distinguishing tumors with prominent clear cell morphology from metastatic renal cell carcinoma [74]. Although these tumors are never functional, immunohistochemistry for pancreatic and gastrointestinal hormones may occasionally be positive [76]. Serous cystic lesions and pancreatic neuroendocrine tumors can occur in the same pancreas, and have been reported as occurring intimately admixed with one another. This combination is suggestive of VHL, but has also been described as a sporadic event [77].

Most pancreatic neuroendocrine tumors are associated with VHL germline mutations in exon 3 and 1. Mutation types include missense mutation, nonsense mutation, splice site mutation, small deletion, in-frame insertion and gene rearrangement [78]. An association between metastasis and exon 3 mutation in VHL has been reported but has not been reproduced in other studies [79].

The pathway of tumorigenesis in pancreatic neuroendocrine tumors has been investigated using mRNA expression profiling by Speisky et al. [80]. They found that compared to sporadic PNET, VHL PNET showed different expression of multiple genes which correlate with pVHL inactivation. In VHL PNET there is low pVHL, and upregulation of multiple genes involved in the HIF pathway *(CA9, HIF2A, GLUT2)*, angiogenesis *(VEGFR1, CDH5, EDNRA, ANGPT2, CD34, VEGR2, VEGRA, ANGPT1)*, cell cycle signaling (cyclin D1, CDKN2A), epithelial-mesenchymal transition (vimentin), growth factor and receptors *(PDGFB, IRS1, ERBB1)* and metastasis *(LAMA4, CXCR4)*. In addition, using immunohistochemistry pVHL (low), HIF-1α (high), carbonic anhydrase IX (high), cyclin D1 (high), vimentin (high), E-cadherin (low) have shown similar staining pattern between PNET and microadenomas which is associated with reverse pattern of staining in adjacent normal islet cells. These features support micro-adenomas as precursor lesions of PNET in VHL.

Endolymphatic SAC Tumors

The endolymphatic sac tumor was described as a distinct entity by Heffner [81] in 1989. It was only relatively recently proven to be a manifestation of VHL [28] and can be identified by MRI or computer tomography (CT) imaging in up to 11% of all VHL patients [82]. Bilateral tumors are pathognomonic of VHL disease and occur in one third of cases [28]. The tumors are usually asymptomatic, but patients may present with hearing loss or less commonly, tinnitus and vertigo. Sudden catastrophic hearing loss may occur due to hemorrhage, otic capsule invasion or endolymphatic hydrops. CT and MRI imaging classically show a lesion with destruction of the middle ear structures and petrous temporal bone. It is recommended that symptomatic patients undergo surgical resection via the retrolabyrinthrine posterior petrosectomy approach [34].

Endolymphatic sac tumors arise from the vestibular aqueduct, the intraosseous portion of the sac [83–85]. These tumors are locally aggressive and can invade into the temporal bone and even into the posterior fossa [82]. They can also be symptomatic even if very small. Histologically, the tumor forms papillary, glandular and cystic structures, lined by a single layer of low cuboidal cells showing little nuclear variability [86]. Some cystic structures can contain periodic acid-Schiff reagent (PAS) positive colloid-like material. Clear cell areas may occur, and predominate in some tumors. The stroma contains prominent small-caliber vascular channels. Hemorrhage, hemosiderin deposition and fibrosis are often present. The tumor cells are positive for cytokeratins by immunohistochemistry. Staining for thyroglobulin is negative which helps distinguish them from metastatic papillary thyroid carcinoma [81]. Microscopic lesions have been described in endolymphatic sacs of asymptomatic VHL patients. These show variable morphology, comprising microscopic papillary epithelial proliferations, cystic structures, and foci of clear cell change and are associated with inactivation of the *VHL* gene, suggesting that they represent true precursor lesions.

The rarity of endolymphatic sac tumor has made correlation with VHL genotype difficult and there are only a few case reports with sequencing data. One VHL patient showed a one base pair deletion in exon 1 and loss of heterozygosity (LOH) at the *VHL* locus [87]. In a report of 3 cases (2 of which were sporadic), there was normal VHL-mediated HIF1 regulation in all tumors with no *VHL* mutations being found in the sporadic tumors and no LOH in the VHL-related tumor [88]. In a report of four sporadic cases, two were associated with somatic mutations of *VHL* (one also with gene deletion) and one was associated with *VHL* gene deletion without mutation [89].

Papillary Cystadenoma

The two remaining well-recognized VHL-associated lesions are papillary cystadenomas of the epididymis, and its infrequent female counterpart, papillary cystadenoma of the broad ligament. Both lesions are believed to be of mesonephric origin. Although epididymal cystadenomas occur in up to 60% of male VHL patients, sporadic forms of the epididymal lesions are a more common cause of clinically significant epididymal disease. In contrast, few sporadic broad ligament lesions have been described. In the setting of VHL, bilateral tumors are not uncommon at both locations.

Papillary cystadenoma of the epididymis arises within efferent ductules in the head of the epididymis, while papillary cystadenoma of the broad ligament often arises in the area of the mesosalpinx [90, 91]. Both tumors have similar gross and microscopic findings. They form circumscribed, sometimes encapsulated lesions with a partially cystic cut surface. On histologic examination, papillary structures comprising fibrovascular cores covered by cuboidal to columnar epithelium project into cyst lumina. Some cystic structures contain eosinophilic colloid-like material. Tubular and nested arrangements of cells may also be seen. A significant proportion of cells have clear cytoplasm. A mild degree of nuclear variation may occur. There is a prominent vascular network. The epithelium in the lesions shows EMA and cytokeratin positivity, with a CK7-positive, CK20-negative immunoprofile. Variable staining patterns for other markers have been described, including for vimentin and CD10 [92, 93]. RCCMa is usually negative and, in combination with CK7, may be useful in distinguishing these lesions from metastatic renal cell carcinoma.

Putative precursor lesions termed 'epididymal tumorlets' which show evidence of *VHL* gene inactivation have been described in the epididymal ductular system of the

Table 3. Routine surveillance protocol for VHL disease (modified from Maher [104])

Screen for retinal hemangioblastoma: annual ophthalmic examinations (direct and indirect ophthalmoscopy), beginning in infancy or early childhood
Screen for CNS hemangioblastoma: MRI scans of the head every 12–36 months, beginning in adolescence
Screen for renal cell carcinoma and pancreatic tumors: MRI (or ultrasound) examinations of the abdomen every 12 months, beginning from the age of 16 years
Screen for phaeochromocytoma: annual blood pressure monitoring and 24 hour urine studies for catecholamine metabolites; more intense surveillance (e.g. annual measurement of plasma normetanephrine levels, adrenal imaging, beginning from the age of 8 years should be considered in families at high-risk for pheochromocytomas)

head of the epididymis of patients with VHL. Several different histologic patterns have been described, including complex epithelial change, papillary change, cystic change, and clear cell change [91]. Mesonephric rests have been described adjacent to papillary cystadenoma of the broad ligament [90].

Other Tumors

Rare tumors which have been reported in patients with VHL syndrome include hemangioblastoma-like lesions in other organs such as the adrenal gland and liver, neuroendocrine tumors at other sites including the duodenum and gallbladder, lipid cell tumors of the ovary, microcystic adenoma of the ethmoid sinus, papillary cystadenoma with multifocal microcysts in the lung, cerebellar astrocytoma and chondrosarcoma of the iliac wing [94–102]. However, many of these are single case reports and may represent coincidental associations.

Screening/Prognosis

The median life expectancy for VHL patients is approximately 49 years [103]. The major cause of mortality is metastatic renal cell carcinoma and neurological complications of hemangioblastoma. Because VHL is a multisystem disease a multidiscipline approach to management is essential. All VHL patients and families should enter a screening program from childhood. Currently, the interval for surveillance of VHL neoplasms is every 12 months and a widely accepted screening protocol for VHL disease recommended by Maher [104] is presented in table 3.

With current screening programs and improved genetic counseling, retinal hemangioblastomas are being detected at an early and commonly asymptomatic stage. The mean age of first tumor presentation, however, remains largely unchanged compared to 12 years ago when the data were first presented by Maher. One explanation for this is that although young individuals are now being detected earlier, older asymptomatic family members under surveillance will be picked up with late-onset tumors, hence balancing the shift of the curve to the left [26].

Early detection of retinal hemangioblastoma and renal cell carcinoma due to screening programs is clearly beneficial. Small retinal hemangioblastomas are easier to treat hence lessening the risk of major complications. Renal cell carcinomas can be safely monitored until they reach 3 cm in diameter and then treated by nephron sparing surgery due to the very low metastatic risk of small tumors. Earlier detection of cerebellar hemangioblastomas is currently less useful as most centers will only treat symptomatic lesions. The benefits of early detection, however, may increase with the development of novel targeted therapies.

Future Directions

The improved understanding of the role of the *VHL* gene in the activation or dysregulation of various cellular pathways raises the possibility of targeted therapies in both VHL and in sporadic neoplasms associated with the VHL-HIF pathway. Recently, drugs which modify the VHL-HIF pathway such as the multiple tyrosine kinase inhibitors sunitinib and sorafenib (VEGFRs and PDGFs inhibitors, respectively), and the mTOR inhibitor temsirolimus have been approved by the US Food and Drug Administration for treatment of sporadic and VHL-related renal carcinoma [105–109].

As promising as targeted therapies are, response remains variable from patient to patient, the reasons for which are currently unclear. In a phase II clinical trial, sunitinib was found to be effective in only 17% of patients with pancreatic neuroendocrine tumors, although a follow-up phase III clinical trial demonstrated an improvement in median progression-free survival for responders [110, 111]. Although, the association of response with underlying molecular biology (history of VHL or *VHL* gene inactivation) was not assessed, there is a case report of a VHL patient with metastatic pancreatic neuroendocrine tumor with no demonstrable disease progression after 4 years on sunitinib treatment [112]. In another case report, sunitinib was given to a VHL patient with renal cell carcinoma, pancreatic neuroendocrine tumor and metastatic pheochromocytoma. The patient showed clinical improvement with normalization of blood pressure, a decrease in plasma normetanephrines and chromogranin A level, and shrinkage of all three tumors after 6 months of treatment [113]. Clinical trials assessing the response of hemangioblastoma to multiple tyrosine kinase inhibitors and mTOR inhibitors are yet to be conducted. However, a single case of pazopanib use in hemangioblastoma has been reported [114].

Many other novel therapeutics directly and indirectly targeting the HIF pathway are still being investigated. These may be useful both in tumors and in non-neoplastic conditions where persistent activation of the HIF pathway results in an undesired angiogenic response, such as in cardiovascular ischemia, pre-eclampsia and anemia. These drugs can be divided into those that target upstream regulating signaling pathways (PI3K/Akt inhibitor, Trx-1 inhibitor, Topo-I inhibitor, Topo-II inhibitor, HDAC inhibitor, microtubules inhibitor, Hsp90 inhibitor, PHD activator, p53-MDM2), directly target HIF (antisense to HIF-1α mRNA, DNA intercalator, HIF-DNA binding inhibitor, inhibitor of HIF dimerization) or target downstream transcriptional activity (VEGF inhibitor, hexokinase inhibitor, MCT1 inhibitor, CAIX/CAXII inhibitor) [115]. Unfortunately, few of the direct HIF inhibitors have shown response in preclinical models. Drugs targeting upstream and downstream pathways are currently not entirely specific as these drugs cannot differentiate between different HIF isoforms which have similar gene targets but may have opposing activity. A few of these drugs are currently in phase I and II clinical trials for solid cancers [110]. Clinical trials of combination therapies are also underway to determine if there are synergistic effects of VHL-HIF pathway inhibition with other therapeutic agents (http://clinicaltrials.gov).

Conclusion

VHL syndrome is a multisystem inherited disease associated with mutation of the *VHL* gene. It is characterized by development of multiple solid neoplasms. With recent advances in the understanding of the molecular biology and pathogenesis of VHL neoplasms, it is hoped that novel therapies will pave the way for more effective ways to treat and manage this disease.

References

1 Maher ER, et al: von Hippel-Lindau disease: a genetic study. J Med Genet 1991;28:443–447.
2 Chen F, et al: Germline mutations in the von Hippel-Lindau disease tumor suppressor gene: correlations with phenotype. Hum Mutat 1995;5:66–75.
3 Maher ER, et al: Clinical features and natural history of von Hippel-Lindau disease. Q J Med 1990; 77:1151–1163.
4 Melmon KL, Rosen SW: Lindau's disease. Review of the literature and study of a large kindred. Am J Med 1964;36:595–617.
5 Richards FM, et al: Mapping the von Hippel-Lindau disease tumour suppressor gene: identification of germline deletions by pulsed field gel electrophoresis. Hum Mol Genet 1993;2:879–882.
6 Maher ER, Neumann HP, Richard S: von Hippel-Lindau disease: a clinical and scientific review. Eur J Hum Genet 2011;19:617–623.
7 Beroud C, et al: Software and database for the analysis of mutations in the VHL gene. Nucleic Acids Res 1998;26:256–258.
8 Richards FM, et al: Molecular analysis of de novo germline mutations in the von Hippel-Lindau disease gene. Hum Mol Genet 1995;4:2139–2143.
9 Wu P, et al: Family history of von Hippel-Lindau disease was uncommon in Chinese patients: suggesting the higher frequency of de novo mutations in VHL gene in these patients. J Hum Genet 2012; 57:238–243.
10 Crossey PA, et al: Identification of intragenic mutations in the von Hippel-Lindau disease tumour suppressor gene and correlation with disease phenotype. Hum Mol Genet 1994;3:1303–1308.

11 Franke G, et al: Alu-Alu recombination underlies the vast majority of large VHL germline deletions: molecular characterization and genotype-phenotype correlations in VHL patients. Hum Mutat 2009;30:776–786.
12 McNeill A, et al: Genotype-phenotype correlations in VHL exon deletions. Am J Med Genet A 2009; 149A:2147–2151.
13 Richards FM, et al: Expression of the von Hippel-Lindau disease tumour suppressor gene during human embryogenesis. Hum Mol Genet 1996;5:639–644.
14 Kaelin WG Jr: The von Hippel-Lindau protein, HIF hydroxylation, and oxygen sensing. Biochem Biophys Res Commun 2005;338:627–638.
15 Kibel A, et al: Binding of the von Hippel-Lindau tumor suppressor protein to elongin B and C. Science 1995;269:1444–1446.
16 Kamura T, et al: The Rbx1 subunit of SCF and VHL E3 ubiquitin ligase activates Rub1 modification of cullins Cdc53 and Cul2. Genes Dev 1999;13:2928–2933.
17 Stebbins CE, Kaelin WG Jr, Pavletich NP: Structure of the VHL-ElonginC-ElonginB complex: implications for VHL tumor suppressor function. Science 1999;284:455–461.
18 Lisztwan J, et al: The von Hippel-Lindau tumor suppressor protein is a component of an E3 ubiquitin-protein ligase activity. Genes Dev 1999;13: 1822–1833.
19 Kaelin WG Jr: The von Hippel-Lindau tumour suppressor protein: O_2 sensing and cancer. Nat Rev Cancer 2008;8:865–873.
20 Yang H, et al: pVHL acts as an adaptor to promote the inhibitory phosphorylation of the NF-kappaB agonist Card9 by CK2. Mol Cell 2007;28:15–27.
21 Chitalia VC, et al: Jade-1 inhibits Wnt signalling by ubiquitylating beta-catenin and mediates Wnt pathway inhibition by pVHL. Nat Cell Biol 2008;10: 1208–1216.
22 Nakamura E, et al: Clusterin is a secreted marker for a hypoxia-inducible factor-independent function of the von Hippel-Lindau tumor suppressor protein. Am J Pathol 2006;168:574–584.
23 Richard S: von Hippel-Lindau disease: recent advances and therapeutic perspectives. Expert Rev Anticancer Ther 2003;3:215–233.
24 Niemela M, et al: Hemangioblastomas of the retina: impact of von Hippel-Lindau disease. Invest Ophthalmol Vis Sci 2000;41:1909–1915.
25 Neumann HP, et al: Prevalence, morphology and biology of renal cell carcinoma in von Hippel-Lindau disease compared to sporadic renal cell carcinoma. J Urol 1998;160:1248–1254.
26 Ong KR, et al: Genotype-phenotype correlations in von Hippel-Lindau disease. Hum Mutat 2007;28: 143–149.
27 Maddock IR, et al: A genetic register for von Hippel-Lindau disease. J Med Genet 1996;33:120–127.
28 Manski TJ, et al: Endolymphatic sac tumors. A source of morbid hearing loss in von Hippel-Lindau disease. JAMA 1997;277:1461–1466.
29 Libutti SK, et al: Pancreatic neuroendocrine tumors associated with von Hippel Lindau disease: diagnostic and management recommendations. Surgery 1998;124:1153–1159.
30 Dollfus H, et al: Retinal hemangioblastoma in von Hippel-Lindau disease: a clinical and molecular study. Invest Ophthalmol Vis Sci 2002;43:3067–3074.
31 Aiello LP, et al: Rapid and durable recovery of visual function in a patient with von Hippel-Lindau syndrome after systemic therapy with vascular endothelial growth factor receptor inhibitor su5416. Ophthalmology 2002;109:1745–1751.
32 Girmens JF, et al: Treatment of von Hippel-Lindau retinal hemangioblastoma by the vascular endothelial growth factor receptor inhibitor SU5416 is more effective for associated macular edema than for hemangioblastomas. Am J Ophthalmol 2003;136: 194–196.
33 Wanebo JE, et al: The natural history of hemangioblastomas of the central nervous system in patients with von Hippel-Lindau disease. J Neurosurg 2003; 98:82–94.
34 Wind JJ, Lonser RR: Management of von Hippel-Lindau disease-associated CNS lesions. Expert Rev Neurother 2011;11:1433–1441.
35 Ammerman JM, et al: Long-term natural history of hemangioblastomas in patients with von Hippel-Lindau disease: implications for treatment. J Neurosurg 2006;105:248–255.
36 Jagannathan J, et al: Surgical management of cerebellar hemangioblastomas in patients with von Hippel-Lindau disease. J Neurosurg 2008;108:210–222.
37 Mehta GU, et al: Functional outcome after resection of spinal cord hemangioblastomas associated with von Hippel-Lindau disease. J Neurosurg Spine 2010;12:233–242.
38 Wind JJ, et al: Long-term outcome after resection of brainstem hemangioblastomas in von Hippel-Lindau disease. J Neurosurg 2011;114:1312–1318.
39 Asthagiri AR, et al: Prospective evaluation of radiosurgery for hemangioblastomas in von Hippel-Lindau disease. Neuro-Oncology 2010;12:80–86.
40 Lonser RR, et al: Edema is a precursor to central nervous system peritumoral cyst formation. Ann Neurol 2005;58:392–399.

41 Chan CC, et al: VHL gene deletion and enhanced VEGF gene expression detected in the stromal cells of retinal angioma. Arch Ophthalmol 1999;117: 625–630.
42 Vortmeyer AO, et al: von Hippel-Lindau gene deletion detected in the stromal cell component of a cerebellar hemangioblastoma associated with von Hippel-Lindau disease. Hum Pathol 1997;28:540–543.
43 Hussein MR: Central nervous system capillary haemangioblastoma: the pathologist's viewpoint. Int J Exp Pathol 2007;88:311–324.
44 Hasselblatt M, et al: Cellular and reticular variants of haemangioblastoma revisited: a clinicopathologic study of 88 cases. Neuropathol Appl Neurobiol 2005;31:618–622.
45 Polydorides AD, Rosenblum MK, Edgar MA: Metastatic renal cell carcinoma to hemangioblastoma in von Hippel-Lindau disease. Arch Pathol Lab Med 2007;131:641–645.
46 Carney EM, et al: PAX2(–)/PAX8(–)/inhibin A(+) immunoprofile in hemangioblastoma: a helpful combination in the differential diagnosis with metastatic clear cell renal cell carcinoma to the central nervous system. Am J Surg Pathol 2011;35:262–267.
47 Kennedy M, et al: Development of the hemangioblast defines the onset of hematopoiesis in human ES cell differentiation cultures. Blood 2007;109: 2679–2687.
48 Vortmeyer AO, et al: Developmental effects of von Hippel-Lindau gene deficiency. Ann Neurol 2004; 55:721–728.
49 Shively SB, et al: Developmentally arrested structures preceding cerebellar tumors in von Hippel-Lindau disease. Mod Pathol 2011;24:1023–1030.
50 Jilg CA, et al: Nephron sparing surgery in von Hippel-Lindau associated renal cell carcinoma; clinicopathological long-term follow-up. Fam Cancer 2012.
51 Johnson A, et al: Feasibility and outcomes of repeat partial nephrectomy. J Urol 2008;180:89–93.
52 Steinbach F, Novick AC, Shoskes D: Renal transplantation in patients with renal cell carcinoma and von Hippel-Lindau disease. Urology 1994;44:760–763.
53 Poston CD, et al: Characterization of the renal pathology of a familial form of renal cell carcinoma associated with von Hippel-Lindau disease: clinical and molecular genetic implications. J Urol 1995; 153:22–26.
54 Walther MM, et al: Prevalence of microscopic lesions in grossly normal renal parenchyma from patients with von Hippel-Lindau disease, sporadic renal cell carcinoma and no renal disease: clinical implications. J Urol 1995;154:2010–2014; discussion 2014–2015.
55 Lutz MS, Burk RD: Primary cilium formation requires von Hippel-Lindau gene function in renal-derived cells. Cancer Res 2006;66:6903–6907.
56 Thoma CR, Frew IJ, Krek W: The VHL tumor suppressor: riding tandem with GSK3beta in primary cilium maintenance. Cell Cycle 2007;6:1809–1813.
57 Esteban MA, et al: Formation of primary cilia in the renal epithelium is regulated by the von Hippel-Lindau tumor suppressor protein. J Am Soc Nephrol 2006;17:1801–1806.
58 Plotnikova OV, Pugacheva EN, Golemis EA: Primary cilia and the cell cycle. Methods Cell Biol 2009;94:137–160.
59 Thoma CR, et al: pVHL and GSK3beta are components of a primary cilium-maintenance signalling network. Nat Cell Biol 2007;9:588–595.
60 Montani M, et al: VHL-gene deletion in single renal tubular epithelial cells and renal tubular cysts: further evidence for a cyst-dependent progression pathway of clear cell renal carcinoma in von Hippel-Lindau disease. Am J Surg Pathol 2010;34:806–815.
61 Sourbier C, et al: Targeting the nuclear factor-kappaB rescue pathway has promising future in human renal cell carcinoma therapy. Cancer Res 2007;67: 11668–11676.
62 Morais C, et al: The emerging role of nuclear factor kappa B in renal cell carcinoma. Int J Biochem Cell Biol 2011;43:1537–1549.
63 Hes FJ, Hoppener JW, Lips CJ: Clinical review 155: Pheochromocytoma in von Hippel-Lindau disease. J Clin Endocrinol Metab 2003;88:969–974.
64 Walther MM, et al: Clinical and genetic characterization of pheochromocytoma in von Hippel-Lindau families: comparison with sporadic pheochromocytoma gives insight into natural history of pheochromocytoma. J Urol 1999;162:659–664.
65 Welander J, Soderkvist P, Gimm O: Genetics and clinical characteristics of hereditary pheochromocytomas and paragangliomas. Endocr Relat Cancer 2011;18:R253–R276.
66 Koch CA, et al: Pheochromocytoma in von hippel-lindau disease: distinct histopathologic phenotype compared to pheochromocytoma in multiple endocrine neoplasia type 2. Endocr Pathol 2002;13:17–27.
67 Lee CM, et al: VHL type 2B gene mutation moderates HIF dosage in vitro and in vivo. Oncogene 2009;28:1694–1705.
68 Girelli R, et al: Pancreatic cystic manifestations in von Hippel-Lindau disease. Int J Pancreatol 1997; 22:101–109.
69 Agrawal D, et al: Prevalence and clinical significance of pancreatic cysts associated with cysts in other organs. Dig Liver Dis 2011;43:797–801.

70 Kanno A, et al: Serous cystic neoplasms of the whole pancreas in a patient with von Hippel-Lindau disease. Intern Med 2011;50:1293–1298.
71 Scolari F, et al: von Hippel-Lindau syndrome presenting as pancreatic cysts. Contrib Nephrol. Basel, Karger, 2001, vol 136, pp 325–330.
72 Libutti SK, et al: Clinical and genetic analysis of patients with pancreatic neuroendocrine tumors associated with von Hippel-Lindau disease. Surgery 2000;128:1022–102.
73 Corcos O, et al: Endocrine pancreatic tumors in von Hippel-Lindau disease: clinical, histological, and genetic features. Pancreas 2008;37:85–93.
74 Hoang MP, Hruban RH, Albores-Saavedra J: Clear cell endocrine pancreatic tumor mimicking renal cell carcinoma: a distinctive neoplasm of von Hippel-Lindau disease. Am J Surg Pathol 2001;25:602–609.
75 Perigny M, et al: Pancreatic endocrine microadenomatosis in patients with von Hippel-Lindau disease: characterization by VHL/HIF pathway proteins expression. Am J Surg Pathol 2009;33: 739–748.
76 Lubensky IA, et al: Multiple neuroendocrine tumors of the pancreas in von Hippel-Lindau disease patients: histopathological and molecular genetic analysis. Am J Pathol 1998;153:223–231.
77 Blandamura S, et al: Three cases of pancreatic serous cystadenoma and endocrine tumour. J Clin Pathol 2007;60:278–282.
78 Blansfield JA, et al: Clinical, genetic and radiographic analysis of 108 patients with von Hippel-Lindau disease (VHL) manifested by pancreatic neuroendocrine neoplasms (PNETs). Surgery 2007; 142:814–818.
79 Chung DC, et al: A novel pancreatic endocrine tumor suppressor gene locus on chromosome 3p with clinical prognostic implications. J Clin Invest 1997; 100:404–410.
80 Speisky D, et al: Molecular profiling of pancreatic neuroendocrine tumors in sporadic and von Hippel-Lindau patients. Clin Cancer Res 2012;18: 2838–2849.
81 Heffner DK: Low-grade adenocarcinoma of probable endolymphatic sac origin. A clinicopathologic study of 20 cases. Cancer 1989;64:2292–2302.
82 Joy HM, et al: Radiological considerations in the diagnosis of an endolymphatic sac tumour. Clin Radiol 2002;57:652–654.
83 Lonser RR, et al: The vestibular aqueduct: site of origin of endolymphatic sac tumors. J Neurosurg 2008;108:751–756.
84 Michaels L: Origin of endolymphatic sac tumor. Head Neck Pathol 2007;1:104–111.
85 Glasker S, et al: Effects of VHL deficiency on endolymphatic duct and sac. Cancer Res 2005;65:10847–10853.
86 Bell D, et al: Endolymphatic sac tumor (aggressive papillary tumor of middle ear and temporal bone): sine qua non radiology-pathology and the University of Texas MD Anderson Cancer Center experience. Ann Diagn Pathol 2011;15:117–123.
87 Kawahara N, et al: VHL gene inactivation in an endolymphatic sac tumor associated with von Hippel-Lindau disease. Neurology 1999;53:208–210.
88 Jensen RL, et al: Endolymphatic sac tumors in patients with and without von Hippel-Lindau disease: the role of genetic mutation, von Hippel-Lindau protein, and hypoxia inducible factor-1alpha expression. J Neurosurg 2004;100:488–497.
89 Vortmeyer AO, et al: Somatic von Hippel-Lindau gene mutations detected in sporadic endolymphatic sac tumors. Cancer Res 2000;60:5963–5965.
90 Nogales FF, et al: An analysis of five clear cell papillary cystadenomas of mesosalpinx and broad ligament: four associated with von Hippel-Lindau disease and one aggressive sporadic type. Histopathology 2012;60:748–757.
91 Glasker S, et al: Epididymal cystadenomas and epithelial tumourlets: effects of VHL deficiency on the human epididymis. J Pathol 2006;210:32–41.
92 Aydin H, et al: Clear cell papillary cyst adenoma of the epididymis and mesosalpinx: immunohistochemical differentiation from metastatic clear cell renal cell carcinoma. Am J Surg Pathol 2005;29: 520–523.
93 Odrzywolski KJ, Mukhopadhyay S: Papillary cystadenoma of the epididymis. Arch Pathol Lab Med 2010;134:630–633.
94 Browning L, Parker A: Bilateral adrenal haemangioblastoma in a patient with von Hippel-Lindau disease. Pathology 2008;40:429–431.
95 Rojiani AM, et al: Hepatic hemangioblastoma. An unusual presentation in a patient with von Hippel-Lindau disease. Am J Surg Pathol 1991;15:81–86.
96 Sinkre PA, et al: Clear cell carcinoid tumor of the gallbladder: another distinctive manifestation of von Hippel-Lindau disease. Am J Surg Pathol 2001; 25:1334–1339.
97 Karasawa Y, et al: Duodenal somatostatinoma and erythrocytosis in a patient with von Hippel-Lindau disease type 2A. Intern Med 2001;40:38–43.
98 Wagner M, et al: Lipid cell tumors in two women with von Hippel-Lindau syndrome. Obstet Gynecol 2010;116(suppl 2):535–539.
99 Xu DS, et al: A von Hippel-Lindau disease-associated microcystic adenoma of the ethmoid sinus: case report. Neurosurgery 2011;69:E1017–E1021; discussion E1021–E1022.
100 Klein J, et al: Multifocal microcysts and papillary cystadenoma of the lung in von Hippel-Lindau disease. Am J Surg Pathol 2007;31:1292–1296.

101 Ng HK, Tse JY, Poon WS: Cerebellar astrocytoma associated with von Hippel-Lindau disease: case report with molecular findings. Br J Neurosurg 1999; 13:504–507.
102 Marinozzi A, et al: Chondrosarcoma of the iliac wing in von Hippel-Lindau disease. J Exp Clin Cancer Res 2007;26:599–601.
103 Lonser RR, et al: von Hippel-Lindau disease. Lancet 2003;361(9374):2059–2067.
104 Maher ER: von Hippel-Lindau disease. Curr Mol Med 2004;4:833–842.
105 Arjumand W, Sultana S: Role of VHL gene mutation in human renal cell carcinoma. Tumour Biol 2012;33:9–16.
106 Motzer RJ, et al: Sunitinib efficacy against advanced renal cell carcinoma. J Urol 2007;178:1883–1887.
107 Escudier B, et al: Sorafenib for treatment of renal cell carcinoma: final efficacy and safety results of the phase III treatment approaches in renal cancer global evaluation trial. J Clin Oncol 2009;27:3312–3318.
108 Escudier B: Sunitinib for the management of advanced renal cell carcinoma. Expert Rev Anticancer Ther 2010;10:305–317.
109 Hudes G, et al: Temsirolimus, interferon alfa, or both for advanced renal-cell carcinoma. N Engl J Med 2007;356:2271–2281.
110 Bajetta E, Guadalupi V, Procopio G: Activity of sunitinib in patients with advanced neuroendocrine tumors. J Clin Oncol 2009;27:319–320; author reply 320.
111 Kulke MH, et al: Activity of sunitinib in patients with advanced neuroendocrine tumors. J Clin Oncol 2008;26:3403–3410.
112 Ali T, Kandil D, Piperdi B: Long-term disease control with sunitinib in a patient with metastatic pancreatic neuroendocrine tumor (NET) associated with von Hippel-Lindau syndrome (VHL). Pancreas 2012;41:492–493.
113 Jimenez C, et al: Use of the tyrosine kinase inhibitor sunitinib in a patient with von Hippel-Lindau disease: targeting angiogenic factors in pheochromocytoma and other von Hippel-Lindau disease-related tumors. J Clin Endocrinol Metab 2009;94: 386–391.
114 Kim BY, Jonasch E, McCutcheon IE: Pazopanib therapy for cerebellar hemangioblastomas in von Hippel-Lindau disease : Case report. Target Oncol 2012.
115 Jones DT, Harris AL: Small-molecule inhibitors of the HIF pathway and synthetic lethal interactions. Expert Opin Ther Targets 2012.

Anthony J. Gill
Department of Anatomical Pathology, Royal North Shore Hospital
Pacific Highway
St Leonards, NSW 2065 (Australia)
E-Mail affgill@med.usyd.edu.au

Stratakis CA (ed): Endocrine Tumor Syndromes and Their Genetics.
Front Horm Res. Basel, Karger, 2013, vol 41, pp 50–62 (DOI: 10.1159/000345669)

Carney Complex

Stéphanie Espiard[a] · Jérôme Bertherat[a–c]

[a]Inserm U1016, CNRS UMR 8104, Institut Cochin, [b]Department of Endocrinology and National Reference Center for Rare Adrenal Disorders, Hôpital Cochin, APHP, and [c]Faculté de Médecine Paris Descartes, Université René Descartes, Paris, France

Abstract

Carney complex is a rare, dominantly inherited multiple endocrine neoplasia syndrome, affecting endocrine glands as the adrenal cortex (causing Cushing's syndrome), the pituitary and the thyroid. It is associated with many other nonendocrine tumors, including cardiac myxomas, testicular tumors, melanotic schwannoma, breast myxomatosis, and abnormal pigmentation (lentiginosis) or myxomas of the skin. The gene located on the CNC1 locus was identified 12 years ago as the regulatory subunit 1A (R1A) of the protein kinase A *(PRKAR1A)* located at 17q22–24. Inactivating heterozygous germline mutations of *PRKAR1A* are observed in about two thirds of Carney complex patients with some genotype-phenotype correlation useful for follow-up and prognosis. More rarely, mutations of phosphodiesterase genes have been reported in patients presenting mainly with Cushing's syndrome. In vitro and in vivo studies help to understand how R1A inactivation leads to tumorigenesis. *PRKAR1A* appears to be a relatively weak tumorigenic signal which can cooperate with other signaling pathways and tumor suppressors.

Carney complex (CNC) was described for the first time in 1985 as 'the complex of myxomas, spotty pigmentation and endocrine overactivity' by J. Aidan Carney [1]. Patients previously diagnosed as LAMB (lentigineses, atrial myxoma, mucocutaneous myxoma, blu nevi) or NAME (nevi, atrial, myxoma, myxoid neurofibroma, ephelide) could be considered as having CNC. About 70% are familial cases with an autosomal dominant transmission [2]. Other cases are considered as sporadic. The prevalence of CNC is unknown due to the rarity of the disease. It is probably underestimated because of the difficulty of its diagnosis. About 750 cases of diverse ethnicity have been reported by the NIH-Mayo clinic, the Cornell center (USA) and Cochin Hospital (France). In the largest genotyped series of patients 63% are females and 37% are males [3].

Diagnosis and Clinical Manifestations

The endocrine and nonendocrine manifestations of CNC can be numerous and vary between patients. In general, families with CNC tend to have similar groupings of manifestations, although some intrafamilial variability exists. Also, some CNC families can exhibit predominantly with primary pigmented adrenocortical disease (PPNAD) [3].

The diagnostic criteria for CNC were reviewed in 2001 and are provided in table 1 [2]. Diagnosis is based on the presence of two or more cardinal manifestations confirmed by histology, biochemical testing or imaging. If the patient has a demonstrated germline *PRKAR1A* gene mutation and/or a first-degree relative affected by CNC, a single manifestation is sufficient for the diagnosis (cf. table 1).

Cardiac Myxomas

Cardiac myxomas are benign neoplasms found in about 20–40% of Carney patients. Unlike sporadic tumors, CNC-associated myxomas occur at a young age, can be multiple in a third of the cases, and can be located in any cardiac chamber. They can grow rather rapidly [2, 3]. They can be the cause of stroke due to embolism, and may lead to cardiac insufficiency and/or sudden death. They require surgical removal. Historically, these tumors are likely to have been the most frequent cause of death (including sudden death) in CNC patients, either related to the complications of the myxoma or its surgery. Early diagnosis is important and should start in the first year of life with annual screening by cardiac ultrasound. In patients with a history of cardiac myxomas, screening should be performed every 6 months. In difficult cases, transesophageal ultrasound and cardiac magnetic resonance imaging can be helpful.

Skin Lesions

Identification of skin manifestations is very important because three of the major criteria are cutaneous, they are easily recognizable, and they present early in life. The most common clinical manifestation of CNC is lentiginosis, observed in about 70 80% of CNC patients. Other pigmented lesions such as multiple blue nevi or café-au-lait spots are reported in about 50% of the cases and cutaneous tumors (myxomas or fibromas) are reported in 20–31% [3, 4].

Lentiginosis is a condition that presents with hamartomatous melanocytic lesions. They look like flat, poorly circumscribed, brownish to black, small (<5 mm) macules. They are typically located around the lips, on the eyelids, ears and the genital area. The recognition of this distribution is important because it is specific for CNC. The density of pigmented spots varies from a few lesions to profuse pigmentation. Lentiginosis often appears during childhood and during the prepubertal period. It usually does not acquire its typical intensity and distribution until the peripubertal period and tends to fade after the fourth decade. CNC lentigines may

Table 1. Diagnosis criteria of CNC defined by Stratakis et al. [2] and other findings suggestive of a possible association with CNC

Major diagnostic criteria for CNC
Spotty skin pigmentation (lentiginosis) with typical distribution (lips, cunjunctiva and inner or outer canthi, vaginal mucosa)
Myxoma (cutaneous and mucosa)*
Cardiac myxoma*
Breast myxomatosis* or fat-suppressed MRI findings suggestive of this diagnosis
PPAD* or paradoxical positive response of urinary glucocorticosteroid excretion to dexamethasone administration during Liddle's test.
Acromegaly due to GH-producing adenoma*
Large-cell calcifying Sertoli cell tumor* or characteristic calcification on testicular ultrasound
Thyroid carcinoma* or multiple, hypoechoic nodules on thyroid ultrasound in a young patient
Psammomatous melanotic schwannomas*
Blue nevus, epithelioid blue nevus*
Breast ductal adenoma*
Osteochondromyxoma*
Supplementary criteria
Affected first-degree relative
Inactivating mutation of the *PRKAR1A* gene
Findings suggestive of or possibly associated with CNC but not diagnosis for the disease
Intense freckling (without darkly pigmented spots or typical distribution)
Blue nevus, common type (if multiple)
Café-au-lait spots or other birthmarks
Elevated IgF-1 levels, abnormal GTT or paradoxical GH response to TRH testing in the absence of clinical acromegaly
Cardiomyopathy
Pilonidal sinus
History of CS, acromegaly or sudden death in extended family
Multiple skin tags or other skin lesions; lipomas
Colonic polyps (usually mild and almost always combined with clinical or subclinical acromegaly)
Hyperprolactinemia (usually mild and almost always combined with clinical or subclinical acromegaly)
Single, benign thyroid nodule in a young patient; multiple thyroid nodules in an older patient (detected on ultrasound)
Family history of carcinoma, in particular of the thyroid, colon, pancreas and ovary; other multiple benign or malignant tumors

* After histological confirmation.

be detectable until the eighth decade and their distinction from solar lentigines is also more difficult. However, lentiginosis lesions do not change with sun exposure [4].

Blue nevi are the second most frequent skin lesions in patients with CNC as they are observed in about 40% of patients. They are small, blue to black-colored marks with circular or star-shaped appearance and their distribution is variable [4].

Cutaneous myxomas, the third most common skin manifestation, are reported in 20–31% of patients but this incidence may be an underestimate because not every skin lesion is biopsied [3, 4]. Clinically, they can be misdiagnosed as cutaneous papillomas or fibromas. They typically appear before the age of 18 years and have a tendency to recur in older patients. The lesions vary between asymptomatic, sessile, small (rarely exceeding 1 cm in diameter), opalescent or dark pink papules and large finger-like pedunculated lesions. They can be located anywhere but usually affect the eyelids, ears, nipples, external ear canal, trunk and perineum. Early diagnosis is essential since it is estimated that approximately 80% of the CNC patients with cardiac myxomas present with cutaneous myxomas earlier in life [3, 4]. Thus, in case of clinical suspicion, a biopsy must be performed.

Finally, other pigmented lesions (café-au-lait spots, spitz and compound nevi) or depigmented lesions can also be observed. They are rarely present as isolated skin manifestations of CNC and may be present at birth [2, 3].

No malignant transformation of these skin lesions has been reported and patients with CNC do not appear to have a significant predisposition for skin cancers. However, it can be difficult to clinically differentiate an atypical nevus frequently found in CNC patients from a melanoma and dermatological examination may be necessary.

Endocrine Glands and Gonads

Cushing Syndrome and PPNAD

The most common endocrine manifestation of CNC is PPNAD, a cause of ACTH-independent Cushing's syndrome (CS). It is detected in about 60% of cases with a female predominance (71% female, 29% male) [3]. A minority of CNC patients present with PPNAD during the first 2–3 years of life, whereas the majority are young adults, with a peak during the second and third decades of life [2]. Histological evidence of PPNAD has been found in every CNC patient who underwent an autopsy. The macroscopic appearance of the adrenal cortex is characterized by small pigmented nodules less than 10 mm in their greatest diameter most often surrounded by atrophic cortex. Adrenal glands usually remain normal in size and weight [1]. The disease is bilateral with primary involvement of both adrenals. Clinical signs are those of ACTH-independent CS which may be obvious or subclinical with insidious development. Cyclic forms of hypercortisolism can also be observed with a large and rapid burst of cortisol excess, which might regress spontaneously. Cortisol hypersecretion is special because of its variable level of urinary cortisol over time and a possible paradoxical rise of cortisol after high-dose dexamethasone administration [2]. This test may be used diagnostically for the identification of PPNAD, even in patients that have normal baseline cortisol levels and do not have clinical stigmata of CS. Computed tomography (CT) scan typically reveals bilateral micronodules (<10 mm), much more often than macronodules that can be observed in older patients. However, in a third of the cases the adrenal might appear normal on CT scan.

Recently, 2 cases of adrenocortical cancer in CNC were described. In both cases, cosecretion of androgen and cortisol and rapid occurrence of metastasis or local recurrence was observed [5].

For patients with CS, bilateral adrenalectomy is the most common treatment. Anticortisolic drugs such as ketoconazole or mitotane have been rarely used and might not be appropriate for long-term treatment.

Pituitary

Pituitary tumors in CNC patients are GH- or mixed GH-PRL-secreting pituitary adenomas. The incidence of acromegaly is about 12% [3]. It usually appears during or after the third decade of life and clinical acromegaly is uncommon. Biochemical abnormality of the GH axis may be present without pituitary adenoma. Alterations of the dynamics of GH secretion might be observed in two thirds of the patients. In addition, mild elevation of prolactin level is noted in 64% of the cases. Rare prolactinomas have been described. In operated acromegalic patients histological investigation can reveal somatomammotroph hyperplasia. At immunostaining GH-secreting tumors frequently stain also for PRL or α-subunit. TSH, LH and occasionally FSH staining have be seen only in foci of normal pituitary cells entrapped within the tumor or the hyperplasia [6].

Patients can be followed by GH levels, oral glucose tolerance test, and IGF-1 levels. If a tumor develops it is usually operated. Somatostatin analogs as a primary or adjuvant treatment have been used with variable results. If no clear tumor can be detected by MRI, somatostatin analogs and/or GH antagonist treatment can be discussed.

Thyroid Tumors

Benign thyroid adenomas were observed in 25% of cases, mostly follicular type [3]. In contrast to the mouse model, hyperthyroidism is usually not observed [7]. Cystic or nodular disease is observed in 75% of the patients when sonographic systematic examination is done, a prevalence higher than in the general population [2]. Thyroid cancer (papillary carcinomas or follicular carcinomas or both) has been reported in 2.5% of patients [3]. Chronic surveillance of the thyroid is also required. Thus, for postpubertal pediatric and adult patients, an annual clinical examination and less frequently thyroid ultrasound are recommended. Fine-needle cytology analysis of the suspicious thyroid nodules is very helpful.

Testicular Lesions

The testicular tumors can be of three types: large cell calcifying Sertoli tumors (LCCST), Leydig cell tumors and of adrenal origin (PPNAD).

LCCST is a rare stromal benign tumor. It is observed in 41% of male affected by CNC [3]. It appears in the first decade of life and is usually bilateral and multifocal. It progress gradually with age to replace the normal testicular tissue. LCCST is frequently asymptomatic. In most examined adults with CNC, LCCST are detected by ultrasound investigation as bilateral microcalcifications. Malignant changes have been reported very rarely. LCCST can cause replacement and obstruction of seminiferous tubules leading to reduce fertility. CNC patients have morphologically abnormal sperm and reduced sperm number [8].

Leydig cell tumors and nodular adrenocortical rests, which can lead to recurrent CS after adrenalectomy, seem possible but are quite rare also.

Ovarian Tumors

Ovarian lesions have been reported in 14% of affected women [3, 9]. Lesions are commonly ovarian cysts and tumors of the ovarian surface epithelium including serus cystadenomas and cystic teratomas [9]. These lesions are easily found by sonographic examination as multiple hypoechoic lesions. Although usually asymptomatic, they can grow or may rarely progress to ovarian carcinoma (mucinous adenocarcinoma or endometrioid carcinoma). Thus, sonography of the ovaries may be part of the initial evaluation in women with CNC and follow-up of any identified lesion is recommended.

Psammomatous Melanotic Schwannoma

Pigmented melanotic schwannoma, derived from the Schwann cells of the nervous system, can be observed in 8% of patients with CNC [3]. It differs from other schwannomas by its heavy pigmentation, frequent calcification and multicentricity. They can be observed anywhere in the central or peripheral system but their most frequent sites are the gastrointestinal tract (esophagus, liver, stomach and rectum) and the paraspinal sympathetic chain. Malignancy may be observed in 10% of the psammomatous melanotic schwannoma with frequent metastasis to the lung, liver or brain [2]. Because of their location in or around the spinal column and the risk of malignancy, these tumors are a significant cause of morbidity and mortality for CNC patients.

They are the most difficult tumors to treat because of spinal location and inoperable metastases. There is a need for effective medical for metastatic schwannoma.

Breast Lesions

Breast tissue characteristic lesions in CNC include lobular or nodular myxomatosis, myxoid fibroadenomas or ductal adenomas. They are often bilateral and occur in 20% of the female patients [3]. However, this percentage is likely to represent an underestimate of the true incidence of these lesions because breast magnetic resonance imaging was performed in only a small number of the patients. Treatment and follow-up of these lesions by ultrasonography or MRI is recommended.

Bone Lesions: Osteochondromyxoma

Osteochondromyxoma are a rare component of CNC that occur early in life, usually before the age of two. Clinically, tumors were painless masses that occurred in distal

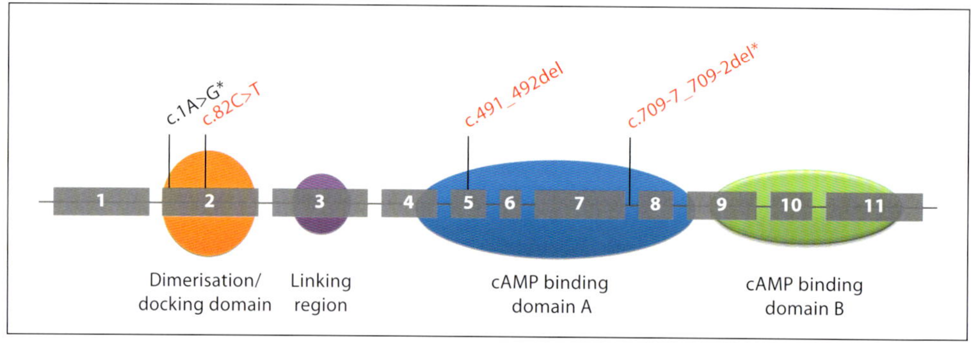

Fig. 1. *PRKAR1A* gene. Schematic illustration of the gene. Domains of the encoded protein are denoted with ovals. The three hot-spot mutations are indicated in red. The star indicates mutations associated with isolated PPNAD. Adapted from: http://prkar1a.nichd.nih.gov/.

long bones (diaphyseal) and small flat bones (nasal). Osteochondromyxoma are usually benign but local invasiveness or recurrence has often been observed. Complete excision of the lesion, when possible, should be curative.

Others Lesions

Pancreatic neoplasms may be observed in 2.5% of CNC patients [3]. They include acinar cell carcinoma, adenocarcinoma, intraductal pancreatic mucinous neoplasm. These tumors may be aggressive and are the major cause of death by cancer for CNC patients [10]. It remain to be determined if screening by magnetic resonance cholangiopancreatogram should be performed.

Others tumors like parotid mixed tumor, bronchogenic cyst, hepatocellular adenoma and carcinoma, colonic, gastric carcinomas and retroperitoneal fibrous histiocytomas have been rarely described [2].

Molecular Genetics

Genetic linkage analysis identified two independent loci for CNC, located respectively on chromosome 17p22–24 and 2p16. The gene located at 17q has been identified as the protein kinase A regulatory subunit 1-alpha (*PRKAR1A*) [11, 12]. Alterations on chromosome 2 are loss of heterozygoty and copy numbers gains and currently no candidate gene has been found [13].

PRKAR1A

The *PRKAR1A* gene contains 11 exons, 10 of whom are coding, with a coding region of a total size of 1143pb (fig. 1). About one-hundred and seventeen different mutations have been identified (online database: http://prkar1a.nichd.nih.gov) in 284 unrelated families of various ethnic origins [14]. 62% of CNC index cases carried a *PRKAR1A* defect [3]. These germline mutations are all inactivating heterozygous mutations. They are spread along the whole coding sequence, in exons as well as adjacent intronic sequences. They may involve more frequently exons 2, 3, 5, 7 and 8. Molecular alterations are point mutations or small deletions involving up to 15 bp although larger gene deletions have been described in small number of cases. Most of them are private, identified in only single families, except three mutations which have been found in more than three pedigrees: c.82C>T, c.491_492del and c.709–7_709–2del. The c.491_492delTG in exon 5 and c.709–7_709–2del in intron 7 were observed in 11 and 14 families, respectively, and are considered as hot spot mutation [3] (fig. 1).

These mutations may be categorized into 2 groups according to their molecular consequences. The first group includes about 80% of mutations, which leads to a premature stop codon by nonsense, frame shift or splice variants. The mutant mRNA is degraded by the mechanism of nonsense-mediated mRNA decay [14]. A second hit in the tumors is frequently observed. Indeed, loss of the normal allele adding to the constitutional loss of the other allele by functional germline mutations is often observed in CNC tumors. *PRKAR1A* is for these reasons considered as a tumor-suppressor gene.

The second group of mutations escape nonsense-mediated mRNA decay and lead to a mutant mRNA. These mutations lead to premature stop codons in the 3′ end of the gene or an altered sequence without premature stop codons. Produced protein may be defective, shorter in case of large deletion. Longer protein can be predicted when a frameshift mutation occurs in the last coding exon. The encoded mutant proteins could have an altered function due to conformational changes and could exert a dominant negative effect over the wild type protein [14]. Somatic allelic loss of the wild-type allele is not always required with these mutants. This second group tends to be associated with a higher number of CNC manifestations [3]. Recently, a mechanism of proteasomal degradation leading to haploinsufficiency by mutations located in the last exons leading to a longer protein has been described [15].

PRKAR1A defects are found in 37% of CNC sporadic cases, namely without family history and 85% of these would be de novo. For other sporadic cases, neither *PRKAR1A* mutation nor large gene deletion can be demonstrated. In about 20% of familial cases also no *PRKAR1A* mutations or gene deletion can be found. CNC patients without *PRKAR1A* genetic defects present less tumors and later disease than the patients with *PRKAR1A* mutation.

The overall penetrance of *PRKAR1A* mutation is above 95% by the age of 50 years [14]. Only two mutations (c.709–7del6 and c.1A>G) have been reported with an incomplete penetrance. Interestingly, they are associated mostly with isolated PPNAD. Some genotype/phenotype correlations have been found. Exonic mutations were more often associated with acromegaly, cardiac myxomas, lentigines and psammomatous melanotic schwannoma. Cardiac myxoma, lentigines and thyroid tumors are more frequent in patients presenting the hot spot mutation c.491–492del [3].

Phosphodiesterases Genes

Genomewide SNP genotyping of tumor and germline DNA of young patients with isolated PPNAD and/or micronodular adrenocortical hyperplasia led to the identification of mutations in two phosphodiesterase genes [16, 17]. Thus, a germline-inactivating mutation of *PDE8B* on chromosome 5 has been described in a young girl who had a CS at the age of 2 years [17]. Germline-inactivating mutations of *PDE11A*, located at chromosome 2, have been found in patients with adrenal micronodular hyperplasia including PPNAD [16]. Besides, inactivation of *PDE11A* appears to predispose to testicular germ cell and prostatic tumors. *PDE11A* variants may play a role in predisposition to PPNAD. Recently, a high frequency of *PDE11A* variants in a large cohort of CNC patients with *PRKAR1A* mutations has been demonstrated. Men with CNC due to *PRKAR1A* mutation carrying *PDE11A* variants develop significantly more PPNAD and large-cell calcifying Sertoli cell tumor [18].

Pathogenesis

cAMP Pathway

The cAMP pathway is a ubiquitous signaling pathway regulating various cellular functions like proliferation and differentiation. In endocrine tissues, hormonal activity is tightly regulated by cAMP signaling. Ligands activating the cAMP pathway bind to their specific seven transmembrane receptors coupled to Gs protein. Activation of Gs protein leads to stimulation of adenyl cyclase which synthetizes the second messenger, cAMP. cAMP in turn activates the protein kinase A (PKA). PKA is a heterotetramer formed by 2 regulatory subunits and 2 catalytic subunits. In human, four different regulatory subunits (RIalpha, RIbeta, RIIalpha, RIIbeta), and four catalytic subunits (Calpha, Cbeta, Cgamma and PRKX) have been identified. Regulatory subunit 1 alpha (R1A) protein is organized in a dimerization domain at the amino-terminal, a PKA inhibitor site, two tandem-binding domains for cAMP and a linker region containing a docking site for the C subunit. Regulatory subunits of PKA bind cAMP, which lead to their dissociation from catalytic subunits. Catalytic subunits are then activated and phosphorylate many cytoplasmic and nuclear targets like the transcription factor CREB (cAMP response-binding protein). R1A inactivation stimulates PKA activity [19]. Therefore, inactivating mutations of *PRKAR1A* increases cAMP signaling [11]. It also alters the ratio of R1alpha to R2beta, and this alteration might contribute to tumorigenesis [12] (fig. 2).

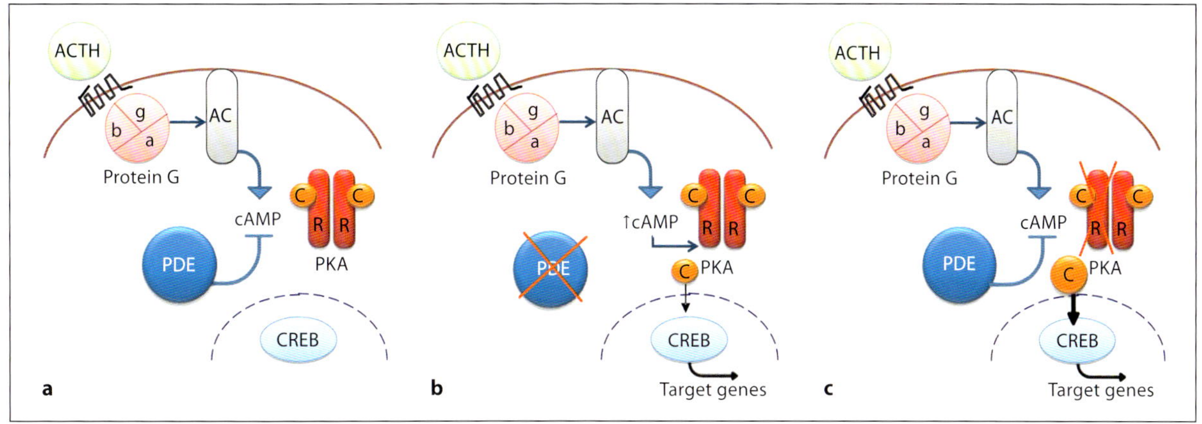

Fig. 2. The cAMP signaling pathway and the molecular defects leading its activation in CNC and PPNAD. **a** Regulation of normal cAMP pathways. ACTH = Adrenocorticotropic hormone; AC = adenylate cyclase; PKA = protein kinase A; PDE = phosphodiesterase; R = regulatory subunits of protein kinase A; C = catalytic subunits of protein kinase A; CREB = cAMP response binding protein. **b** Phosphodiesterases gene *(PDE11A* or *PDE8B)* mutations leading to reduced enzymatic activity and subsequently increased cAMP production. **c** *PRKAR1A* inactivating mutations leading to PKA activity increased. The activated PKA catalytic subunits phosphorylates the various PKA targets (i.e. in the nucleus the transcription factor CREB = cAMP-responsive element-binding protein).

Animal Models

Various transgenic mouse models have been develop to study the consequences of the inactivation of *PRKAR1A* on tumors development. *Prkar1a* homozygous knockout mice died during embryonic development due to a defect in the development of a functional heart tube. To bypass the embryonic lethality, transgenic mice carrying an inducible antisense transgene for *prkar1a* exon 2 were established. These mice develop different tumors: thyroid follicular hyperplasia and adenomas, adrenocortical hyperplasia, lymphomas, hepatocellular carcinomas and others mesenchymal tumors including sarcomas with myxomatous differentiation [21]. *Prkar1a*(+/–) mice survive and develop schwannomas and fibro-osseous bone lesions [20]. This data reinforce that complete loss a *PRKAR1A* is necessary for the development of the majority of tumors. Mice with tissue-specific inactivation of *prkar1a* with cre-lox technology have been generated. Depending on the targeted tissue, these mice develop pituitary [22], heart [23], thyroid [7] and neural crest [24] tumors (table 2). AdKO mice, which harbor adrenal specific inactivation, develop adrenal cortex hyperactivity and bilateral hyperplasia as observed in PPNAD, apparently caused by improper maintenance and proliferation of foetal adrenal cells [19].

To confirm that *PRKAR1A* inactivation is a general tumorigenic signal, *Prkar1a*(+/–) mice were cross with Trp53(+/–) or Rb(+/–) mice or treated with skin oncogenic toxic. These mice had overall reduced survival and develop more sarcomas, pituitary and thyroid tumors, as well as skin papillomas [25].

Table 2. Summary of main transgenic mice models developed to study the consequences of the inactivation of *PRKAR1A*

Mouse models	Phenotype	References
General knockout/down		
Prkar1a–/–	death at E9.5 no functional heart tube development growth retardation	Amieux et al. [21]
Prkar1a+/–	nonpigmented schwannomas fibro-osseous bone lesions thyroid tumors liver tumor reduced fertility in male (sperm abnormality)	Kirschner et al. [20] Burton et al. [8]
Prkar1a X2AS–/– (*tTA/X2AS* line)	thyroid follicular hyperplasia and adenomas adrenocortical hyperplasia lymphomas other mesenchymal tumors	Griffin, Cancer Res [2004]
Tissue-specific knockout		
Adrenal cortex *(Akr1b7-cre)*	ACTH independent Cushing's syndrome adrenal tumors	Sahut-Barnola, Plos Genet [2010]
Cardiac *(aMHC-Cre)*	death at ED 11.5–12.5 thin-walled, dilated hearts cardiac myxomatous degeneration	Yin et al. [23]
Pituitary *(GHRHR-Cre)*	alterations of the GH axis pituitary tumors with GH, prolactin, and TSH immunostaining	Yin et al. [22]
Neural crest precursor *(TEC3KO)*	schwannomas	Jones et al. [28]
Thyroid *(Tpo-cre)*	hyperthyroidism benign and malignant follicular thyroid neoplasms	Pringle et al. [7]

Other Pathways

Observations in transgenic mice suggest that *PRKAR1A* haploinsufficiency is a general and relatively low tumorigenic signal, which need the additive effects of other oncogene or inactivation of other tumor suppressors and/or tissue-specific factors. Evidence of activation of the Wnt/β-catenin signaling pathway by *PRKAR1A* inactivation has been observed in CNC tumors as well as in vitro and in vivo studies. Activation of the MAPK signaling pathway (mitogen-activated protein kinase), mTOR pathway and dysregulation of cyclins and E2F family members have been also demonstrated [19, 25]. Alterations of the TGFß signaling pathway due to reduced smad3 expression have been shown in adrenocortical cells [19].

Conclusion

CNC is a rare genetic endocrine neoplasia syndrome. PPNAD is the most frequent endocrine manifestation and leads to frank or insidious CS. It is associated with non-endocrine lesions that may allow early diagnosis, like the skin manifestations, or that may have dramatic consequences, like cardiac myxomas and some rare malignant tumors. Multidisciplinary management of this disease is important as well as follow-up in reference centers. Analysis of large series of genotyped CNC patients with careful phenotype analysis is important to improve diagnosis, treatment and follow-up guidelines. Recent mouse studies gave new insights in the mechanisms of tumor development in CNC. In the long-term this will be very important for the development of targeted therapies.

References

1 Carney JA, Gordon H, Carpenter PC, Shenoy BV, Go VL: The complex of myxomas, spotty pigmentation, and endocrine overactivity. Medicine (Baltimore) 1985;64:270–283.

2 Stratakis CA, Kirschner LS, Carney JA: Clinical and molecular features of the Carney complex: diagnostic criteria and recommendations for patient evaluation. J Clin Endocrinol Metab 2001;86:4041–4046.

3 Bertherat J, Horvath A, Groussin L, Grabar S, Boikos S, Cazabat L, et al: Mutations in regulatory subunit type 1A of cyclic adenosine 5′-monophosphate-dependent protein kinase (PRKAR1A): phenotype analysis in 353 patients and 80 different genotypes. J Clin Endocrinol Metab 2009; 94:2085–2091.

4 Mateus C, Palangié A, Franck N, Groussin L, Bertagna X, Avril M-F, et al: Heterogeneity of skin manifestations in patients with Carney complex. J Am Acad Dermatol 2008;59:801–810.

5 Bertherat J: Adrenocortical cancer in Carney complex: a paradigm of endocrine tumor progression or an association of genetic predisposing factors? J Clin Endocrinol Metab 2012;97:387–390.

6 Kirschner LS: PRKAR1A and the evolution of pituitary tumors. Mol Cell Endocrinol 2010;326:3–7.

7 Pringle DR, Yin Z, Lee AA, Manchanda PK, Yu L, Parlow AF, et al: Thyroid-specific ablation of the Carney complex gene, PRKAR1A, results in hyperthyroidism and follicular thyroid cancer. Endocr Relat Cancer 2012;19:435–446.

8 Burton KA, McDermott DA, Wilkes D, Poulsen MN, Nolan MA, Goldstein M, et al: Haploinsufficiency at the protein kinase A RI alpha gene locus leads to fertility defects in male mice and men. Mol Endocrinol 2006;20:2504–2513.

9 Stratakis CA, Papageorgiou T, Premkumar A, Pack S, Kirschner LS, Taymans SE, et al: Ovarian lesions in Carney complex: clinical genetics and possible predisposition to malignancy. J Clin Endocrinol Metab 2000;85:4359–4366.

10 Gaujoux S, Tissier F, Ragazzon B, Rebours V, Saloustros E, Perlemoine K, et al: Pancreatic ductal and acinar cell neoplasms in Carney complex: a possible new association. J Clin Endocrinol Metab 2011;96:E1888–E1895.

11 Kirschner LS, Carney JA, Pack SD, Taymans SE, Giatzakis C, Cho YS, et al: Mutations of the gene encoding the protein kinase A type I-alpha regulatory subunit in patients with the Carney complex. Nat Genet 2000;26:89–92.

12 Casey M, Vaughan CJ, He J, Hatcher CJ, Winter JM, Weremowicz S, et al: Mutations in the protein kinase A R1alpha regulatory subunit cause familial cardiac myxomas and Carney complex. J Clin Invest 2000;106:R31–R38.

13 Matyakhina L, Pack S, Kirschner LS, Pak E, Mannan P, Jaikumar J, et al: Chromosome 2 (2p16) abnormalities in Carney complex tumours. J Med Genet 2003;40:268–277.

14 Horvath A, Bertherat J, Groussin L, Guillaud-Bataille M, Tsang K, Cazabat L, et al: Mutations and polymorphisms in the gene encoding regulatory subunit type 1-alpha of protein kinase A (PRKAR1A): an update. Hum Mutat 2010;31:369–379.

15 Patronas Y, Horvath A, Greene E, Tsang K, Bimpaki E, Haran M, et al: In vitro studies of novel PRKAR1A mutants that extend the predicted RIα protein sequence into the 3′-untranslated open reading frame: proteasomal degradation leads to RIα haploinsufficiency and Carney complex. J Clin Endocrinol Metab 2012;97:E496–E502.
16 Horvath A, Boikos S, Giatzakis C, Robinson-White A, Groussin L, Griffin KJ, et al: A genome-wide scan identifies mutations in the gene encoding phosphodiesterase 11A4 (PDE11A) in individuals with adrenocortical hyperplasia. Nat Genet 2006; 38:794–800.
17 Horvath A, Mericq V, Stratakis CA: Mutation in PDE8B, a cyclic AMP-specific phosphodiesterase in adrenal hyperplasia. N Engl J Med 2008;358: 750–752.
18 Libé R, Horvath A, Vezzosi D, Fratticci A, Coste J, Perlemoine K, et al: Frequent phosphodiesterase 11A gene (PDE11A) defects in patients with Carney complex (CNC) caused by PRKAR1A mutations: PDE11A may contribute to adrenal and testicular tumors in CNC as a modifier of the phenotype. J Clin Endocrinol Metab 2011;96:E208–E214.
19 Yu B, Ragazzon B, Rizk-Rabin M, Bertherat J: Protein kinase A alterations in endocrine tumors. Horm Metab Res 2012;44:741–748.
20 Kirschner LS, Kusewitt DF, Matyakhina L, Towns WH 2nd, Carney JA, Westphal H, et al: A mouse model for the Carney complex tumor syndrome develops neoplasia in cyclic AMP-responsive tissues. Cancer Res 2005;65:4506–4514.
21 Amieux PS, Howe DG, Knickerbocker H, Lee DC, Su T, Laszlo GS, et al: Increased basal cAMP-dependent protein kinase activity inhibits the formation of mesoderm-derived structures in the developing mouse embryo. J Biol Chem 2002;277:27294–27304.
22 Yin Z, Williams-Simons L, Parlow AF, Asa S, Kirschner LS: Pituitary-specific knockout of the Carney complex gene Prkar1a leads to pituitary tumorigenesis. Mol Endocrinol 2008;22:380–387.
23 Yin Z, Jones GN, Towns WH 2nd, Zhang X, Abel ED, Binkley PF, et al: Heart-specific ablation of Prkar1a causes failure of heart development and myxomagenesis. Circulation 2008;117:1414–1422.
24 Jones GN, Tep C, Towns WH 2nd, Mihai G, Tonks ID, Kay GF, et al: Tissue-specific ablation of Prkar1a causes schwannomas by suppressing neurofibromatosis protein production. Neoplasia 2008;10: 1213–1221.
25 Almeida MQ, Stratakis CA: How does cAMP/protein kinase A signaling lead to tumors in the adrenal cortex and other tissues? Mol Cell Endocrinol 2011;336:162–168.

Jérôme Bertherat
Service des Maladies Endocriniennes et Métaboliques
Centre de Référence des Maladies Rares de la Surrénale, Hôpital Cochin
27, rue du Fg St Jacques, FR–75014 Paris (France)
E-Mail jerome.bertherat@cch.aphp.fr

Stratakis CA (ed): Endocrine Tumor Syndromes and Their Genetics.
Front Horm Res. Basel, Karger, 2013, vol 41, pp 63–78 (DOI: 10.1159/000345670)

Multiple Endocrine Neoplasia Type 4

Misu Lee · Natalia S. Pellegata
Institute of Pathology, Helmholtz Zentrum München, Neuherberg, Germany

Abstract
A few years ago a novel multiple endocrine neoplasia syndrome, named multiple endocrine neoplasia type 4 (MEN4), was discovered thanks to studies conducted on a MEN syndrome in the rat (named MENX). The rat and the human syndromes are both caused by germline mutations in the *Cdkn1b*/*CDKN1B* gene, respectively. This gene encodes p27Kip1, a putative tumor suppressor which binds to and inhibits cyclin/cyclin-dependent kinase complexes, thereby preventing cell cycle progression. MEN4 patients carry heterozygous mutations at various residues of p27Kip1 and present with endocrine lesions mainly belonging to a MEN1-like spectrum: their most common phenotypic features are parathyroid and pituitary adenomas. Recently, germline mutations in p27kip1 were also identified in patients with a sporadic parathyroid disease presentation. In vitro functional analysis of several *CDKN1B* sequence changes identified in MEN4 patients detected impaired activity of the encoded p27Kip1 variant proteins (e.g. reduced expression, mislocalization or poor binding to interaction partners), thereby highlighting the characteristics of the protein which are critical for tumor suppression. Although the number of MEN4 patients is low, the discovery of this syndrome has demonstrated a novel role for *CDKN1B* as a tumor susceptibility gene for neuroendocrine tumors. Here, we review the clinical characteristics of the MEN4 syndrome and the molecular phenotype of the associated p27Kip1 mutations.

Multiple endocrine neoplasia type 4 (MEN4) is the latest member to join the family of MEN syndromes. These syndromes are autosomal dominant disorders characterized by the occurrence of tumors involving two or more endocrine glands, although tumors can also develop in nonendocrine organs. MEN type 1 (MEN1) and type 2 (MEN2) syndromes are the 'classical' MEN syndromes, whose clinical characteristics, tumor spectrum and molecular genetics have been elucidated. MEN1 is characterized by tumors of the parathyroid, endocrine pancreas and anterior pituitary and is caused by loss-of-function mutations of the *MEN1* gene [1, 2]. MEN2 is a syndrome of medullary thyroid carcinoma (MTC) occurring in association with pheochromocytoma and multigland parathyroid adenoma. Three variants are recognized: MEN2a, the most common, characterized by all three above-mentioned tumors; MEN2b, where parathyroid is not involved and pheochromocytoma develops together with marfanois habitus, gastrointestinal disorders and multiple mucosal ganglioneuromas; FMTC, where MTC is the only manifestation. MEN2 is caused by activating mutations of the *RET* proto-oncogene [1, 2].

While *RET* mutations virtually explain all MEN2 cases, in approximately one third of the clinically suspected MEN1 patients *MEN1* mutations are not found. While this might be due to the mutation lying outside the regions tested, it also suggests that other predisposing genes may play a role in causing this phenotype. Our recent work on a rat strain that spontaneously developed a MEN-like phenotype (named MENX syndrome) demonstrated that a germline mutation in the *Cdkn1b* gene, encoding the cell cycle inhibitor p27Kip1 (hereafter p27), is responsible for this syndrome [3]. Thus, we decided to check whether mutations in the human homologue *CDKN1B* could explain some of the MEN1-like cases without mutations in *MEN1*. We screened for the presence of *CDKN1B* germline mutations, several patients fulfilling the above criteria and we identified a germline heterozygous nonsense mutation at codon 76 in a female proband with pituitary adenoma and primary hyperparathyroidism. This mutation segregated with the predisposition to a MEN1-like phenotype in the proband's family [3]. Subsequently, we and other groups have identified additional index cases presenting with a MEN1-like phenotype and carrying heterozygous *CDKN1B* gene mutations. Altogether, these findings identified *CDKN1B* as a novel tumor susceptibility gene for multiple endocrine neoplasia and led to the recognition of a novel MEN syndrome named MEN4 caused by mutations in p27 (OMIM No. 610755). Recently, *CDKN1B* mutations were also identified in patients with a sporadic presentation of endocrine tumors [4]. The overall number of MEN4 patients is still too low to allow us to formulate guidelines for the clinical diagnosis of the disease or for patient management. However, since new mutation-positive cases keep being discovered, *CDKN1B* needs to be considered as the predisposing gene in cases presenting with multiple endocrine tumors and no mutations in other tumor susceptibility genes.

In this chapter, we summarize the clinical features of the MEN4 cases described so far and we compare them with other familial endocrine tumors syndromes (table 1). We also present the functional characterization of the associated germline *CDKN1B* mutations in an attempt to better understand the role of p27 in the susceptibility to neuroendocrine tumors.

Phenotypic Features of Patients Carrying *CDKN1B* Germline Mutations

Primary Hyperparathyroidism

To date, 12 index cases having germline nucleotide substitutions in *CDKN1B* have been reported in the literature. The phenotypic features of these patients are summarized in table 2. The most common feature is primary hyperparathyroidism (PHPT), which was observed in 10 of the 12 patients (incidence 81%). In the majority of the

Table 1. Tumor spectrum of the various MEN syndromes; the main clinical features of MEN1, MEN2A, MEN2B and MEN4 are tabulated

	MEN1	MEN2A	MEN2B	MEN4
Pituitary adenoma	+			+
Parathyroid adenoma	+	+		+
Medullary thyroid tumors		+	+	
Pheochromocytoma		+	+	
Paragangliomas		+		
Insulinoma	+			
Neuroma			+	

Table 2. Germline changes in the *CDKN1B* gene and the clinical characteristics of the mutation-positive patients

CDKN1B mutation	Parathyroid adenoma	Pituitary tumor	Other manifestations
MEN4 (MEN1-like)			
ATG-32–29del	PHPT		gastric carcinoid tumor
ATG-7G>C	PHPT		bilateral adrenal mass non-functioning uterine fibroid
K25fs	PHPT	ACTH-secreting	
A55T	PHPT (hepatic metastasis)		Zollinger-Ellison syndrome gastrinoma
P69L	PHPT	nonfunctioning	bronchial carcinoids, papillary thyroid carcinoma, multiple lung metastases
W76X	PHPT	GH-secreting (acromegaly)	
P95S	PHPT (2 para-thyroid tumors)		Zollinger-Ellison syndrome mass in duodenum and tail of pancreas
Stop>Q	PHPT (3 para-thyroid tumors)		
MEN4 (others)			
G9R	PHPT		
K96Q		PRL-secreting	breast tumor
I119T		GH-secreting	
P133T	PHPT (1 para-thyroid tumors)		

Mutations are numbered with reference to the cDNA sequence AY890407 (GenBank).
ACTH = Adrenocorticotropic hormone; GH = growth hormone; PHPT = primary hyperparathyroidism; PRL = prolactin.

Table 3. Genes predisposing to hereditary PHPT and pituitary adenoma

Gene	Tumor type
PHPT	
CaSR	parathyroid hyperplasia/adenoma
CDKN1B	parathyroid hyperplasia/adenoma
HRPT2	parathyroid adenoma/carcinoma
MEN1	parathyroid hyperplasia/adenoma
RET	parathyroid hyperplasia/adenoma
Pituitary Adenoma	
AIP	GH-secreting GH/PRL-secreting
CDKN1B	PRL-secreting GH-secreting ACTH-secreting nonfunctioning
MEN1	PRL-secreting GH-secreting GH/PRL-secreting TSH-secreting ACTH-secreting
PRKAR1	GH-secreting

ACTH = Adrenocorticotropic hormone; GH = growth hormone; PRL = prolactin; TSH = thyroid-stimulating hormone.

mutation-positive patients the presence of a parathyroid tumor as the underlying cause of PHPT was confirmed by surgical resection. The age of onset was quite variable, ranging from 46 to 74 years of age.

PHPT is the most common feature of the MEN1 syndrome too, occurring in more than 90% of patients [5]. In addition to *CDKN1B* mutations, nucleotide substitutions in *RET*, *CaSR* (calcium-sensing receptor) and *HRPT2* (parafibromin) genes are known to predispose to PHPT (table 3) [6]. Biochemical analysis of these patients usually detects hypercalcemia, which is associated with increased circulating levels of parathyroid hormone. Currently there is no medical treatment for PHPT and surgical removal of the affected parathyroid gland(s) is the only available option for a definitive treatment.

Pituitary Adenoma

The second most common tumor type occurring in *CDKN1B* mutation carriers is pituitary adenoma, observed in 5 of 12 (41.6%) index cases. Pituitary adenomas are common tumors of the anterior lobe of the pituitary gland and account for about 15% of intracranial neoplasm. These tumors are usually classified based on the hormone secreted by the tumor cells or because these cells do not produce any hormone (nonfunctioning tumors) [7]. Thus, there are lactotroph adenomas which secrete prolactin

(PRL), somatotroph adenomas producing growth hormone (GH), corticotroph adenomas secreting adrenocorticotropic hormone (ACTH), and thyrotroph adenomas secreting thyroid-stimulating hormone (TSH). Gonadotroph adenomas may secrete follicle-stimulating hormone (FSH) and/or luteinizing hormone (LH), but many of them are not associated with hormone excess and are therefore nonfunctioning tumors. The clinical manifestations of pituitary tumors depend upon the secreted hormone or the size of the tumor in the case of nonfunctioning adenomas. MEN4 patients develop various types of pituitary adenomas, as summarized in table 2. Two patients developed a GH-secreting tumor and had features of acromegaly, 1 patient with ACTH-secreting tumor had Cushing's disease. One patient had a nonfunctioning tumor and another a suspected prolactinoma (elevated prolactin levels in blood). Age of onset was sometimes earlier than typical sporadic cases, although highly variable (from 30 to 79 years).

Pituitary adenomas are a component tumor feature of MEN1 and of other inherited tumor syndromes, such as Carney complex and familial isolated pituitary adenoma (FIPA). The vast majority of MEN1-associated pituitary adenomas are prolactinomas (60% of cases), followed by GH-secreting tumors (25%). Mutations in the protein kinase A regulatory subunit-1-alpha *(PRKAR1A)* gene cause Carney complex, a familial multiple neoplasia syndrome having multifocal hyperplasia of the somato-mammotropic pituitary cells as a component feature [8]. More recently, the aryl hydrocarbon receptor interacting protein (AIP) was identified as a pituitary adenoma predisposing gene. *AIP* gene mutations explain up to 30% of FIPA families. FIPA-associated pituitary adenomas are usually GH- or GH/PRL-secreting adenomas, with few prolactinomas or other tumor subtypes (table 3) [9]. Being that the number of mutation carriers identified so far is small, it is not possible to ascertain whether *CDKN1B* variants do indeed equally affect the various pituitary cell lineages or they preferentially target a specific one. MEN1-associated pituitary tumors tend to be more aggressive than their sporadic counterpart, usually respond poorly to conventional therapy and tend to recur [10]. We do not yet know whether the pituitary adenomas developing in the context of *CDKN1B* mutations are also more aggressive. Interestingly, the GH-secreting adenoma associated to the p27W76X mutation (table 2) showed sella and cavernous sinus invasion, and, at histopathological examination, displayed cell atypia and a quite elevated mitotic activity, suggesting aggressive tumor behavior [3].

Although usually benign, pituitary adenomas may cause severe morbidity secondary to excessive hormone production or, in nonfunctioning adenomas, due to local invasion of adjacent neuroanatomical structures. Transsphenoidal surgery is currently the treatment of choice for pituitary adenomas, but it is not always curative. If residual tumor is discovered or if the tumor recurs, radiation therapy is performed, but this approach is associated with serious long-term complications [11]. Receptor-mediated pharmacological therapy is also used but the response varies greatly among patients and tumor subtypes [12].

Associated Tumors
MEN4 patients may develop tumors involving organs other than parathyroid and pituitary glands. Indeed, neuroendocrine carcinomas of the cervix, carcinoids in the bronchi and stomach, and a gastrinoma have also been observed (table 2). Two MEN4 patients presented with masses in the pancreas or in the adrenal glands, but the precise nature of these lesions is currently unknown. Interestingly, endocrine pancreatic tumors and adrenal tumors are also observed in MEN1 patients, and so are lung carcinoids, which in MEN1 patients occur with a frequency of about 36% [13].

The *CDKN1B* Tumor Susceptibility Gene

The identification of *CDKN1B* as a tumor susceptibility gene for multiple endocrine tumors originated from studies of MENX, a MEN-like syndrome in the rat. This multitumor syndrome was discovered about 10 years ago when a Sprague-Dawley-derived rat colony spontaneously started to develop multiple neuroendocrine tumors at a young age, including anterior pituitary adenoma, adrenal and extra-adrenal pheochromocytoma, thyroid C-cell hyperplasia, and parathyroid hyperplasia [14]. The MENX syndrome was reported to be inherited as a recessive trait. Linkage studies finally mapped the *MENX* locus to a 3-Mb region containing several genes, including *Cdkn1b*, encoding the cell cycle inhibitor p27. This gene was selected as a putative candidate gene for the rat syndrome because p27 knockout mice develop pituitary gland tumors [15], an organ also affected by the MENX syndrome, and p27 is a putative tumor suppressor, which is consistent with the recessive mode of inheritance observed in MENX rats. Upon sequencing of the *Cdkn1b* gene in affected and unaffected littermates, a tandem duplication of eight nucleotides in exon 2 (c.520–528dupTTCAGAC; RefSeq: NM_031762.3), which causes a frameshift, was identified in all the affected rats. The mutated allele encodes a protein having a C-terminal sequence different from that of the wild-type protein, which was later found to be highly unstable and therefore absent, or present at very low level, in the tissues of affected rats [3]. Capitalizing on this finding, we then sequenced *CDKN1B* in patients with a MEN1-like phenotype and no MEN1 gene mutations and we identified the first germline mutation in a patient with PHPT and pituitary adenoma.

The *CDKN1B* gene has two coding exons resulting in a 2.5-kb-long coding region. *CDKN1B* is located on chromosome 12p13, a chromosomal region known to undergo hemizygous loss in hematological malignancies. The MEN4-associated germline mutations identified in the coding sequence of *CDKN1B* are for the vast majority missense mutations (8/12) although also a nonsense mutation and an insertion (duplication) were detected (fig. 1). Two nucleotide changes occur in the 5′ untranslated region of the transcript (one missense and one deletion). Each index case presents with a distinct germline mutation. The p27 variants which were characterized at the func-

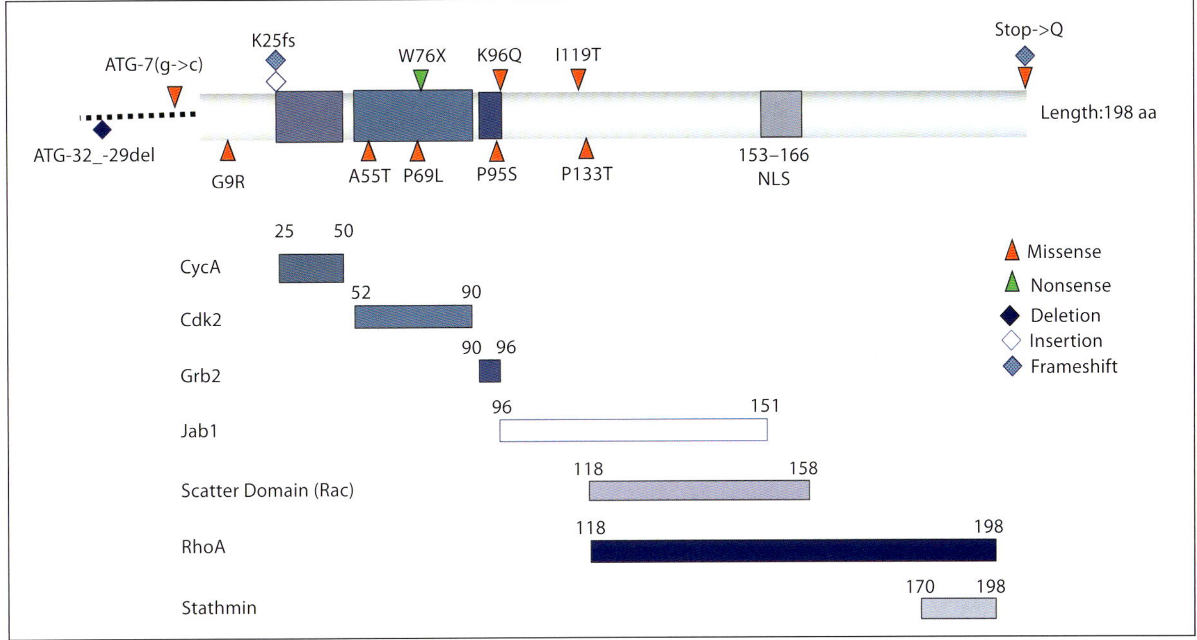

Fig. 1. Schematic structure of the p27 protein. The p27 protein is composed of several protein-binding domains and contains a nuclear localization signal (NLS). The position of the germline mutations is indicated by colored symbols. CycA = Cyclin A; Cdk2 = cyclin-dependent kinase 2; Grb2 = growth factor receptor-bound protein 2; Jab1 = c-jun activation domain binding protein 1; RhoA = Ras homolog gene family, member A.

tional level seem to be inactivating, and this is consistent with the tumor suppressive role of the protein (see below).

Somatic *CDKN1B* mutations are extremely rare in human tumors and to date only a handful has been reported in the literature, namely: a nonsense mutation in an adult T-cell leukemia/lymphoma (p27W76X) [16]; a nonsense mutation in a breast cancer sample (p27Q104X) [17]; a missense change in an unclassified myeloproliferative disorder (p27I119T) [18]. Lately, a somatic missense change (p27P133T) and a 25 nucleotide deletion starting at codon 25 (c.582del25) in *CDKN1B* were identified in sporadic parathyroid adenomas [4]. The tumor tissue carrying the c.582del25 change showed loss of heterozygosity of the wild-type allele and no immunoreactivity for p27. Interestingly, 3 of 4 of these somatic changes (p27W76X, p27I119T, p27P133T) were also identified in the germline of individuals with neuroendocrine tumors. Since the p27 protein is so rarely mutated, the finding that the same mutation arose independently in somatic and germline settings seems to suggest that these variant proteins have a pro-oncogenic effect.

Several single nucleotide polymorphisms (SNPs) have been identified in the human *CDKN1B* gene (http://www.ncbi.nlm.nih.gov/snp), including three which are potentially functional: –838C>A (rs36228499), –79C>T (rs34330) and 326T>G (V109G, rs2066827). Several studies have demonstrated a significant association between coding SNP rs2066827 (V109G) and a variety of cancers including those of the prostate, ovary, breast and, recently, also medullary thyroid carcinoma [19]. Whether this amino acid substitution affects p27 levels or function is currently unknown. Recently, SNP –79C>T (rs34330) was associated to the risk of developing papillary thyroid carcinoma (follicular variant) [20]. The authors went on to demonstrate that the variant allele associates with reduced gene transcription and, consequently, with lower p27 protein levels.

CDKN1B Germline Mutations in Patients with a MEN1-Like Phenotype (MEN4)

To date, 8 germline base substitutions in *CDKN1B* have been identified in association with a MEN1-like phenotype. Most of them were missense mutations, thus it is intrinsically difficult to assign these variants a pathological role. However, several of them are usually not found in control unaffected individuals and they affect the protein's function (see below), thus they have been classified as potentially pathogenic. We refer to them as 'mutations' throughout the text. The changes with no detectable molecular phenotype and/or observed in control individuals are considered genetic variants of unknown significance. Since for most index cases only a few first-degree relatives were available for genetic analysis, if at all, segregation with the disease phenotype in these families was not used as the main criterion for assigning a possible pathogenic role to *CDKN1B* variants. All the identified changes occur in heterozygosity, thereby suggesting a dominant inheritance of the tumor predisposition. We here present these changes following their position along the gene sequence (from 5′ to 3′).

Two mutations have been found in the 5′ UTR region of the *CDKN1B* gene. One of them is a heterozygous GAGA deletion at the –29 position (c.–32/–29del; RefSeq: AY890407), which was identified in a Spanish female patient with gastric carcinoid tumor (at age 69) and PHPT (at age 74). In peripheral blood leukocytes from this patient, the *CDKN1B* mRNA was significantly reduced compare to a normal healthy control [21]. In a study of American patients with a MEN1-like phenotype and no MEN1 gene mutations, Agarwal et al. [22] discovered a mutation at the –7 position in the Kozak sequence (ATG–7G>C) in a patient with a parathyroid tumor, bilateral adrenal masses and uterine fibroids. No loss of heterozygosity was found in the tumor but protein expression could not be assessed.

The remaining 6 mutations occur in the coding sequence of the *CDKN1B* gene. A 19-bp duplication (c.59–77dup19) in exon 1, which causes a frameshift after codon 25, was identified in a Dutch patient diagnosed with three lesions compatible with MEN1: ACTH-secreting pituitary adenoma (Cushing's disease; age 46 years), small-cell neuroendocrine cervical carcinoma (age 45 years), and hyperparathyroidism (age 47 years). The resulting variant transcript is predicted to encode a p27 protein having an amino acid sequence different from that of the wild-type protein after the site of the insertion, and being 69 amino acids shorter (p.K25fs). The cervical carcinoma of the patient showed loss of the wild-type *CDKN1B* allele and no p27 protein expression, while the other tumor tissues could not be analyzed [23].

Recently, a cohort of familial and sporadic Spanish patients with a MEN1 phenotype was screened for mutations in *MEN1*, *CDKN1B* and *AIP*, and a novel missense mutation in *CDKN1B* (c.163G>A; p. Ala55Thr, A55T) was found in a lady presenting with Zollinger-Ellison syndrome with gastrinoma and hepatic metastases (at age 42 years) and PHPT (at age 51 years) [24].

The screening of a series of Italian patients with suspected MEN1 identified a *CDKN1B* germline mutation in a 79-year-old Caucasian female patient diagnosed with PHPT caused by a parathyroid adenoma (at age 67 years) and a papillary thyroid carcinoma (at age 64 years). Magnetic resonance imaging (MRI) revealed a nonfunctioning pituitary microadenoma in this lady (at age 79 years). She also developed bilateral multiple lung metastases of a bronchial carcinoid and type 2 diabetes mellitus. This index case carries a missense mutation at codon 69 of p27 which results in a proline to threonine amino acid substitution (c.678C>T, p.P69L) [25].

The heterozygous TGG>TAG (c.227G>A) nonsense mutation at codon 76, which determines the premature truncation of the protein (p.W76X), was the first *CDKN1B* mutation to be detected in a 48-year-old Caucasian female presenting with GH-secreting pituitary tumor (acromegaly; at age 30 years) and PHPT (at age 46 years). In the family of the index case, this mutation is inherited together with the predisposition to MEN1-like tumors. Indeed, a mutation-carrier sister of the proband presented with renal angiomyolipoma (at age 55 years), a MEN1-associated tumor [3]. The normal renal tissue of this woman showed cytoplasmic immunoreactivity for p27, while her angiomyolipoma had no p27 staining [25].

An individual affected by PHPT and displaying masses in both duodenum and pancreas was found to carry a CCC>TCC missense mutation at codon 95, leading to a proline to serine amino acid change (P95S). Another sequence variant was found in a patient with a family history of PHPT. This change transforms the stop codon in glutamine (TAA>CAA; stop>Q), thereby leading to a protein predicted to be 60 amino acids longer than the wild-type one [22].

The analysis of family members of the mutation-positive index cases (when possible) showed that some *CDKN1B* sequence changes are also found in a few of their nonsymptomatic first-degree relatives, suggesting that some mutated alleles may have incomplete penetrance.

CDKN1B Germline Mutations in Endocrine Disease

In addition to patients with a MEN1-like phenotype, also patients with a FIPA phenotype and no mutations in the *AIP* gene were found to occasionally carry germline *CDKN1B* gene variants. In 88 AIP mutation-negative FIPA families (for a total of 124 affected subjects) the *CDKN1B* gene was sequenced and two point mutations were found in two patients: c.286A>C (p.K96Q) and c.356T>C (p.I119T) (table 2; fig. 1). These sequence changes led to functional or conformational alterations in the encoded p27 proteins in vitro (see below). Additional variants were identified in this FIPA patients cohort (p.S56T, p.T142T, c.605 + 36C>T) but are likely to be nonpathogenic because they were occasionally observed in control unaffected individuals and were not predicted to affect p27 function by in silico modeling [26].

So far, we presented *CDKN1B* mutations occurring in patients selected because of a familial presentation of neuroendocrine disease, either MEN1-like or FIPA-like. However, it was recently demonstrated that germline p27 changes can be identified also in patients with an apparently sporadic presentation of neuroendocrine tumors. Indeed, we discovered two novel germline *CDKN1B* variants in a study of 90 single gland parathyroid adenomas, presumed to be sporadic [4]. Specifically, one patient carried a heterozygous germline single nucleotide change at base 25 in *CDKN1B* exon 1 (c.25G>A), which would result in a glycine to arginine substitution at codon 9 (G9R) of the translated p27 protein product. This patient, a 68-year-old man, had a typical single-gland, mildly symptomatic tumor presentation. The germline DNA of another patient, a 53-year-old woman presenting with fatigue, slightly elevated serum calcium and parathyroid hormone levels, carried a heterozygous single nucleotide substitution (c.397C>A), directing a proline to threonine substitution at position 133 (P133T) of the encoded p27 protein [4].

Function of the p27 Protein

To fully appreciate the effect of the different *CDKN1B* mutations on the function of the encoded variant p27 proteins, it is important to briefly summarize the most relevant functions of wild-type p27. It is a ubiquitously expressed protein, member of the KIP1 family of cyclin-dependent kinase (CDK) inhibitors [27], together with p21 and p57. The wild-type p27 protein is 198 amino acids long and possesses a nuclear localization signal (NLS) between amino acids 153 and 166, which targets the protein to the cell nucleus (fig. 1). The most important function of p27 is to regulate the progression from the G1 to the S phase of the cell cycle by inactivating the cyclin A,E/ CDK2 complexes. The substrate of CDK2 is the retinoblastoma protein (pRb). Upon phosphorylation by CDK2, pRb releases members of the E2F family of transcription factors which in turn activate the transcription of genes required for the progression into the S phase. Thus, in the presence of p27, cell cycle progression is blocked, and this is an important mechanism regulating tissue homeostasis in most adult organs [28]. Due to the important role of p27 in cell growth, its function is tightly regulated through different mechanisms modulating the intracellular level of the protein, its localization or posttranslational modifications. The best known mechanism regulating the amount of p27 is ubiquitin-mediated proteasomal degradation of the protein

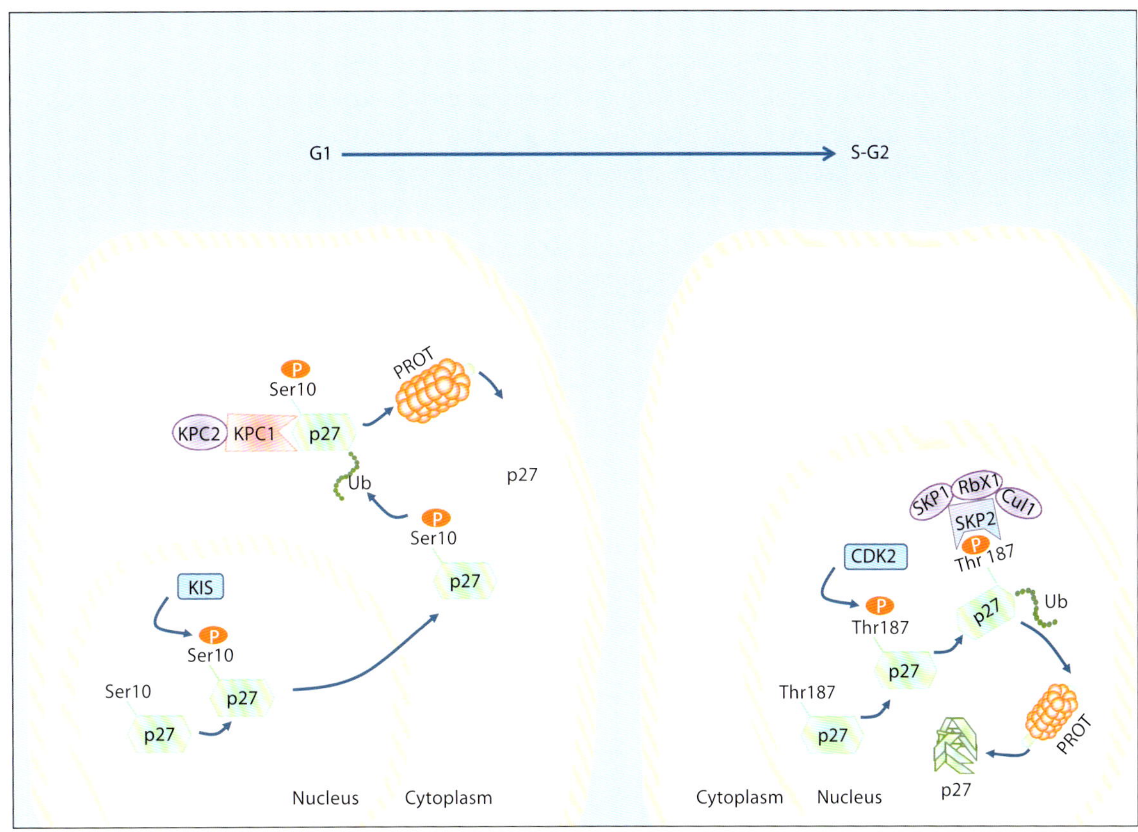

Fig. 2. Diagram illustrating the known p27 degradation pathways. After the dissociation of p27 from the cyclin E/Cdk2 complex in early G1, a portion of p27 is phosphorylated on Ser10 by kinase-interacting stathmin (KIS) and then exported to the cytoplasm. Once in the cytoplasm, p27 interacts with the KPC1/KPC2 complex that promotes p27 ubiquitylation and degradation of the protein by the proteasome (PROT). Upon mitogenic stimulation, p27 becomes a substrate of the Cdk2 complex which phosphorylates the protein at the Thr187 residue. Phosphorylation at Thr187 allows the interaction with Skp2 and the subsequent ubiquitylation-mediated degradation by the proteasome.

[29]. Two main pathways involved in p27 degradation have been identified (fig. 2). At the beginning of the G1 phase, after the dissociation from the cyclinE-CDK2 complex, p27 is phosporylated at serine 10 (Ser10), the major phosphorylation residue of p27. Phosphorylation at Ser10 increases the binding affinity of p27 to CRM1 (or exportin 1) via the nuclear export signal of p27. This association promotes the export of p27 to the cytoplasm, where it is then ubiquitylated and degraded by the ubiquitylation-promoting complex KPC1 [30].

The second mechanism involved in p27 degradation occurs in late G1 and requires the phosphorylation of the protein at the threonine (Thr) 187 residue by CDK2, which creates a recognition site for the nuclear SKP2 ubiquitin ligase. SKP2 induces polyubiquitylation of p27 and its subsequent degradation by the proteasome (fig. 2) [31].

The subcellular localization of p27 indirectly regulates the protein's activity by rendering the protein available, or unavailable, to various interacting partners (such as cyclin/CDK complexes) or to degradation pathways. In addition, recent evidence suggests that p27 exerts different functions while in the nucleus or in the cytoplasm, so that the subcellular localization of the protein may also directly affect its function. For instance, while in the nucleus p27 inhibits cyclin/CDK complexes, in the cytoplasm p27 is a necessary assembly factor for cyclin D/CDK4,6 complexes, which in turn promote cell proliferation. Recently, based on genetic studies on mutant mouse strains, it has been suggested that cytoplasmic p27 may have oncogenic properties (see below) [32].

p27 and Tumorigenesis

CDKN1B has been considered an atypical tumor suppressor gene for many years because it is not mutated (or extremely rarely) in human cancers. In contrast, the level of expression of the encoded p27 protein is reduced in the vast majority of human neoplasms. Downregulation of p27 associates with poor clinical outcome in several malignancies, including cancers of the breast, colon, prostate, and ovary, among others [33]. Several studies in various tumor entities demonstrated that *CDKN1B* mRNA levels are similar among samples with high or low p27 protein levels. Therefore, it is believed that the decrease of p27 expression in human tumors is mainly due to post-transcriptional or posttranslational mechanisms. Indeed, in tumors such as colorectal carcinoma and lymphomas, it could be shown that enhanced proteasome-mediated degradation of p27 is responsible for p27 downregulation.

Animal models have significantly contributed to our understanding of the role of p27 in tumorigenesis. p27 knockout mice were generated and analyzed: they develop normally, are usually bigger than their wild-type littermates and show pituitary adenoma of the intermediate lobe as sole tumor phenotype (frequency 100%) [15]. These observations further supported the tumor suppressive role of p27 in tumor formation. Our work on the MENX syndrome demonstrated that a homozygous *Cdkn1b* mutation, causing extreme reduction of the p27 protein levels [34], renders rats susceptible to multiple neuroendocrine tumors formation. Interestingly, heterozygous knockout mice, upon γ-irradiation or treatment with carcinogens, develop tumors at higher frequency and multiplicity compared with their wild-type littermates, indicating that the loss of one *Cdkn1b* allele already predisposes mice to tumor formation [35]. In conclusion, it seems that the amount of p27 protein plays an important role in promoting tumor formation in both humans and rodents.

Recently, many studies have demonstrated a relationship between the mislocalization of p27 and tumorigensis. Indeed, cytoplasmic immunoreactivity for p27 has been observed in several tumor types, including breast cancer and clear renal cell carcinoma, and it is usually associated with high tumor grades and poorer patient survival. Sequestration of p27 in the cytoplasm impairs the protein's ability to inhibit cyclin/CDK complexes. Mice homozygous for a mutant p27 protein unable to bind to cyclin/CDK complexes (p27 CK–/CK–) show increased tumor multiplicity (lung, retina, pituitary, ovary, adrenals, spleen, and lymphomas) and aggressiveness when compared with homozygous p27 knockout mice p27 (p27–/–), suggesting that p27CK- plays a pro-oncogenic role. Interestingly, in p27CK–/CK– mice the tissues susceptible to tumor formation abundantly express p27 in the cytoplasm not only in the nucleus, thereby leading to the speculation that the oncogenic role of protein may depend on its cytoplasmic localization [32].

Functional Effects of p27 Mutations

Most of the *CDKN1B* germline mutations identified in patients have been cloned and studied in vitro to try and elucidate how they associate with tumor predisposition. Only the K25fs and the most recent A55T change have yet to be studied in transfection experiments. The most common molecular phenotypes associated with these allelic variants are a reduced amount of the *CDKN1B* transcript or of the encoded p27 protein. These features are in agreement with the tumor suppressive role of p27 in tumor formation.

U-rich elements in the 5′-UTR region of *CDKN1B* regulate mRNA stability and p27 translation. In vitro transcription/translation assays performed using the c-32_–29del mutation in 5′-UTR region of the gene showed a decreased rate of transcription of the variant transcript and a reduced level of the encoded p27 protein [21]. In contrast to the c-32_–29del mutation, cells transfected with the ATG-7 variant showed a reduction of the expression level of the encoded p27 protein, but no changes at the mRNA level [22].

Concerning the p27G9R mutation, glycine at position 9 in p27 protein is highly conserved among vertebrates, and this amino acid substitution mimics a phosphorylation event on the adjacent Ser10 residue, the most important phosphorylation site of p27. The G9R change makes the protein less stable then wild-type p27, which may explain why that parathyroid tumor tissue of the mutation-positive patient has a low level of expression of p27 [4].

Proline at position 69 of p27 is located in the CDK2 binding domain of the protein (amino acids 52–93) (fig. 1) and we could demonstrate that the mutant p27P69L protein does not bind to CDK2 in vitro. In addition, the P69L change made the protein more unstable than wild-type p27. Our observation that the overexpression of p27P69L associates with reduced growth suppression when compared to expression of wild-type p27 is likely explained by the lower expression level of the mutant protein and by its inability to bind to CDK2 [25].

In contrast to the other mutations so far described, the truncated p27W76X mutant protein lacks the nuclear localization signal and indeed is localized in the cytoplasm in vitro, in the normal tissues of a mutation-positive patient [25]. The inability of p27W76X to enter the nucleus, the cell compartment where p27 exerts its function as a cell cycle inhibitor, abolishes its ability to inhibit the growth of GH3 cells both by clonogenic assay and by stable expression of this variant p27 protein.

The missense mutations p27P95S and p27K96Q are situated in the proline rich domain (amino acids 90–96) of p27 which mediates the binding to the adaptor molecule Grb2, which in turn recruits and leads to the activation of Ras. Both mutant p27 proteins fail to bind to Grb2 in vitro, and this is assumed to affect the ability of p27 to impair the activation of the Ras pathway [22].

The p27I119T protein displays an abnormal migration pattern by polyacrylamide gel electrophoresis, in that it migrates slower than the wild-type protein [26]. The unique migration pattern of p27I119T, suggestive of noncanonical posttranslational modifications, is not due to increased phosphorylation at the newly created threonine residue. Since glycosylation occurs at serine, threonine or aspartic acid residues, the migration shift associated with the 119T residue could be caused by glycosylation of the protein, thereby conferring greater stability. In agreement with this finding, p27I119T is more stable than wild-type p27 in vitro [26].

The p27P133T variant, observed both as germline and somatic change in patients with PHPT, was analyzed in vitro using various assays but no differences in behavior when compared with the wild-type p27 protein could be identified, so this is a change of unknown pathogenic significance [4].

In one patient, a missense mutation changed the stop codon of the protein into Glutamine (p27stop>Q), and this lead to a frameshift and to an encoded protein which is 60 amino acids longer than wild-type p27. When this variant was analyzed in vitro, the p27stop>Q protein was expressed at lower level than wild-type p27 and treatment with a proteasome inhibitor drug rescued protein levels. Thus, it seems that this mutation makes the p27 protein more unstable [22].

Conclusions

Mutations in *CDKN1B,* although rare, are responsible for a subset of patients with various combinations of endocrine tumors and with no mutations in other susceptibility genes. The most common feature of MEN4 is PHPT followed by pituitary adenomas, most resembling MEN1. However, single endocrine tumors, such as pituitary or parathyroid adenomas, may also be associated with germline *CDKN1B* mutations. The changes so far studied at the functional level reduce the final amount of *CDKN1B* transcript and/or p27 protein, alter the protein's intracellular localization or its ability to interact with partner proteins such as CDK2 or Grb2. Whether complete inactivation of p27 function is required to promote tumor formation in patients is still not clear as only some tumor tissues of mutation-positive patients were examined and some of them show loss of p27 expression while others only have reduced expression.

Clinical follow-up and genetic analysis of the extended families of p27 mutation-positive probands might help us assess the role of *CDKN1B* genotyping in individualized risk assessment and management of MEN4 patients.

Acknowledgments

We thank all members of the laboratory for stimulating discussions. We apologize for not being able to cite many relevant original papers, replaced by reviews, due to space limitation. This work was supported by SFB 824 (DFG Sonderforschungsbereich 824) from the Deutsche Forschungsgemeinschaft, Bonn, Germany.

References

1 Brandi ML, Gagel RF, Angeli A, Bilezikian JP, Beck-Peccoz P, Bordi C, Conte-Devolx B, Falchetti A, Gheri RG, Libroia A, Lips CJ, Lombardi G, Mannelli M, Pacini F, Ponder BA, Raue F, Skogseid B, Tamburrano G, Thakker RV, Thompson NW, Tomassetti P, Tonelli F, Wells SA Jr, Marx SJ: Guidelines for diagnosis and therapy of men type 1 and type 2. J Clin Endocrinol Metab 2001;86:5658–5671.

2 Marx SJ: Molecular genetics of multiple endocrine neoplasia types 1 and 2. Nat Rev Cancer 2005;5: 367–375.

3 Pellegata NS, Quintanilla-Martinez L, Siggelkow H, Samson E, Bink K, Hofler H, Fend F, Graw J, Atkinson MJ: Germ-line mutations in p27kip1 cause a multiple endocrine neoplasia syndrome in rats and humans. Proc Natl Acad Sci USA 2006;103:15558–15563.

4 Costa-Guda J, Marinoni I, Molatore S, Pellegata NS, Arnold A: Somatic mutation and germline sequence abnormalities in cdkn1b, encoding p27kip1, in sporadic parathyroid adenomas. J Clin Endocrinol Metab 2011;96:E701–E706.

5 Thakker RV: Multiple endocrine neoplasia type 1 (MEN1). Best Pract Res Clin Endocrinol Metab 2010;24:355–370.

6 Marx SJ: Hyperparathyroid genes: sequences reveal answers and questions. Endocr Pract 2011;3:18–27.

7 Melmed S: Mechanisms for pituitary tumorigenesis: the plastic pituitary. J Clin Invest 2003;112: 1603–1618.

8 Rothenbuhler A, Stratakis CA: Clinical and molecular genetics of Carney complex. Best Pract Res Clin Endocrinol Metab 2010;24:389–399.

9 Daly AF, Tichomirowa MA, Beckers A: The epidemiology and genetics of pituitary adenomas. Best Pract Res Clin Endocrinol Metab 2009;23;543–554.

10 Verges B, Boureille F, Goudet P, Murat A, Beckers A, Sassolas G, Cougard P, Chambe B, Montvernay C, Calender A: Pituitary disease in MEN type 1 (MEN1): data from the France-Belgium MEN1 multicenter study. J Clin Endocrinol Metab 2002; 87:457–465.

11 Platta CS, Mackay C, Welsh JS: Pituitary adenoma: a radiotherapeutic perspective. Am J Clin Oncol 2010;33:408–419.

12 Hofland LJ, Feelders RA, de Herder WW, Lamberts SW: Pituitary tumours: the sst/d2 receptors as molecular targets. Mol Cell Endocrinol 2010;326:89–98.

13 Debelenko LV, Brambilla E, Agarwal SK, Swalwell JI, Kester MB, Lubensky IA, Zhuang Z, Guru SC, Manickam P, Olufemi SE, Chandrasekharappa SC, Crabtree JS, Kim YS, Heppner C, Burns AL, Spiegel AM, Marx SJ, Liotta LA, Collins FS, Travis WD, Emmert-Buck MR: Identification of men1 gene mutations in sporadic carcinoid tumors of the lung. Hum Mol Genet 1997;6:2285–2290.

14 Fritz A, Walch A, Piotrowska K, Rosemann M, Schaffer E, Weber K, Timper A, Wildner G, Graw J, Hofler H, Atkinson MJ: Recessive transmission of a multiple endocrine neoplasia syndrome in the rat. Cancer Res. 2002;62:3048–3051.

15 Fero ML, Rivkin M, Tasch M, Porter P, Carow CE, Firpo E, Polyak K, Tsai LH, Broudy V, Perlmutter RM, Kaushansky K, Roberts JM: A syndrome of multiorgan hyperplasia with features of gigantism, tumorigenesis, and female sterility in p27(kip1)-deficient mice. Cell 1996;85:733–744.

16 Morosetti R, Kawamata N, Gombart AF, Miller CW, Hatta Y, Hirama T, Said JW, Tomonaga M, Koeffler HP: Alterations of the p27kip1 gene in non-hodgkin's lymphomas and adult T-cell leukemia/lymphoma. Blood 1995;86.1924–1930.

17 Spirin KS, Simpson JF, Takeuchi S, Kawamata N, Miller CW, Koeffler HP: P27/kip1 mutation found in breast cancer. Cancer Res 1996;56:2400–2404.
18 Pappa V, Papageorgiou S, Papageorgiou E, Panani A, Boutou E, Tsirigotis P, Dervenoulas J, Economopoulos T, Raptis S: A novel p27 gene mutation in a case of unclassified myeloproliferative disorder. Leukemia Res. 2005;29:229–231.
19 Pasquali D, Circelli L, Faggiano A, Pancione M, Renzullo A, Elisei R, Romei C, Accardo G, Coppola VR, De Palma M, Ferolla P, Grimaldi F, Colao A, Colantuoni V: Cdkn1b v109g polymorphism a new prognostic factor in sporadic medullary thyroid carcinoma. Eur J Endocrinol 2011;164:397–404.
20 Landa I, Montero-Conde C, Malanga D, De Gisi S, Pita G, Leandro-Garcia LJ, Inglada-Perez L, Leton R, De Marco C, Rodriguez-Antona C, Viglietto G, Robledo M: Allelic variant at –79 (c>t) in cdkn1b (p27kip1) confers an increased risk of thyroid cancer and alters mRNA levels. Endocr Relat Cancer 2010;17:317–328.
21 Malanga D, De Gisi S, Riccardi M, Scrima M, De Marco C, Robledo M, Viglietto G: Functional characterization of a rare germline mutation in the gene encoding the cyclin-dependent kinase inhibitor p27kip1 (cdkn1b) in a Spanish patient with multiple endocrine neoplasia-like phenotype. Eur J Endocrinol 2012;166:551–560.
22 Agarwal SK, Mateo CM, Marx SJ: Rare germline mutations in cyclin-dependent kinase inhibitor genes in multiple endocrine neoplasia type 1 and related states. J Clin Endocrinol Metab 2009;94: 1826–1834.
23 Georgitsi M, Raitila A, Karhu A, et al: Germline cdkn1b/p27kip1 mutation in multiple endocrine neoplasia. J Clin Endocrinol Metab 2007;92:3321–3325.
24 Belar O, De La Hoz C, Perez-Nanclares G, Castano L, Gaztambide S: Novel mutations in MEN1, CDKN1B and AIP genes in patients with multiple endocrine neoplasia type 1 syndrome in Spain. Clin Endocrinol 2012;76:719–724.
25 Molatore S, Marinoni I, Lee M, Pulz E, Ambrosio MR, degli Uberti EC, Zatelli MC, Pellegata NS: A novel germline CDKN1B mutation causing multiple endocrine tumors: clinical, genetic and functional characterization. Hum Mut 2010;31:E1825–E1835.
26 Tichomirowa MA, Lee M, Barlier A, et al: Cyclin-dependent kinase inhibitor 1b (CDKN1B) gene variants in AIP mutation-negative familial isolated pituitary adenoma kindreds. Endocr Relat Cancer 2012;19:233–241.
27 Marinoni I, Pellegata NS: p27kip1: a new multiple endocrine neoplasia gene? Neuroendocrinology 2011;93:19–28.
28 Sherr CJ, Roberts JM: CDK inhibitors: positive and negative regulators of G1-phase progression. Genes Dev 1999;13:1501–1512.
29 Pagano M, Tam SW, Theodoras AM, Beer-Romero P, Del Sal G, Chau V, Yew PR, Draetta GF, Rolfe M: Role of the ubiquitin-proteasome pathway in regulating abundance of the cyclin-dependent kinase inhibitor p27. Science 1995;269:682–685.
30 Kamura T, Hara T, Matsumoto M, Ishida N, Okumura F, Hatakeyama S, Yoshida M, Nakayama K, Nakayama KI: Cytoplasmic ubiquitin ligase KPC regulates proteolysis of p27(kip1) at G1 phase. Nat Cell Biol 2004;6:1229–1235.
31 Carrano AC, Eytan E, Hershko A, Pagano M: Skp2 is required for ubiquitin-mediated degradation of the CDK inhibitor p27. Nat Cell Biol 1999;1:193–199.
32 Besson A, Hwang HC, Cicero S, Donovan SL, Gurian-West M, Johnson D, Clurman BE, Dyer MA, Roberts JM: Discovery of an oncogenic activity in p27kip1 that causes stem cell expansion and a multiple tumor phenotype. Genes Dev 2007;21:1731–1746.
33 Chu IM, Hengst L, Slingerland JM: The CDK inhibitor p27 in human cancer: Prognostic potential and relevance to anticancer therapy. Nat Rev Cancer 2008;8:253–267.
34 Molatore S, Kiermaier E, Jung CB, Pulz E, Höfler H, Atkinson MJ, Pellegata NS: Characterization of a naturally-occurring p27 mutation predisposing to multiple endocrine tumors. Mol Cancer 2010;9:116.
35 Payne SR, Kemp CJ: P27(kip1) (CDKN1B)-deficient mice are susceptible to chemical carcinogenesis and may be a useful model for carcinogen screening. Toxicol Pathol 2003;31:355–363.

Natalia S. Pellegata
Institute of Pathology, Helmholtz Zentrum München
Ingolstaedter Landstrasse 1
D–85764 Neuherberg (Germany)
E-Mail natalia.pellegata@helmholtz-muenchen.de

Stratakis CA (ed): Endocrine Tumor Syndromes and Their Genetics.
Front Horm Res. Basel, Karger, 2013, vol 41, pp 79–91 (DOI: 10.1159/000345671)

Novel Hereditary Forms of Pheochromocytomas and Paragangliomas

Patricia L.M. Dahia[a, b]

[a]Division of Hematology and Medical Oncology, Department of Medicine and [b]Cancer Therapy and Research Center, University of Texas Health Science Center at San Antonio, San Antonio, Tex., USA

Abstract

Pheochromocytomas and paragangliomas are catecholamine-secreting tumors of neural crest origin that arise from the adrenal medulla or extra-adrenal sympathetic paraganglia, respectively. Over the last decade, the extensive genetic heterogeneity of these tumors came to light with the identification of multiple susceptibility genes. These mutations account for at least one-third of pheochromocytomas and paragangliomas, the highest inheritable proportion of any known human tumor. This chapter will present an overview of genetic and molecular features of the most recently identified hereditary forms of pheochromocytoma and paraganglioma: those caused by mutations in five genes of the succinate dehydrogenase (SDH) complex, the transmembrane-encoding gene *TMEM127* and the MYC-binding partner, *MAX*. Initial genotype-phenotype correlations, as well as emerging functional data, have aligned the new mutants either with defects in hypoxic-angiogenic signaling (SDH-related) or kinase receptor/mTOR pathways (TMEM127 and MAX). These findings, in combination with those of the more well-established syndromes, have been relevant for guiding clinical follow-up. The progress of recent years in understanding the pathogenesis of pheochromocytomas and paragangliomas is expected to continue to improve patient screening and to become, in the long term, the catalyst for development of new therapeutic options for surgically untreatable tumors.

Pheochromocytoma is a tumor arising from the chromaffin cells of the adrenal medulla, and its counterpart, paraganglioma, originates from sympathetic ganglia outside the adrenals [1]. Clinical features are driven by excess catecholamines produced by the tumors. The majority of them are benign but approximately 15% are defined as malignant by the identification of metastases in nonchromaffin tissues. Early detection of malignant tumors poses a clinical challenge as they cannot be clinically or histologically distinguished from benign lesions.

Perhaps the most striking feature of these tumors is their genetic diversity. The majority of pheochromocytomas and paragangliomas develop sporadically, but a significant number of cases, currently estimated at more than one-third, are inherited as part of familial syndromes [2]. These syndromes include multiple endocrine neoplasia type 2 (MEN2), von Hippel Lindau (VHL) disease, neurofibromatosis type 1, and a group of familial paraganglioma/pheochromocytoma syndromes (PGLs), characterized by mutations in the *RET, VHL, NF1,* and the succinate dehydrogenase (*SDH*) genes *SDHB, SDHC* and *SDHD*, respectively. In the past 3 years, novel susceptibility genes associated with pheochromocytoma and/or paraganglioma have been identified, *SDHAF2, SDHA, TMEM127* and *MAX* [3–6]. The focus of this review will be the emerging clinical, genetic and functional features that are recognized in the new hereditary tumor forms, with emphasis on their similarities or contrasts with more well-established familial pheochromocytoma and paraganglioma syndromes, MEN2, VHL and neurofibromatosis (listed and summarized in table 1). We also offer a brief discussion on future perspectives for this field.

SDH-Related Mutations and Familial Paraganglioma Syndromes

Paraganglioma syndromes (PGLs) encompass a group of inherited syndromes which involve mutations in the genes that encode components of the succinate dehydrogenase (SDH) mitochondrial enzyme complex II [7]. SDH is a mitochondria-located tricarboxylic acid (TCA) cycle enzyme that converts succinate to fumarate; it also acts as complex II of the electron transport chain [8, 9].

SDH is comprised of four subunits, A, B, C and D. Subunits A and B represent the catalytic portion of complex II, while subunits C and D anchor the complex to the mitochondrial membrane [8, 9]. Until recently, only mutations encoding subunits B, C, and D of the SDH complex had been implicated in the development of paraganglial tumors[10–12]. Loss-of-function mutations in *SDHA* have now been reported to be a rare cause of paraganglioma, as discussed below [4].

Four PGL syndromes have been categorized: types 1, 2, 3 and 4, caused by *SDHD, SDHAF2, SDHC* and *SDHB*, respectively. However, additional forms of familial PGLs are known to exist (i.e. SDHA-related PGLs). While these mutations are inherited in an autosomal dominant pattern, the associated disease penetrance is variable and there is a parent-of-origin effect on clinical expression of the disease [13].

PGL type 1 disease results most often in multiple benign head and neck paragangliomas [10, 14–16], although malignancies have also been reported in patients with *SDHD* mutations [10, 14–19]. Pheochromocytomas can also occur in association with this entity [19]. The mode of inheritance seen in PGL type 1 disease follows a parent of origin pattern of transmission (table 1). This has been associated with imprinting of other target genes on the same chromosome, rendering the maternal *SDHD* allele transcriptionally silent. The rare occurrence of maternal transmission of an *SDHD* mutation has been attributed to recombination of the maternal allele [20].

PGL type 3 disease, caused by mutations in the *SDHC* subunit gene, is rare and predominantly associated with benign parasympathetic paraganglia of the head and

Table 1. Clinical, genetic and functional features of pheochrompocytoma/paraganglioma hereditary forms

Syndrome	Paraganglial features	Nonparaganglial tumors	Relative frequency*, %	Predisposition gene(s)	Gene product function	Transcription cluster
Familial PGL1	multiple head and neck paraganglioma, less frequent adrenal, moderate rate of family history, predominant paternal transmission	thyroid tumors?	5–6	*SDHD*	succinate dehydrogenase, mitochondria respiratory chain; tricyclic acid cycle	1
Familial PGL2	multiple head and neck paraganglioma, moderate rate of family history, no malignancy described yet , paternal transmission	none recurrently observed	<1	SDHAF2	succinate dehydrogenase, mitochondria respiratory chain; tricyclic acid cycle	1
Familial PGL3	multiple paraganglioma, low rate of family history, rare malignancy	none recurrently observed	1	SDHC	succinate dehydrogenase, mitochondria respiratory chain; tricyclic acid cycle	1
Familial PGL4	single paraganglioma, occasional adrenal, frequent malignancy, low penetrance	renal cell carcinoma	6–8	SDHB	succinate dehydrogenase, mitochondria respiratory chain; tricyclic acid cycle	1
Carney-Stratakis syndrome	paraganglioma (sympathetic and parasympathetic); gastrointestinal stromal tumors	gastrointestinal stromal tumors	rare	*SDHB/ SDHC/ SDHD*	succinate dehydrogenase, mitochondria respiratory chain; tricyclic acid cycle	1
Familial pheochromocytoma 2q	predominant adrenal disease, relatively late onset, moderate rate of family history	other tumors?	1.7–2	*TMEM127*	endosomal trafficking? mTOR regulation?	2
Undetermined familial pheochrompocytoma and/or paraganglioma syndrome (*MAX*-related)	predominant adrenal disease, paternal transmission, moderate rate of malignancy, moderate positive family history	other tumors?	1.2	MAX	transcription factor	2
Undetermined familial pheochrompocytoma and/or paraganglioma syndrome (*SDHA*-related)	predominant extraadrenal disease, low penetrance	gastrointestinal stromal tumors	rare	SDHA	succinate dehydrogenase, mitochondria respiratory chain; tricyclic acid cycle	1
Undetermined familial pheochrompocytoma and/or paraganglioma (*KIF1β*-related)	predominant adrenal disease, Other malignancies (two index families only)	neuroblastoma, medulloblastoma, other tumors?	rare	*KIF1Bβ*	kinesin family member involved in apoptosis	2
Undetermined familial pheochrompocytoma and/or paraganglioma (*PHD2*-related)	single case reported (family segregation unclear)	erythrocytosis?	rare	*PHD2*	2-oxoglutarate-dependent prolyl hydroxylase	?
Multiple endocrine neoplasia type 2A (MEN2) and 2B (MEN2B)	predominant adrenal disease, occasional bilaterality, benign, family history common	medullary thyroid carcinoma;para-thyroid hyperplasia or adenoma)	5–6	*RET*	kinase receptor	2
von Hippel-Lindau	predominant adrenal disease, early onset, family history common	clear cell RCC; CNS hemangioblastomas	9–12	*VHL*	ubiquitin ligase complex component	1

Table 1. Continued

Syndrome	Paraganglial features	Nonparaganglial tumors	Relative frequency*, %	Predisposition gene(s)	Gene product function	Transcription cluster
Neurofibromatosis type 1	predominant adrenal, family history common	neurofibromas; malignant peripheral nerve sheath tumors; gliomas, leukemia; pheochrompocytoma	1–2	*NF1*	Ras-GTPase activating protein-GAP	2

* From multiple multiinstitutional studies, if available.

neck (HNPs) [11, 15, 21, 22]. The mutations seen in PGL type 3 disease are classic single base substitutions or more complex, large deletions that had previously been undetected by standard sequencing procedures.

PGL type 4, characterized genetically by mutations or deletions in SDH subunit B, typically presents clinically with single tumors, frequently paragangliomas. Due to its low penetrance compared to other pheochromocytoma/paraganglioma susceptibility genes mutations in *SDHB* account for the largest part of 'apparently sporadic' tumors found to carry a germline mutation [12, 23, 24]. However, HNP and adrenal pheochromocytoma may also be seen. Patients harboring *SDHB* mutations are at increased risk of malignant disease [25] and have shortened survival when compared to other patients with malignant disease at presentation [26]. Germline *SDHB* mutations have also been rarely detected in patients with renal cell carcinoma, either alone or in association with paragangliomas [27]. Of additional translational relevance, SDHB immunohistochemistry of tumor material has been shown to function as an effective marker of SDH function. Negative SDHB staining of pheochromocytoma/paraganglioma strongly suggests the presence of a mutation in one of the SDH genes [28, 29] and can thus guide genetic testing to these genes.

The *SDHAF2* gene, mapped to 11q12.2, was identified as the elusive PGL2 susceptibility gene through the characterization of its yeast ortholog, known as *SDH5* [3]. The function of SDH5/SDHAF2 is the flavination of the SDHA protein, a step required for the assembly of a functional mitochondrial complex II. Germline mutation of *SDHAF2* in the original PGL2 kindred linked to this locus segregates with the disease in a pattern consistent with a dominant trait with paternal transmission [3]. Only a few cases of familial *SDHAF2* mutation have been reported and are characterized by multiple head and neck paragangliomas transmitted through the paternal line [30]. The emerging clinical features associated with germline *SDHAF2* mutations are a young age at onset, multifocal tumors and low penetrance within families. The current recommendation is that *SDHAF2* genotyping should be considered in a patient with head and neck PGL and negative *SDHD, SDHB, SDHC* screening [31].

Previously, *SDHA* loss-of-function mutations had been associated with a recessive form of childhood encephalomyopathy, a disease associated with high morbidity [8].

This gene has multiple polymorphisms and highly homologous pseudogene sequences, which explains in part the limitations in successful screening in other disorders. More recently, the first *SDHA* mutation was found in the context of pheochromocytoma/paraganglioma [4]. The mutant tumor, in addition to the expected loss of SDH function, had a unique profile of negative staining for both SDHA and SDHB by immunohistochemistry. An independent study of SDHA immunohistochemistry screening of a large series of PGL/PCC led to the identification of five new SDHA mutation carriers in six tumors with negative staining for this protein [32]. All had loss of heterozygosity of the wild-type allele at the tumor DNA level. It is suggested that *SDHA* genotyping might be considered in patients with hereditary pheochromocytoma/paraganglioma accompanied by loss of immunostaining for the SDHB and SDHA proteins in tumoral tissue.

In addition to the PGL syndromes, *SDHB, SDHC* and *SDHD* mutations have also been detected in patients with Carney-Stratakis syndrome, a disorder in which paragangliomas co-occur with gastrointestinal stromal tumors (GISTs) [33]. Dysfunction in SDH function, regardless of the mutation status of GISTs, is a common feature of these tumors and indicates a broader effect of SDH in tumorigenesis beyond paraganglial disease [34].

The tumorigenic mechanism associated with SDH mutations is still not fully understood. It has been extensively shown that mutant tumors express high levels of hypoxia-inducible factor (HIF) [29, 35, 36]. This HIF stabilization occurs through accumulation of succinate which then inhibits the prolyl hydroxylation of HIF, a step necessary to target HIF for degradation by pVHL [37, 38]. HIF accumulation leads to a state of pseudohypoxia in the cell, a condition shared by many cancers which results in increased angiogenesis and enhanced growth factor signaling [39]. A similar profile has been observed in tumors that lack fumarate hydratase (FH) [40]. More recent work has revealed that prolyl hydroxylase inactivation is but one of the targets of SDH loss of function. The accumulation of succinate caused by loss or mutations in SDHA or B, and also FH, competitively leads to reduced α-ketoglutarate availability and consequently, diminished function of a group of enzymes that are dependent on this metabolite [41, 42]. Amongst these are histone demethylases, collagen prolyl-4 hydroxylases, and the TET family of 5-methlycytosine hydroxylases. The extensive epigenetic changes caused by dysfunction of these dioxygenases bring about an array of downstream events that likely account for the tumorigenic effects of *SDH* mutations.

Critical questions involving the pathogenesis of pheochromocytomas derived from SDH mutations still remain unanswered: the reasons for the preferential association of *SDHB* mutations and malignant or aggressive pheochromocytomas or paragangliomas are unclear at present. In vitro work based on short-interfering (si) RNA has suggested that cells with downregulated *SDHB* display increased adhesion properties and activation of genes involved in the epithelial to mesenchymal transition [43, 44]. Future studies should address whether these features affect the intrinsic aggressiveness of mutant *SDHB* tumors or other yet unidentified targets of the mutation account for this unique phenotype.

TMEM127

The *TMEM127* gene, located on chromosome 2q11, encodes for a transmembrane protein of 238 amino acids. This previously unknown gene was identified as a susceptibility gene to pheochromocytoma through integrative genomics, involving a combination of linkage analysis, transcription expression profiling and high-density copy number mapping [5]. Tumor samples from patients with a *TMEM127* mutation align with pheochromocytomas with kinase signaling receptor activation and consistently exhibit loss of heterozygosity, suggesting that this gene functions as a tumor suppressor [5, 45, 46]. Genetic studies of pheochromocytoma patients carrying *TMEM127* mutations indicate low prevalence of these variants and genotype-phenotype associations delineated a profile of *TMEM127* mutation carriers that stands out for an average age at presentation similar to that of sporadic cases and older than most other susceptibility mutation carriers, an almost exclusive adrenal location of the tumors and familial history recognizable in only one quarter of the cases [45]. All mutations reported so far have been identified in the germline and are preferentially mapped within or around transmembrane-encoding domains of the gene (62.5%). In vitro testing of some of these mutations revealed loss of the characteristic membrane distribution of TMEM127, which underscores the relevance of the membrane localization for its tumor suppressive activities [45].

Little is known about the function of the TMEM127 product apart from its intracellular localization to multiple endomembrane pools, including early and recycling endosome [5]. This subcellular distribution is dynamic and responsive to nutrient levels, such as amino acids. These data are consistent with a potential role of TMEM127 as a component of the protein recycling endocytic machinery. In vitro and primary tumor analyses have indicated an effect of TMEM127 in inhibition of mTOR function [5], but the mechanisms underlying this interaction have not yet been defined. Recently, a subdomain spanning the transmembrane regions of TMEM127 was found to share structural homology with claudins. These are a large family of proteins involved in tight junction and intercellular signaling [47]. This structural clue may provide insights into the functional properties of TMEM127 and mechanism of tumor suppression.

MAX

The MYC-associated factor X *(MAX)* gene is the most recently recognized pheochromocytoma/paraganglioma susceptibility gene [6]. It was identified by exome sequencing of germline DNA from three independent patients with familial pheochromocytoma who did not carry mutations in any of the other known susceptibility genes and whose tumors shared transcriptional similarities with *TMEM127, RET* and *NF1* mutant pheochromocytomas or paragangliomas (the kinase signaling activated or 'cluster 2' by transcription classification, discussed below). Segregation of MAX mutations with the clinical phenotype in these families, absence of MAX protein in the tumors, and loss of heterozygosity of the wild-type allele in tumor DNA, suggested that *MAX* behaves as a classic tumor suppressor gene. Similar to *SDHD* and *SDHAF2*-related cases, mutations in *MAX* are transmitted via the paternal line. A large recent multicenter study provided insights into the clinical features shared by patients with *MAX* mutations: all tumors had an adrenal location, although in some cases co-occurrence of paragangliomas was also found. More than half of tumors were multicentric, either bilateral or multifocal and approximately 10% were malignant [48]. Familial history of pheochromocytoma/paraganglioma was noted in more than one-third of patients, and it is presently unclear whether other neoplasms are causally linked to these mutations.

MAX is a key member of the MYC-MAX-MXD1 network of basic helix-loop-helix leucine zipper (bHLHZ) transcription factors that regulate cell growth, proliferation, and stem cell biology during normal development and tissue homeostasis [reviewed in ref., 49]. MYC heterodimerizes with MAX, and binds DNA at specific recognition sites of MYC target genes, and thus promotes their transactivation or repression. MAX can also form homodimers or heterodimers with other bHLHZ proteins in this network (MXD1, MXI1, MXD3, MXD4, MNT and MGA). These dimers bind the same DNA sequences as MYC-MAX dimers, acting as antagonists of MYC-dependent cell transformation by transcriptional repression. Whether there are tissue-specific or developmentally specific targets of the MYC-MAX or MAX-other bHLHZ pairs is yet to be defined, along with the potential relevance of this information for therapeutic purposes.

Overlapping Signals in Pheochromocytoma/Paraganglioma

An intriguing outstanding question in the field of pheochromocytoma-paraganglioma remains the genetic diversity (at least ten susceptibility tumors at this time) contrasted with relative homogeneity in clinical phenotype. This pattern implies that the apparent genetic distinction may translate into overlapping signals or pathway crosstalk. Using expression profiling in a large series of hereditary and sporadic pheochromocytomas and paragangliomas, we and others identified two main transcription groups o 'clusters' [29, 36, 50, 51]. 'Cluster 1' includes those tumors with *VHL* and SDH mutations suggesting that hypoxia, extracellular matrix components, and angiogenic factors unify this group. In contrast, 'cluster 2' encompasses *RET, NF1, TMEM127* and *MAX* mutations, indicating gene transcription associated with tyrosine kinase signaling, RNA synthesis and processing and protein translation. This transcription classification was instrumental in the identification of two susceptibility genes, *TMEM127* and *MAX*, and provides an approach for recognition of other potential candidate genes in these tumors.

The prominent inherited nature of pheochromocytomas and paragangliomas was addressed by Lee et al. [52], who unveiled a common molecular mechanism underlying the development of all forms of familial pheochromocytoma, in which the physiological apoptosis that targets neural precursor cells during embryonic development is disrupted by pheochromocytoma susceptibility mutations. This apoptotic process is c-Jun dependent but can be antagonized by JunB. EglN3, a proapoptotic protein which is also prolylhydroxylase, acts downstream of c-Jun to promote death of outcompeted neurons. Egln3 function appears to be antagonized, through distinct mechanisms, by the various mutations that cause pheochromocytoma [52]. When families carry germline mutations in *RET, VHL, SDH* or *NF1*, apoptosis is limited during embryogenesis of neuronal precursors. It is presumed that the abnormally surviving cells may become the original focus for neoplastic transformation later in life [52].

Following up on the key role of Egln3 in sympathetic precursor survival, another gene was found to be associated with pheochromocytoma, *KIF1Bβ*, which maps to chromosome 1p36.2, a region commonly deleted in neural crest-derived tumors [53]. KIF1Bβ has been shown to mediate Egln3-related apoptosis, and loss-of-function germline mutations of *KIF1Bβ* have been identified in both familial and isolated cases of pheochromocytoma, as well as in other neural tumors, neuroblastoma and medulloblastoma [53, 54]. While the *KIF1Bβ* gene is presumed to act as a tumor suppressor, loss of heterozygosity was not consistently seen in mutant cases, a deviation from the classic two-hit model that is known to function in all other instances of inherited mutations of pheochromocytoma due to tumor suppressor genes. The confirmation of its true action as a haploinsufficient gene and additional, independent validation is needed prior to establishing a definitive causal relationship between the *KIF1Bβ* gene and pheochromocytoma.

A report of a germline mutation in the gene encoding for PHD2/EGLN1, one of the HIF prolyl hydroxylases and a gene which has previously been shown to cause familial eryhtrocytosis [55], was detected in one patient with concurrent sympathetic paraganglioma and congenital erythrocytosis and considered to be related to the paraganglial phenotype in this case [56]. No additional cases have been reported with PHD2 mutations and it remains to be determined whether this gene is causally linked to paragangliomas.

Sporadic Pheochromocytoma/Paraganglioma

While at least 30% of pheochromocytoma cases are familial, the majority appear to arise sporadically [31]. This figure may, however, be an underestimate of the proportion of inherited disease, since germline mutations in the known susceptibility genes of *RET, VHL, SDHB*, and *SDHD* may be seen in 8–16% of 'sporadic-appearing' cases [31, 57]. Recently, the issue of somatic mutations in pheochromocytoma has been reexamined in a large and well-annotated series of pheochromocytoma. Guided by transcriptional clustering distribution, 14% of sporadic pheochromocytomas were found to carry a somatic mutation in *RET* or *VHL* [51]. A small number of somatic mutations have also been identified in a large screen of the *MAX* gene [48], but not in any *SDH*-related or the *TMEM127* genes [45, 51].

Despite the low frequency of somatic mutations in the pheochromocytoma and paraganglioma susceptibility genes, the homogenous alignment of sporadic tumors with hereditary counterparts by transcription profiling supports the notion that these tumors carry mutations in genes involved in the main pathways disrupted by the germline mutations [29, 51]. A comprehensive, high-resolution analysis of somatic events in pheochromocytomas has not yet been performed to address the frequency of somatic mutations beyond those in pheochromocytoma susceptibility genes.

Challenges and Future Perspectives

As discussed extensively above, a growing number of pheochromocytomas and paragangliomas are linked to inherited mutations. The current incidence of 30% is likely an underestimation given the addition of several novel susceptibility genes in the past few years. Transcriptional clustering, which has facilitated the identification of *TMEM127* and *MAX*, can continue to be explored for discovery of additional susceptibility genes, the existence of which is supported by the existence of genetically undetermined familial or early-onset pheochromocytomas and/or paragangliomas. Recognition of a high prevalence of hereditary disease among pheochromocytoma patients, including unsuspected familial cases, has already changed current clinical practice and has broadened the applicability of genetic screening [58–60], which have benefitted patients and at-risk relatives. *RET* screening in MEN2 is emblematic of the high degree of success that can be achieved when genetic-based evidence is applied to patient care. With the rapid decrease in costs and broader accessibility, genomewide next generation sequencing methods are bound to replace conventional techniques for diagnosis of susceptibility mutations, enabling the simultaneous screen of the current as well as any novel susceptibility genes [61]. While these broad sequencing strategies will obviate the need for stepwise screening, common variants and/or variants of unknown significance within and outside each susceptibility gene will be exposed by these methods [31]. Interpretation of their clinical relevance will impose the implementation of new guidelines for patient surveillance.

The current view of the genetic profiling of pheochromocytoma and paraganglioma is that mutations in the susceptibility genes are mutually exclusive, suggesting that these genetic disruptions target overlapping pathways that would not impart additional selective advantage to the growth of these tumors. This view however, might be naïve and born out of our yet limited analysis of high-resolution, nucleotide-level sequencing of pheochromocytomas and paragangliomas. This comprehensive sequence landscape may lead us to reconsider some of the current concepts on the genetics of these tumors.

As our understanding of the intracellular consequences of the various disrupted signals deepens, it is estimated that the possibility of using this information for development of novel strategies for targeted therapies will become a reality. This information will be of particular relevance for malignant and/or inoperable tumors [62]. Emerging data from small patient cohorts suggest that the use of angiogenic inhibitors may have clinical utility for this patient group [63, 64]. In vitro findings support the benefit of combination therapies with kinase inhibitors to overcome compensatory feedback that might result in monotherapy [65]. Undoubtedly, genetic advances have provided fertile ground for new hypothesis formulation that can advance the field further.

Acknowledgments

The author is grateful to Dr. Elizabeth King for her assistance. P.L.M.D. is supported by funds from the Department of Defense CMRP (PR110571), the Cancer Prevention and Research Institute of Texas (CPRIT), the Voelcker Fund, the Alex Lemonade Stand Foundation, the Concern Foundation, the Greehey Children's Cancer Research Institute and the Institute of Integrated Medical Sciences (IIMS)-CTSA-NIH.

References

1 Bravo EL: Pheochromocytoma. Cardiol Rev 2002;10:44–50.
2 Welander J, Soderkvist P, Gimm O: Genetics and clinical characteristics of hereditary pheochromocytomas and paragangliomas. Endocr Relat Cancer 2011;18:R253–R276.
3 Hao HX, Khalimonchuk O, Schraders M, Dephoure N, Bayley JP, Kunst H, Devilee P, Cremers CW, Schiffman JD, Bentz BG, Gygi SP, Winge DR, Kremer H, Rutter J: SDH5, a gene required for flavination of succinate dehydrogenase, is mutated in paraganglioma. Science 2009;325:1139–1142.
4 Burnichon N, Briere JJ, Libe R, Vescovo L, Riviere J, Tissier F, Jouanno E, Jeunemaitre X, Benit P, Tzagoloff A, Rustin P, Bertherat J, Favier J, Gimenez-Roqueplo AP: SDHA is a tumor suppressor gene causing paraganglioma. Hum Mol Genet 2010;19:3011–3020.
5 Qin Y, Yao L, King EE, Buddavarapu K, Lenci RE, Chocron ES, Lechleiter JD, Sass M, Aronin N, Schiavi F, Boaretto F, Opocher G, Toledo RA, Toledo SP, Stiles C, Aguiar RC, Dahia PL: Germline mutations in TMEM127 confer susceptibility to pheochromocytoma. Nat Genet 2010;42:229–233.
6 Comino-Mendez I, Gracia-Aznarez FJ, Schiavi F, et al: Exome sequencing identifies MAX mutations as a cause of hereditary pheochromocytoma. Nat Genet 2011;43:663–667.
7 Dahia PL: Evolving concepts in pheochromocytoma and paraganglioma. Curr Opin Oncol 2006;18:1–8.
8 Ackrell BA: Cytopathies involving mitochondrial complex II. Mol Aspects Med 2002;23:369–384.
9 Gottlieb E, Tomlinson IP: Mitochondrial tumour suppressors: a genetic and biochemical update. Nat Rev Cancer 2005;5:857–866.
10 Baysal BE, Ferrell RE, Willett-Brozick JE, Lawrence EC, Myssiorek D, Bosch A, van der Mey A, Taschner PE, Rubinstein WS, Myers EN, Richard CW 3rd, Cornelisse CJ, Devilee P, Devlin B: Mutations in SDHD, a mitochondrial complex II gene, in hereditary paraganglioma. Science 2000;287:848–851.
11 Niemann S, Muller U: Mutations in SDHC cause autosomal dominant paraganglioma, type 3. Nat Genet 2000;26:268–270.
12 Astuti D, Latif F, Dallol A, Dahia PL, Douglas F, George E, Skoldberg F, Husebye ES, Eng C, Maher ER: Gene mutations in the succinate dehydrogenase subunit SDHB cause susceptibility to familial pheochromocytoma and to familial paraganglioma. Am J Hum Genet 2001;69:49–54.
13 Gimenez-Roqueplo AP, Dahia PL, Robledo M: An update on the genetics of paraganglioma, pheochromocytoma, and associated hereditary syndromes. Horm Metab Res 2012;44:328–333.
14 Neumann HP, Pawlu C, Peczkowska M, Bausch B, McWhinney SR, Muresan M, Buchta M, Franke G, Klisch J, Bley TA, Hoegerle S, Boedeker CC, Opocher G, Schipper J, Januszewicz A, Eng C: Distinct clinical features of paraganglioma syndromes associated with SDHB and SDHD gene mutations. JAMA 2004;292:943–951.

15 Schiavi F, Boedeker CC, Bausch B, et al: Predictors and prevalence of paraganglioma syndrome associated with mutations of the SDHC gene. JAMA 2005; 294:2057–2063.

16 Benn DE, Gimenez-Roqueplo AP, Reilly JR, Bertherat J, Burgess J, Byth K, Croxson M, Dahia PL, Elston M, Gimm O, Henley D, Herman P, Murday V, Niccoli-Sire P, Pasieka JL, Rohmer V, Tucker K, Jeunemaitre X, Marsh DJ, Plouin PF, Robinson BG: Clinical presentation and penetrance of pheochromocytoma/paraganglioma syndromes. J Clin Endocrinol Metab 2006;91:827–836.

17 Timmers HJ, Pacak K, Bertherat J, Lenders JW, Duet M, Eisenhofer G, Stratakis CA, Niccoli-Sire P, Tran BH, Burnichon N, Gimenez-Roqueplo AP: Mutations associated with succinate dehydrogenase D-related malignant paragangliomas. Clin Endocrinol (Oxf) 2008;68:561–566.

18 Burnichon N, Rohmer V, Amar L, Herman P, Leboulleux S, Darrouzet V, Niccoli P, Gaillard D, Chabrier G, Chabolle F, Coupier I, Thieblot P, Lecomte P, Bertherat J, Wion-Barbot N, Murat A, Venisse A, Plouin PF, Jeunemaitre X, Gimenez-Roqueplo AP: The succinate dehydrogenase genetic testing in a large prospective series of patients with paragangliomas. J Clin Endocrinol Metab 2009;94:2817–2827.

19 Buffet A, Venisse A, Nau V, Roncellin I, Boccio V, Le Pottier N, Boussion M, Travers C, Simian C, Burnichon N, Abermil N, Favier J, Jeunemaitre X, Gimenez-Roqueplo AP: A decade (2001–2010) of genetic testing for pheochromocytoma and paraganglioma. Horm Metab Res 2012;44:359–366.

20 Yeap PM, Tobias ES, Mavraki E, Fletcher A, Bradshaw N, Freel EM, Cooke A, Murday VA, Davidson HR, Perry CG, Lindsay RS: Molecular analysis of pheochromocytoma after maternal transmission of SDHD mutation elucidates mechanism of parent-of-origin effect. J Clin Endocrinol Metab 2011; 96:E2009–E2013.

21 Neumann HP, Erlic Z, Boedeker CC, et al: Clinical predictors for germline mutations in head and neck paraganglioma patients: cost reduction strategy in genetic diagnostic process as fall-out. Cancer Res 2009;69:3650–3656.

22 Pigny P, Cardot-Bauters C: Genetics of pheochromocytoma and paraganglioma: new developments. Ann Endocrinol (Paris) 2010;71:76–82.

23 Cascon A, Cebrian A, Ruiz-Llorente S, Telleria D, Benitez J, Robledo M: SDHB mutation analysis in familial and sporadic phaeochromocytoma identifies a novel mutation. J Med Genet 2002;39:E64.

24 Gimenez-Roqueplo AP, Favier J, Rustin P, Rieubland C, Kerlan V, Plouin PF, Rotig A, Jeunemaitre X: Functional consequences of a SDHB gene mutation in an apparently sporadic pheochromocytoma. J Clin Endocrinol Metab 2002;87:4771–4774.

25 Gimenez-Roqueplo AP, Favier J, Rustin P, Rieubland C, Crespin M, Nau V, Khau Van Kien P, Corvol P, Plouin PF, Jeunemaitre X: Mutations in the SDHB gene are associated with extra-adrenal and/or malignant phaeochromocytomas. Cancer Res 2003;63:5615–5621.

26 Amar L, Baudin E, Burnichon N, Peyrard S, Silvera S, Bertherat J, Bertagna X, Schlumberger M, Jeunemaitre X, Gimenez-Roqueplo AP, Plouin PF: Succinate dehydrogenase B gene mutations predict survival in patients with malignant pheochromocytomas or paragangliomas. J Clin Endocrinol Metab 2007;92:3822–3828.

27 Ricketts C, Woodward ER, Killick P, Morris MR, Astuti D, Latif F, Maher ER: Germline SDHB mutations and familial renal cell carcinoma. J Natl Cancer Inst 2008;100:1260–1262.

28 van Nederveen FH, Gaal J, Favier J, et al: An immunohistochemical procedure to detect patients with paraganglioma and phaeochromocytoma with germline SDHB, SDHC, or SDHD gene mutations: a retrospective and prospective analysis. Lancet Oncol 2009;10:764–771.

29 Dahia PL, Ross KN, Wright ME, CY et al: A HIF1alpha regulatory loop links hypoxia and mitochondrial signals in pheochromocytomas. PLoS Genet 2005;1:72–80.

30 Bayley JP, Kunst HP, Cascon A, et al: SDHAF2 mutations in familial and sporadic paraganglioma and phaeochromocytoma. Lancet Oncol 2010;11:366–372.

31 Gimenez-Roqueplo AP, Dahia PL, Robledo M: An update on the genetics of paraganglioma, pheochromocytoma, and associated hereditary syndromes. Horm Metab Res 2012;44:328–333.

32 Korpershoek E, Favier J, Gaal J, Burnichon N, van Gessel B, Oudijk L, Badoual C, Gadessaud N, Venisse A, Bayley JP, van Dooren MF, de Herder WW, Tissier F, Plouin PF, van Nederveen FH, Dinjens WN, Gimenez-Roqueplo AP, de Krijger RR: SDHA immunohistochemistry detects germline SDHA gene mutations in apparently sporadic paragangliomas and pheochromocytomas. J Clin Endocrinol Metab 2011;96:E1472–E1476.

33 Stratakis CA, Carney JA: The triad of paragangliomas, gastric stromal tumours and pulmonary chondromas (Carney triad), and the dyad of paragangliomas and gastric stromal sarcomas (Carney-Stratakis syndrome): molecular genetics and clinical implications. J Intern Med 2009;266:43–52.

34 Janeway KA, Kim SY, Lodish M, Nose V, Rustin P, Gaal J, Dahia PL, Liegl B, Ball ER, Raygada M, Lai AH, Kelly L, Hornick JL, O'Sullivan M, de Krijger RR, Dinjens WN, Demetri GD, Antonescu CR, Fletcher JA, Helman L, Stratakis CA: Defects in succinate dehydrogenase in gastrointestinal stromal tumors lacking KIT and PDGFRA mutations. Proc Natl Acad Sci USA 2011;108:314–318.

35 Gimenez-Roqueplo AP, Favier J, Rustin P, Mourad JJ, Plouin PF, Corvol P, Rotig A, Jeunemaitre X: The R22X mutation of the SDHD gene in hereditary paraganglioma abolishes the enzymatic activity of complex II in the mitochondrial respiratory chain and activates the hypoxia pathway. Am J Hum Genet 2001;69:1186–1197.

36 Lopez-Jimenez E, Gomez-Lopez G, Leandro-Garcia LJ, et al: Research resource: Transcriptional profiling reveals different pseudohypoxic signatures in SDHB and VHL-related pheochromocytomas. Mol Endocrinol 2010;24:2382–2391.

37 Selak MA, Armour SM, Mackenzie ED, Boulahbel H, Watson DG, Mansfield KD, Pan Y, Simon MC, Thompson CB, Gottlieb E: Succinate links TCA cycle dysfunction to oncogenesis by inhibiting HIF-alpha prolyl hydroxylase. Cancer Cell 2005;7:77–85.

38 King A, Selak MA, Gottlieb E: Succinate dehydrogenase and fumarate hydratase: linking mitochondrial dysfunction and cancer. Oncogene 2006;25: 4675–4682.

39 Semenza GL: Targeting HIF-1 for cancer therapy. Nat Rev Cancer 2003;3:721–732.

40 Isaacs JS, Jung YJ, Mole DR, Lee S, Torres-Cabala C, Chung YL, Merino M, Trepel J, Zbar B, Toro J, Ratcliffe PJ, Linehan WM, Neckers L: HIF overexpression correlates with biallelic loss of fumarate hydratase in renal cancer: novel role of fumarate in regulation of HIF stability. Cancer Cell 2005;8:143–153.

41 Smith EH, Janknecht R, Maher LJ 3rd: Succinate inhibition of {alpha}-ketoglutarate-dependent enzymes in a yeast model of paraganglioma. Hum Mol Genet 2007;16:3136–3148.

42 Xiao M, Yang H, Xu W, Ma S, Lin H, Zhu H, Liu L, Liu Y, Yang C, Xu Y, Zhao S, Ye D, Xiong Y, Guan KL: Inhibition of alpha-KG-dependent histone and DNA demethylases by fumarate and succinate that are accumulated in mutations of FH and SDH tumor suppressors. Genes Dev 2012;26:1326–1338.

43 Cervera AM, Apostolova N, Crespo FL, Mata M, McCreath KJ: Cells silenced for SDHB expression display characteristic features of the tumor phenotype. Cancer Res 2008;68:4058–4067.

44 Loriot C, Burnichon N, Gadessaud N, Vescovo L, Amar L, Libe R, Bertherat J, Plouin PF, Jeunemaitre X, Gimenez-Roqueplo AP, Favier J: Epithelial to mesenchymal transition is activated in metastatic pheochromocytomas and paragangliomas caused by SDHB gene mutations. J Clin Endocrinol Metab 2012;97:E954–E962.

45 Yao L, Schiavi F, Cascon A, et al: Spectrum and prevalence of FP/TMEM127 gene mutations in pheochromocytomas and paragangliomas. JAMA 2010;304:2611–2619.

46 Burnichon N, Lepoutre-Lussey C, Laffaire J, Gadessaud N, Molinie V, Hernigou A, Plouin PF, Jeunemaitre X, Favier J, Gimenez-Roqueplo AP: A novel TMEM127 mutation in a patient with familial bilateral pheochromocytoma. Eur J Endocrinol 2011; 164:141–145.

47 Simske JS, Hardin J: Claudin family proteins in *Caenorhabditis elegans*. Methods Mol Biol 2011; 762:147–169.

48 Burnichon N, Cascon A, Schiavi F, et al: MAX mutations cause hereditary and sporadic pheochromocytoma and paraganglioma. Clin Cancer Res 2012;18:2828–2837.

49 Cascon A, Robledo M: MAX and MYC: A Heritable Breakup. Cancer Res 2012;72:3119–3124.

50 Eisenhofer G, Huynh TT, Pacak K, Brouwers FM, Walther MM, Linehan WM, Munson PJ, Mannelli M, Goldstein DS, Elkahloun AG: Distinct gene expression profiles in norepinephrine- and epinephrine-producing hereditary and sporadic pheochromocytomas: activation of hypoxia-driven angiogenic pathways in von Hippel-Lindau syndrome. Endocr Relat Cancer 2004;11:897–911.

51 Burnichon N, Vescovo L, Amar L, Libe R, de Reynies A, Venisse A, Jouanno E, Laurendeau I, Parfait B, Bertherat J, Plouin PF, Jeunemaitre X, Favier J, Gimenez-Roqueplo AP: Integrative genomic analysis reveals somatic mutations in pheochromocytoma and paraganglioma. Hum Mol Genet 2011; 20:3974–3985.

52 Lee S, Nakamura E, Yang H, Wei W, Linggi MS, Sajan MP, Farese RV, Freeman RS, Carter BD, Kaelin WG Jr, Schlisio S: Neuronal apoptosis linked to EglN3 prolyl hydroxylase and familial pheochromocytoma genes: developmental culling and cancer. Cancer Cell 2005;8:155–167.

53 Schlisio S, Kenchappa RS, Vredeveld LC, George RE, Stewart R, Greulich H, Shahriari K, Nguyen NV, Pigny P, Dahia PL, Pomeroy SL, Maris JM, Look AT, Meyerson M, Peeper DS, Carter BD, Kaelin WG Jr: The kinesin KIF1Bbeta acts downstream from EglN3 to induce apoptosis and is a potential 1p36 tumor suppressor. Genes Dev 2008;22:884–893.

54 Yeh IT, Lenci RE, Qin Y, Buddavarapu K, Ligon AH, Leteurtre E, Do Cao C, Cardot-Bauters C, Pigny P, Dahia PL: A germline mutation of the KIF1B beta gene on 1p36 in a family with neural and nonneural tumors. Hum Genet 2008;124:279–285.

55 Percy MJ, Zhao Q, Flores A, Harrison C, Lappin TR, Maxwell PH, McMullin MF, Lee FS: A family with erythrocytosis establishes a role for prolyl hydroxylase domain protein 2 in oxygen homeostasis. Proc Natl Acad Sci USA 2006;103:654–659.

56 Ladroue C, Carcenac R, Leporrier M, Gad S, Le Hello C, Galateau-Salle F, Feunteun J, Pouyssegur J, Richard S, Gardie B: PHD2 mutation and congenital erythrocytosis with paraganglioma. N Engl J Med 2008;359:2685–2692.

57 Neumann HP, Bausch B, McWhinney SR, et al: Germ-line mutations in nonsyndromic pheochromocytoma. N Engl J Med 2002;346:1459–1466.

58 Waguespack SG, Rich T, Grubbs E, Ying AK, Perrier ND, Ayala-Ramirez M, Jimenez C: A current review of the etiology, diagnosis, and treatment of pediatric pheochromocytoma and paraganglioma. J Clin Endocrinol Metab 2010;95:2023–2037.

59 Erlic Z, Hoffmann MM, Sullivan M, Franke G, Peczkowska M, Harsch I, Schott M, Gabbert HE, Valimaki M, Preuss SF, Hasse-Lazar K, Waligorski D, Robledo M, Januszewicz A, Eng C, Neumann HP: Pathogenicity of DNA variants and double mutations in multiple endocrine neoplasia type 2 and von Hippel-Lindau syndrome. J Clin Endocrinol Metab 2010;95:308–313.

60 Mannelli M, Castellano M, Schiavi F, et al: Clinically guided genetic screening in a large cohort of Italian patients with pheochromocytomas and/or functional or nonfunctional paragangliomas. J Clin Endocrinol Metab 2009;94:1541–1547.

61 Morgan JE, Carr IM, Sheridan E, Chu CE, Hayward B, Camm N, Lindsay HA, Mattocks CJ, Markham AF, Bonthron DT, Taylor GR: Genetic diagnosis of familial breast cancer using clonal sequencing. Hum Mutat 2010;31:484–491.

62 Ayala-Ramirez M, Feng L, Habra MA, Rich T, Dickson PV, Perrier N, Phan A, Waguespack S, Patel S, Jimenez C: Clinical benefits of systemic chemotherapy for patients with metastatic pheochromocytomas or sympathetic extra-adrenal paragangliomas: insights from the largest single-institutional experience. Cancer 2012;118:2804–2812.

63 Amar L, Fassnacht M, Gimenez-Roqueplo AP, Januszewicz A, Prejbisz A, Timmers H, Plouin PF: Long-term postoperative follow-up in patients with apparently benign pheochromocytoma and paraganglioma. Horm Metab Res 2012;44:385–389.

64 Favier J, Igaz P, Burnichon N, Amar L, Libe R, Badoual C, Tissier F, Bertherat J, Plouin PF, Jeunemaitre X, Gimenez-Roqueplo AP: Rationale for anti-angiogenic therapy in pheochromocytoma and paraganglioma. Endocr Pathol 2012;23:34–42.

65 Nolting S, Garcia E, Alusi G, Giubellino A, Pacak K, Korbonits M, Grossman A: Combined blockade of signalling pathways shows marked anti-tumour potential in phaeochromocytoma cell lines. J Mol Endocrinol 2012;49:79–96.

Note Added in Proof

Two recent papers have described frequent loss-of-function-type mutations of the *NF1* gene in more than one-quarter of sporadic pheochromocytomas, supporting a major and unanticipated role for *NF1* in nonhereditary forms of these tumors [1, 2].

References

1 Welander J, Larsson C, Bäckdahl M, Hareni N, Sivlér T, Brauckhoff M, Söderkvist P, Gimm O: Integrative genomics reveals frequent somatic *NF1* mutations in sporadic pheochromocytomas. Hum Mol Genet 2012;21:5406–5416.

2 Burnichon N, Buffet A, Parfait B, Letouzé E, Laurendeau I, Loriot C, Pasmant E, Abermil N, Valeyrie-Allanore L, Bertherat J, Amar L, Vidaud D, Favier J, Gimenez-Roqueplo AP: Somatic *NF1* inactivation is a frequent event in sporadic pheochromocytoma. Hum Mol Genet 2012;21:5397–5405.

Patricia L.M. Dahia, MD, PhD
Department of Medicine, UTHSCSA
7703 Floyd Curl Drive, MC7880
San Antonio, TX 78229 (USA)
E-Mail dahia@uthscsa.edu

Stratakis CA (ed): Endocrine Tumor Syndromes and Their Genetics.
Front Horm Res. Basel, Karger, 2013, vol 41, pp 92–110 (DOI: 10.1159/000345672)

Carney Triad

J. Aidan Carney

Department of Laboratory Medicine and Pathology and College of Medicine, Mayo Clinic, Rochester, Minn., USA

Abstract

Carney triad is a rare multitumoral syndrome of unknown etiology that was first described in 1977. The neoplasms affect the stomach, lungs, paraganglionic system, adrenal cortex, and esophagus. Approximately 150 cases have been identified. The disorder occurs in young women primarily and is not familial. Multifocal tumors develop in the organs affected. No patient has had tumors in all 5 organs. One patient had tumor in 4 organs; most patients have them in 2. Thus, the syndrome is usually only partially expressed. The gastric tumors are malignant and metastasize to the liver, peritoneum, and lymph nodes. The lung, adrenal, and esophageal tumors are benign. The paraganglionic tumors are usually benign. Long-term follow-up shows that the syndrome is a chronic, persistent, and generally indolent condition whose outcome is largely dependent on the behavior of the metastases of the gastric sarcoma. Among the 79 affected patients described in 1999 (average follow-up 8 years, 64 were alive, 19 were apparently free of tumors, 45 had residual or metastatic disease, and 15 were dead (10 died of causes related to the syndrome).

The multitumoral syndrome referred to as Carney triad (CTr) was described in 1977 under the rubric 'The triad of gastric leiomyosarcoma, functioning extra-adrenal paraganglioma and pulmonary chondroma' [1]. The article was based on findings in 7 patients; 4 were patients at Mayo Clinic, Rochester, Minn., USA, and 3 were patients whose cases were reported in the literature. In 1981, Grace et al. [2] presented the first subsequent case of the disorder and referred to it as 'Carney's triad.'

Definition

CTr is a syndrome of neoplasms that affect the stomach, lungs, paraganglionic system, adrenal cortex, and esophagus. Multiple tumors develop in affected organs. The disorder affects young women primarily. It is not familial. The gastric lesions are malignant; the lung, adrenal, and esophageal tumors are benign; and the paragangliomas are usually benign.

Background

Patients with 2 different tumors, each occurring singly, are not uncommon. Patients with 3 different tumors, each occurring singly, are infrequent. Patients with 3 uncommon or rare tumors each occurring multifocally would be extraordinary indeed, especially if all the patients were young women. On the basis of those extraordinary circumstances, the syndrome described in this chapter was initially suspected.

In 1977, Carney et al. [1] reported the cases of 7 young women, with combinations of intramural stromal gastric tumors, pulmonary cartilaginous tumors, and extra-adrenal paragangliomas. The 3 neoplasms were unusual or rare – one, pulmonary chondroma, was unfamiliar or unknown even to pathologists.

Since 1977, over 140 cases of the condition with different combinations of the 3 neoplasms have been described or have come to my attention; all but 2 are single case reports [3, 4].

Historical

Recognition of the syndrome stemmed from my interest in the multiple endocrine neoplasia (MEN) syndromes, disorders that feature multifocal tumors in 2 or more endocrine organs, affect young patients of both sexes, and are familial with transmission by autosomal dominant inheritance. One of the syndromes, MEN2B, includes a nonendocrine tumor component (ganglioneuromatosis).

In August 1975, I was presented a case for pathologic diagnosis: a young woman (case 1) had 2 types of endocrine tumors (paraganglioma and adrenocortical adenoma) and a nonendocrine tumor (gastric leiomyosarcoma). The findings caught my attention because of their general resemblance to the tumor pattern of MEN2B: 1 of the endocrine tumors, the paraganglioma, was multicentric and the other, the adrenal adenoma, was single. The patient also had nonendocrine gastric tumors.

These findings immediately came to mind 3 months later when I encountered a somewhat similar patient. This patient (case 2), a 25-year-old woman, had an endocrine tumor (carotid body paraganglioma) excised at age 11 and, as an adult, had surgery for multiple nonendocrine gastric tumors (leiomyosarcomas) followed by excision several months later of 5 calcified lung lesions (clinically thought to be metastases from the gastric sarcoma). The patient had bilateral congenital abnormalities of her external and middle ears.

Table 1. Clinical and pathologic findings in 7 patients with multitumoral syndrome

Patient No.[a]	Sex	Age, years	Gastric epithelioid leiomyosarcoma[b]	Pulmonary chondroma[b]	Para-ganglioma[b]
1	F	12	+(5)	+(1)	+(1)
2	F	17	+(5)	+(5)	+(2)
3	F	24	+(12)	+(2)	+(1)
4	F	17	+(10)	–[c]	+(3)
5	F	12	+(multiple)	+(1)	–[c]
6	F	16	+(3)	+(1)	–[c]
7	F	20	+(2)	+(3)	–[c]

– = Absent; + = present.

[a] Patients 1–4 were patients at Mayo Clinic. Patients 5–7 were patients whose cases were reported in the literature.

[b] Number of tumors is shown in parentheses.

[c] Pulmonary chondroma developed subsequent to report.

Cases 1 and 2 were similar in that each had endocrine and nonendocrine tumors. I wondered whether the resemblance might not coincidental and considered the possibility that they had a disorder similar to the MEN2B. Neither patient had a similarly affected relative; thus there was no support for a familial disorder, but the combination of tumors was intriguing.

At a chance meeting in August 1976 with S. G. Sheps MD, the Mayo Clinic clinician most experienced with paraganglioma, I mentioned the 2 cases and inquired whether he had encountered similar ones. He sent me a list of 8 Mayo Clinic patients who had paraganglioma and other tumors. The list included 2 with paragangliomas and gastric sarcomas (cases 3 and 4).

Summaries of the findings in the 4 Mayo Clinic patients are presented in table 1.

Cases 1–4

Case 1

A 15-year-old adolescent girl (fig. 1) was found to have hypertension at a school physical examination. At age 16, she had upper gastrointestinal tract bleeding and was treated for anemia. Two years later, abdominal discomfort led to discovery of an epigastric mass. Persistent hypertension prompted measurement of the urinary content of metanephrines, which was elevated. Laparotomy was performed and 3 para-aortic paragangliomas, a small adrenal cortical adenoma, and 10 gastric leiomyosarcomas with an omental metastasis were found and resected. Postoperatively, the patient was still hypertensive and the urinary content of catecholamines and metanephrines remained elevated. Chest imaging findings were normal. No family member had paraganglionic, adrenocortical, or gastric tumors. No family member was similarly affected. The patient was referred to Dr. Sheps at Mayo Clinic.

Case 2

A 25-year-old woman (fig. 2) was born with bilateral anomalies of the external and middle ears that resulted in left-sided deafness and partial deafness in the right ear. An asymptomatic mass was excised from the left carotid bifurcation at age 12; microscopically, it was a paraganglioma (carotid body tumor). At age 24 years, she had massive hematemesis and was comatose on arrival at the hospital. Emergency partial gastrectomy was performed. The resected stomach contained 5 antral leiomyosarcomas, 1 of which was ulcerated and the source of the gastric hemorrhage. Preoperative evaluation had been impractical because of the patient's serious condition but postoperative evaluation revealed 4 left lung masses, which were clinically thought most likely to be metastases from the gastric tumors. The patient was also hypertensive, and urinary content of catecholamines and metanephrines was elevated. The lung lesions were resected (as was a tumor attached to the para-aortic sympathetic chain found incidentally at surgery). The pulmonary tumors were solid with a cartilaginous appearance and were interpreted microscopically as pulmonary hamartomas. The sympathetic chain lesion proved to be a paraganglioma. Postoperatively, the blood pressure and urinary content of pressor amines were normal. No family member had similar tumors.

Case 3

Routine chest imaging revealed a 5-cm tumor in the left lung of a 17-year-old adolescent girl. Because of its rapid growth, it was removed. Histologic examination showed a pulmonary hamartoma. Hematemesis and melena at age 24 led to discovery and resection of 2 gastric tumors. Microscopically, they were leiomyosarcomas. Three years later, melena recurred and gastrectomy was completed for 3 new leiomyosarcomas with lymph node metastasis. At age 32, the patient had tachycardia, nocturnal sweating, and occasional paroxysmal headaches. Four years later, she complained of dyspnea; a mediastinal mass was found that proved to be an aortopulmonary paraganglioma that was only partly resectable. A calcified left lung tumor that had been present for 8 years was not resected. Postoperatively, plasma and urinary catecholamines and their metabolites were elevated. Despite intensive radiotherapy to the paraganglioma, progressive superior vena caval and respiratory obstruction developed and led to the patient's death at age 39 years. No family member was similarly affected.

Case 4

Lymphedema praecox was diagnosed in a 12-year-old girl. During adolescence, Raynaud phenomenon affected her hands. At age 24, investigation of a 4-year history of anemia led to the diagnosis of 12 gastric 'fibrosarcomas', for which total gastrectomy was performed. At that time she was hypertensive. Laparotomy at age 24 revealed multiple hepatic metastases. Resection of a left lower lobe calcified mass at 33 years of age disclosed 2 cartilaginous neoplasms. Paroxysmal hypertension, headaches and sweating led to finding an elevated urinary content of the pressor amines and their metabolites. Nephrotomography showed a mass anterior to the upper pole of the left kidney, consistent with a paraganglioma. The patient declined further surgery. She died at age 41, reportedly of metastatic leiomyosarcoma. No family member was similarly affected.

Cases 5–7

The similarity of the findings among cases 1–4 suggested the likely existence of an unrecognized multitumoral syndrome that was not familial. A search of the international medical literature identified 3 pertinent articles. Summaries of the 3 reports follow, and the findings are included in table 1.

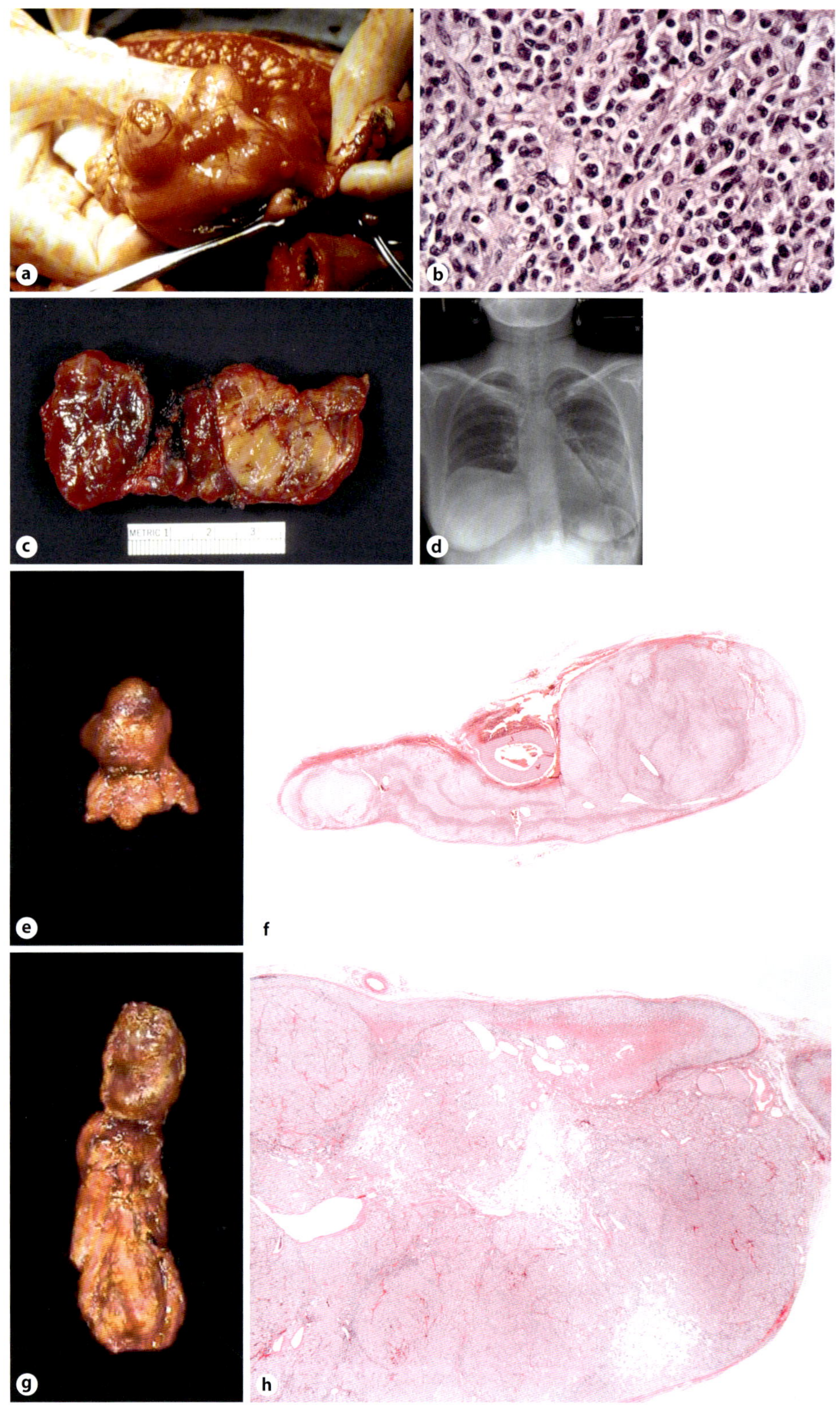
METRIC 1
2
3

Case 5

At age 12, an Italian girl had episodes of hematemesis and melena [5]. An epigastric mass was palpated. Gastric radiographs showed masses in the antrum and body. Subtotal gastrectomy was performed for multiple tumors, interpreted pathologically as leiomyomas. Seven months later, a calcified right lower lobe hamartochondroma was excised. The family history was not mentioned.

Case 6

A 14-year-old American adolescent girl complained of fatigue, pallor and dizzy spells. She was treated for anemia [6]. A firm, nontender upper abdominal mass was palpated at age 16. Gastric radiographs showed a multilobular gastric neoplasm in the lesser curvature and protruding into the gastric lumen. There was a partially calcified 3 × 2 cm lesion in the apex of the left lung. Laparotomy revealed a multilobulated 15 × 8 cm mass in the lesser curvature. A 90% gastrectomy was performed. Pathologically, the tumors were interpreted as leiomyoblastomas. The pulmonary lesion was excised and diagnosed as a chondromatous hamartoma. Hypertension and spells of weakness, tremulousness, and palpitations were present at age 26. Examination revealed a right-sided 12th cranial nerve palsy and a 2-cm mass at the right carotid bifurcation. Carotid angiography showed a glomus jugulare tumor with intracranial extension, a mass behind the internal carotid artery, and a carotid body tumor. Urinary excretion of catecholamine metabolites was increased. The cervical lesions were interpreted as functioning paragangliomas and irradiated. No family member was similarly affected.

Case 7

Iron deficiency anemia in a 20-year-old Swiss woman led to discovery of a lesser curvature gastric tumor [7]. Partial gastrectomy was performed and revealed an ulcerated lesion that was 7 cm in diameter and a second tumor that was 1.5 cm in diameter. The neoplasms were interpreted microscopically as leiomyomas. A chest radiograph 10 months later revealed 2 right-sided masses and 1 left-sided mass that were thought to be probable metastatic leiomyosarcoma.

The Next Case Reported in 1981

Although the 1977 findings were very suggestive if not convincing of a new disorder they needed to be corroborated. Four years passed before the first supporting report appeared. The article reported a case of a young woman who had an aorticopulmonary paraganglioma and gastric leiomyoblastoma [2]. Since then, almost 150 addi-

Fig. 1. Case 1. **a** Several tumors with excrescences were evident on the gastric serosa. **b** Polygonal epithelium-like cells with granular eosinophilic cytoplasm and mildly irregular nuclei. **c** Two paraganglionic tumors formed a dumbbell-shaped mass. **d** Left upper lobe calcified nodule consistent with pulmonary chondroma. **e** Extra-adrenal paraganglioma attached to the right adrenal gland. **f** Right adrenal cortical adenomas. The extratumoral cortex was 0.9 mm thick (normal thickness 1 mm) and was histologically normal. **g** There was a left adrenal pheochromocytoma and an extra-adrenal paraganglioma attached to the adrenal capsule. **h** The left adrenal gland contained a pheochromocytoma. The cortex showed normal zonation.

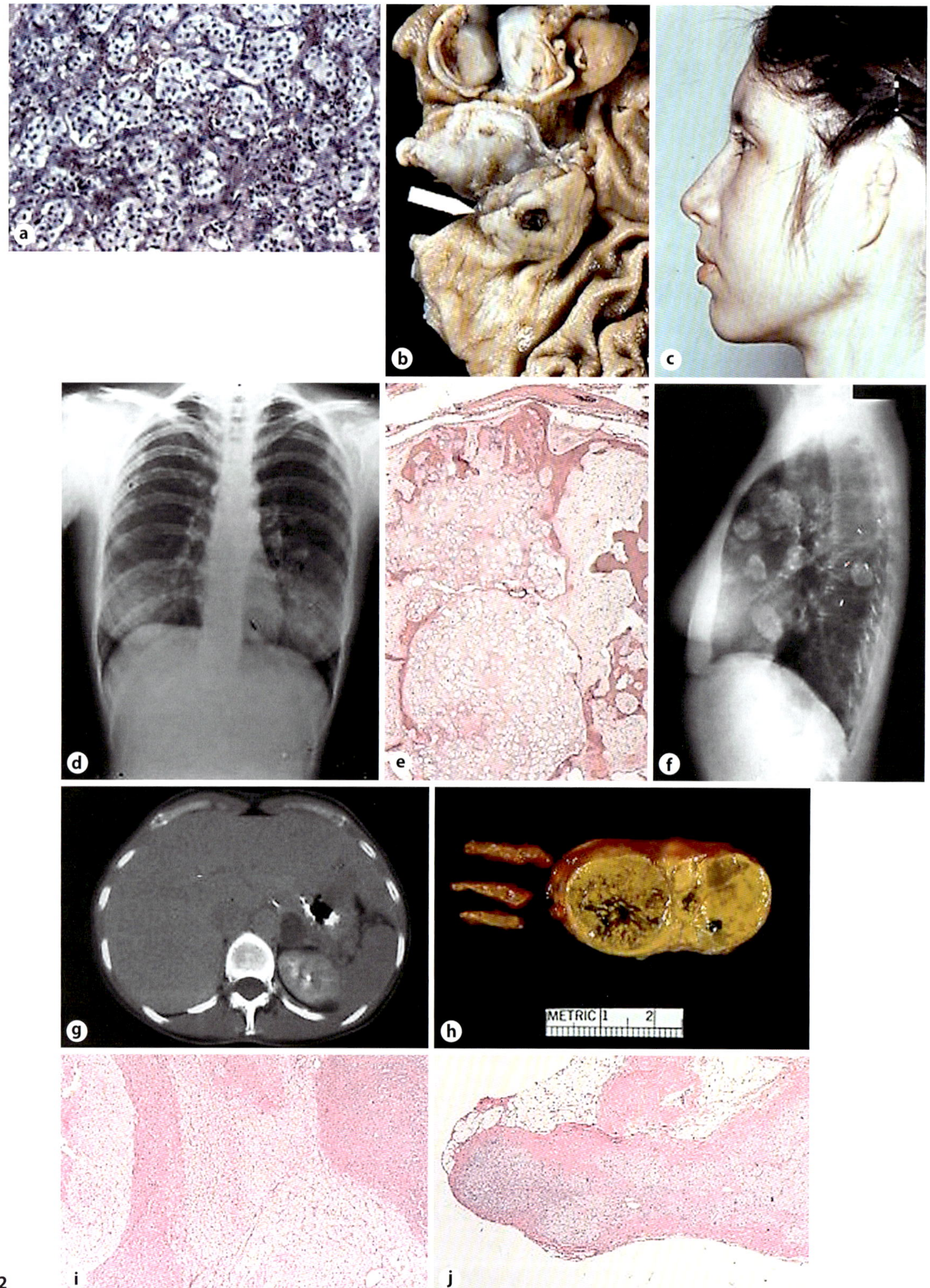

2

tional patients with 3 of the three tumors or 2 of the three have been described or brought to my attention.

Nomenclature of the Gastric and Pulmonary Tumors

Gastric Tumors

Several titles were given to the gastric tumors in the earliest case reports. Virtually all suggested a smooth muscle origin. In 1998, this interpretation was proven to be incorrect; the tumors were shown to arise from the interstitial cells of Cajal, the pacemaker cells of the gut [8].

Before 1960, most intestinal intramural mesenchymal spindle cell tumors were thought to arise in smooth muscle and, consequently, were interpreted as leiomyomas or leiomyosarcomas. Some had a round cell component with clear cells and eccentric nuclei. To distinguish these tumors from pure spindle cell lesions, the terms benign leiomyoblastoma and malignant leiomyoblastoma were introduced. Later, because the round cells simulated epithelial cells, the terms epithelioid leiomyoma and epithelioid leiomyosarcoma were advanced. This terminology [9] was favored at the time of our 1977 article [12].

In 1987, an article by Saul et al. [10] described findings in sporadic (nonsyndromic) intramural alimentary tract spindle cell tumors distributed from the esophagus to the colon. The authors introduced the umbrella term gastrointestinal stromal tumors for these tumors. Subsequently, the abbreviated term GIST was used to refer to the round and spindle cell gastric tumors in CTr. However, because the CTr lesions are different clinically, pathologically, behaviorally, and etiologically from sporadic alimentary tract gastrointestinal stromal tumors of the stomach (table 2), the GIST designation is not appropriate for them. Gastric stromal sarcoma is a more accurate terminology.

Fig. 2. Case 2. **a** The cells in the carotid body tumor had clear cytoplasm and were arranqed in clusters (*zellballen*) supported by vascular stroma. **b** Two submucosal tumors (sectioned), one with ulceration (arrow). **c** Congenital deformity of the left external ear. **d** Imaging revealed multiple calcified lesions in the left lung. **e** Pulmonary chondroma showed benign-appearing cartilage and bone surrounded by a thin pseudocapsule. **f** Multiple calcified pulmonary lesions were seen in chest X-ray. **g** Enlargement of the left adrenal gland was evident on abdominal CT examination. **h** Left adrenal gland featured two juxtaposed neoplasms, one (left) dull yellow with brown and black zones, the other yellow. The slices of the extra-tumoral cortex showed a very thin yellow cortical rim around the medulla. **i** Two populations of cells, one with clear cytoplasm, the second with granular eosinophilic (pink) cytoplasm were seen in the right tumor in **h**. **j** The extratumoral cortex seen in **g** was 0.2 mm thick (normal ~1 mm) and made up of small cells with eosinophilic cytoplasm. A zona reticularis was not seen. There were also two cortical clear-cell nodules. The pink mass outside the adrenal capsule was hypertrophied smooth muscle of tributary of central vein.

Table 2. Comparison of selected findings in sporadic gastric GIST and CTr gastric stromal sarcoma (modified from Zhang et al. [14])

Feature	GIST	CTr gastric stromal sarcoma
Cause	somatic *KIT* or *PDGFRA* mutation	unknown; likely genetic no *KIT, PDGFRA,* or *SDH* mutation
Sex ratio	approximately equal	female predilection
Age, years	>50 (75%); median, 58	range, 6–53; mean, 20
Number of tumors	single	multiple
Location	body > antrum	antrum > body
Immunophenotype	positive for *KIT, PDGFRA,* and *SDHB*	negative for *KIT* and *PDGFRA* positive for *SDHB*
Serial tumor occurrence	no	yes

Pulmonary Tumors

The pulmonary tumors in the reported cases of CTr have almost universally been referred to as pulmonary hamartoma (or chondrohamartoma). Pulmonary hamartoma is the benign cartilaginous tumor of the lung familiar to clinicians and pathologists. It features benign cartilage and bronchial epithelium in 100% of cases, it occurs singly, it occurs in older patients, and is twice as common in men as in women [11]. The cartilaginous tumors in CTr, however, are composed solely of cartilage and have no bronchial epithelial component. Thus, pathologically, they merit the title chondromas. In addition, the CTr lung lesions are multiple and occur in young patients, the great majority of whom are women.

Clinical Features of Carney Triad

The following descriptions are based on reports in 3 articles. The first (published in 1999) described the overall general features of the disorder in 79 patients [12], the second (published in 2007) provided details of the pulmonary tumors in 42 patients [13], and the third (published in 2010) [14] described the gastric tumors in 104 patients.

Patients

The 79 patients in the first article [12] were distributed worldwide. Women predominated, outnumbering men 6:1. None were black. At diagnosis of the first of the 3 tumors, the youngest patient was 7 years old and the oldest was 48 years. The gastric tumor was the commonest presenting finding (73%), followed by the pulmonary tumor (15%) and the paraganglioma (12%). The patients looked and felt well despite a considerable metastatic tumor burden. Symptoms or signs of the tumors were present in 21 patients (27%) for an average of 7 years before diagnosis of the first tumor.

Table 3. Symptoms and signs present in 79 patients with CTr[a] [12]

Tumors	Patients n (%)
Gastric stromal sarcoma	58 (73)
Anemia (with or without melena)	24
Hematemesis (with or without melena)	14
Serendipitous (6 patients) or unknown	7
Epigastric pain, nausea, vomiting	6
Intra-abdominal or intratumoral hemorrhage	4
Asymptomatic abdominal mass	3
Pulmonary chondroma	12 (15)
Asymptomatic radiographically evident pulmonary mass or masses	12
Paraganglioma	8 (10)
Symptomatic or asymptomatic masses	4
Hypertension	4

[a] One patient presented with vomiting due to an esophageal tumor (not resected).

Information on the presence or absence of components of CTr was obtained from 118 parents of the 79 patients, 103 of the parents' children, and 136 of their siblings. Only 2 family members had any of the 3 tumors. Later, it transpired that the 2 sibships had an unrelated familial disorder, the Carney-Stratakis syndrome (familial paraganglioma and gastric stromal sarcoma) [15].

Combinations of Tumors

Tumor occurrence in the 79 patients is shown in table 3. At onset of CTr, the 3 tumors were present in 1 patient (1%), 2 of the 3 tumors were in 27 patients (34%), and 1 of the 3 was in 51 patients (65%). Thus, in most patients, initial expression of the CTr was limited to 1 component. The second tumor was found after an average interval of 8 years. The longest interval between detection of the first and second tumors was 26 years (mean, 8 years), and between the second and third, 18 years (mean, 7 years). Forty-two patients (53%) had gastric and pulmonary tumors, the commonest combination. With the rarity of gastric stromal sarcoma and pulmonary chondroma, it is likely that young patients, especially women, who have multiple gastric stromal sarcomas or multiple pulmonary chondromas have incomplete expression of the CTr. Multiple paragangliomas, although infrequent, occur in several syndromes, and the tumor itself may be familial [14].

Other Tumors

One or more nonfunctioning adrenocortical adenomas were found in 10 of the 79 patients (13%) [12]. Tumor diameter ranged from 0.4 to 4.0 cm. The lesion was bilateral in 1 patient.

Table 4. Combinations of tumors in 104 patients with CTr [14]

Gastric stromal sarcoma	Pulmonary chondroma	Para-ganglioma	Adrenal adenoma	Esophageal leiomyoma	Number of patients
+	+				37
+	+	+			22
+		+			16
+	+			+	10
+	+		+		8
+	+	+	+		4
+		+	+		4
+	+	+	+	+	1
+	+		+	+	1
+		+		+	1

+ = Present.

One or more usually asymptomatic esophageal tumors were present in 7 of the 79 patients (9%) [12]. One patient had vomiting. The lesions were distributed throughout the esophagus and were encountered during investigation of the gastric tumors. They ranged in size from 4 to 12 mm. The lesion was excised in 4 patients and revealed a leiomyoma with positive immunostaining for actin and desmin in 3 and a stromal tumor in 1. One patient had an esophageal carcinoid tumor. There were proximal duodenal stromal tumors in 7 patients (9%); 1 patient had a proximal small intestinal stromal tumor (1%).

Gastric Stromal Sarcoma

Histogenesis

As mentioned earlier, gastrointestinal stromal sarcomas (and gastric gastrointestinal stromal tumors) arise from interstitial cells of Cajal, the pacemaker cells of the gut that mediate impulse transmission from autonomic nerves to gut smooth muscle [8]. They are associated with the myenteric plexus, and they are the only gut cells that show positive immunostaining for CD34 (hematopoietic progenitor cell antigen) and CD117 (transmembrane receptor encoded by the *c-kit* gene). Cells of gastric stromal sarcomas and sporadic gastrointestinal stromal tumors (GISTs) are both immunopositive for CD34 and CD117 (see table 6). On the other hand, the cells of the stromal sarcomas do not stain for SDHB, whereas those of sporadic gastrointestinal stromal tumors (GISTs) do [16].

Symptoms and Signs

The presenting symptom or sign in 104 patients [14] is shown in table 4. The initial sign or symptom of 104 patients (74%) was bleeding from ulceration of the gastric tumors, resulting in 1 or more of the following: anemia, melena, hematemesis, and

Table 5. Location of gastric stromal sarcomas in 62 patients with CTr [12]

Location	Patients n (%)
Antrum or lesser curvature or both	43 (69)
Antrum, lesser curvature, body, with or without cardia	8 (13)
Antrum, body, cardia	2 (3)
Other combinations of locations	9 (15)

Table 6. Immunohistochemical findings in gastric stromal tumors in CTr [14]

Antibody	Number of cases tested	Immuno-positivity, %
*KIT*117	61	100
CD34	40	75
PKCθ	21	21
PDGFRA	10	90
Smooth muscle actin	49	6
Desmin	29	0

acute abdominal symptoms (due to tumor rupture and hemoperitoneum). In occasional patients, an asymptomatic mass was palpated by the patient or a physician (four patients), was found during laparotomy performed for nongastric reasons (one patient), or was discovered at autopsy (2 patients). Although the metastatic spread of the gastric sarcoma occurs early, the metastases usually have a protracted and indolent course.

Imaging

Imaging studies showed smooth or round filling defects, usually in the distal stomach. Gastroscopy revealed sessile, polypoid, ulcerated submucosal masses commonly in the distal stomach. Subserosal tumors were not visualized endoscopically.

Surgery

The initial gastric surgery was subtotal gastric resection in 50 patients, segmental resection in 14, and total gastrectomy in 12.

Pathology

Examination of the resected specimens showed multiple polypoid intramural neoplasms, usually in the antrum and on the lesser curvature (61%) but distributed throughout the stomach (table 5). The size of the neoplasms ranged from 0.4 cm to 8.5 × 5.5 × 4.5 cm.

Two or more tumors were found in each patient. In 1 patient, a single tumor was excised when the patient was 9 years old; a second tumor developed at age 32. The tumors were separate or formed an agglomerated mass of several lesions. They had a soft to hard consistency; some were solid and others were cystic. Microscopically, they were circumscribed and showed little tendency to invade local structures, which was surprising because of the frequent occurrence of metastasis. The tumors were composed of sheets, clusters, and fascicles of polygonal and spindle cells with minimal supporting stroma. On the basis of cell shape, the tumors were classified into 3 types, epithelioid (polygonal) and round (68%), spindle (18%), and mixed epithelioid and spindle (1.4%) [14]. The immunocytochemical staining profile of the neoplasms is shown in table 6. As already mentioned, SDHB immunostaining distinguishes CTr gastric stromal sarcomas (cells unstained) from sporadic stomach gastrointestinal stromal tumors (cells stained) [15].

Development of New Gastric Tumors

New stomach tumors (not recurrences of previously incompletely resected lesions) developed in 23 of 50 patients (46%). The neoplasms occurred in 3 of 12 patients who had 1 or more segmental resections and led to additional gastric resection in 2 patients and total gastrectomy in the third.

Metastasis

Gastric stromal sarcoma metastasis to gastric lesser curvature lymph nodes, liver (14 patients), and peritoneum (8 patients) was found at primary surgery in 28 of 104 patients (27%). Metastasis developed subsequently in an additional 21 patients. The sites affected at primary and subsequent abdominal operations were lymph nodes (30 patients), liver (26 patients), and peritoneum and omentum (14 patients). Intra-abdominal metastasis was found in 22 patients; to the liver (14 patients), peritoneum (10 patients) and gastric lymph nodes (6 patients). The overall metastatic rate was 55%. One patient had liver metastases detected 33 years after primary surgery. Two patients had fatal extra-abdominal metastasis: to lung, bone and skin in 1 and to skeletal muscle in the other. Adenocarcinoma developed in the gastric remnant in 2 patients (aged 39 and 40 years) after subtotal gastric resection.

Treatment and Results

The gastric sarcomas were treated surgically with procedures ranging from local tumor excision to total gastrectomy. Experience has shown that early gastric resection, with removal of as much of the organ as is consistent with preservation of function, is the treatment of choice for gastric sarcomas. Metastases were unresponsive to chemotherapy, radiotherapy, and hyperthermia. In particular, targeted therapy (imatinib and sunitinib) that is successful in treatment of sporadic GIST was ineffective, or had dubiously positive results. This suggests that the molecular mechanism involved in the development of CTr gastric stromal sarcomas is different from those causing the sporadic nonsyndromic sporadic gastrointestinal stromal tumor. Radiofrequency ablation and alcohol injection have been used to control hepatic metastases of the gastric tumor.

Pulmonary Chondroma

Of the 79 patients reported in 1979, 60 (76%) had 1 or more pulmonary cartilaginous tumors [12, 13]. The histogenesis of the lesions is unknown, but presumably they arise from a primitive mesenchymal precursor cell. The lesion was identified histologically in 45 patients and radiologically in 15. Most of the tumors were encountered during the patient's third decade; at tumor detection, the youngest patient was 12 years and the oldest 49 years. The lesions were usually detected during follow-up for the gastric neoplasm and were almost always misinterpreted as metastasis from the stomach sarcoma, and initially treated with chemotherapy. Failure to respond to this resulted in biopsy for pathologic examination, which revealed their cartilaginous nature.

Symptoms, Signs and Imaging Findings

The lung tumors were almost always asymptomatic; 1 patient had dyspnea, atelectasis, and recurrent pulmonary infection, probably related to bronchial compromise by the tumor. The youngest patient age at tumor detection was 12 years and the oldest was 49 years. The tumor was variously interpreted as metastatic gastric sarcoma, indeterminate, pulmonary hamartoma, and metastatic chondrosarcoma (precipitating a search for a bone primary), in decreasing order of frequency.

Treatment

Thoracotomy was performed in 41 of 60 patients (68%), lobectomy (17 patients), segmental or wedge resection (13 patients), tumor enucleation (9 patients) and unspecified procedure (2 patients). Development of additional tumors resulted in 2 thoracotomies in 11 patients and 3 thoracotomies in 3 patients. The pulmonary chondromas in CTr do not need to be excised unless they are causing symptoms.

Pathology

The lesions ranged in size from 0.5 cm to 12 × 10 × 10 cm. The cut surface of the tumors had a cartilaginous, bony, or mucoid appearance. On microscopic examination, they were composed of various amounts of mature cartilage, bone, and undifferentiated mesenchymal cells set in a mucopolysaccharide matrix. None contained bronchial epithelium.

Table 7. Site of origin of 60 paragangliomas in 34 patients [12]

Tumor site and type	Number of tumors
Head and neck	
Glomus tympanicum	5
Glomus jugulare	2
Glomus vagale	2
Carotid body	8
Larynx	2
Thyroid	1
Chest	
Superior mediastinum	3
Aortopulmonary body	9
Sympathetic chain	2
Abdomen	
Retroperitoneum (5 para-adrenal)	7
Adrenal	6
Sympathetic chain	9
Organ of Zuckerkandl	2
Liver (porta hepatis)	2

Results of Surgery

Follow-up ranged from 1 to 30 years (mean, 13 years). One or more additional tumors occurred in 23 of 41 patients (56%). There was no further tumor development in 18 of 41 patients (44%).

Extra-Adrenal Paraganglioma

A total of 60 paragangliomas occurred in 37 of 79 patients (47%), who ranged in age from 12 to 48 years (mean, 27 years) [12]. Paragangliomas are of neuroectodermal origin. The sites of the tumor are presented in table 7. The oldest patient age at discovery of a second paraganglioma was 61 years. Diagnosis was made by pathologic examination of the neoplasm(s) in 34 patients and by combinations of clinical, biochemical, and imaging findings in 3 others. Eight patients had multiple paragangliomas; 5 different sites were affected in 1 patient. Four patients (11%) had intra-adrenal paraganglioma (pheochromocytoma).

Symptoms, Signs, and Laboratory and Imaging Findings

Spells of sweating, palpitations, and tachycardia occurred in 13 patients, accompanied by increased urinary excretion of catecholamines and their metabolites. In 10 patients, a symptomatic or asymptomatic mass was found in the neck, mediastinum, or abdomen. The tumors were imaged with combinations of angiography, computed tomography, and iodine-131 metaiodobenzylguanidine (^{131}I-MIBG) scintiscanning.

Treatment
Fifty paragangliomas were completely or partially excised from 31 patients at 40 operations (1 patient had 5 resections). Adrenalectomy (bilateral in 1 patient) was performed in 5 patients for paraganglioma whose intimate attachment to the adrenal simulated an intra-adrenal tumor. Five patients with inoperable tumors received chemotherapy, radiotherapy, or polyvinyl alcohol particle embolization.

Pathology
The tumors were firm, had a fleshy cut surface, and were very vascular. The eosinophilic cells were arranged in clusters and trabeculae, and were chromogranin positive.

Results of Surgery
Surgical excision cured 45 of the tumors; follow-up ranged from 3 to 20 years (mean, 12 years). Secondary surgery was required in 3 patients because of initial incomplete excision of carotid body, aortopulmonary, and laryngeal paragangliomas, respectively.

Follow-Up

Follow-up information was obtained for the 79 patients in the 1999 study [12]. The length ranged from 1 to 49 years (mean, 26 years) and exceeded 30 years for 15 patients. The age of the oldest surviving patient was 60 years. Of the 79 patients, 64 (81%) were alive; 19 of them (30%) had no residual tumor. Forty-eight of the 79 patients (61%) survived with residual or metastatic neoplasm: 21 (27%) had hepatic metastatic gastric stromal sarcoma, and 4 had recurrent gastric stromal sarcoma that was present and considered to be unresectable for 12 and 15 years in 2 cases.

Twenty-six patients had pulmonary chondroma(s) at last follow-up. From 1 patient, 5 left lung chondromas were excised at age 25; 12 calcified pulmonary nodules, located bilaterally, were found when she was 47 years (she also had hepatic metastatic gastric sarcoma and a nonfunctioning 2.6 cm adrenal mass, likely a cortical adenoma). A single chondroma was found in a 27-year-old man; by the time he succumbed to metastatic gastric stromal sarcoma at age 67, he had 6 chondromas (the largest was 10 cm in diameter).

Seven patients survived with paraganglioma, 4 of whom also had residual or metastatic gastric stromal sarcoma or pulmonary chondroma.

Fifteen of the 79 patients (19%) were dead; 10 (13%) died of CTr, usually metastatic gastric stromal sarcoma, 3 died of other causes but with components of CTr, and 2 of causes unrelated to CTr [11].

Treatment of the Tumors

Based on experience [12, 13, 14], ideal treatment of the gastric and paraganglionic tumors is early surgical removal. Recurrences and metastases of the gastric tumor have not responded to radiotherapy, chemotherapy, or targeted therapy. The pulmonary tumors do not need to be excised unless they become symptomatic. The benign esophageal and adrenal tumors usually do not cause symptoms and management will vary from case to case.

Unusual Features of the Carney Triad

Sex Predeliction
The female sex predeliction in the CTr is unexplained. Possible explanations include the presence of a sex-specific modifier, such as high estrogen levels or an activating gene mutation or amplification on an X chromosome.

Absence of Familial Cases
Development of CTr from a mutation that occurred after zygote formation would explain the absence of familial cases.

Indolent Behavior of Gastric Tumor Metastases
The biological behavior of the gastric tumors is unexpected. Apparent early metastasis is usually followed by slow or very slow metastatic growth. The frequent occurrence of metastases contrasted with the circumscription and lack of local invasiveness of the primary gastric neoplasm.

Juxtaposition of Different Gastric and Esophageal Tumors
A surprising and unexplained finding is the occurrence of two histogenetically different intramural tumors of the alimentary tract (gastric stromal sarcoma and esophageal leiomyoma) in contiguous portions of the intestinal tract.

Congenital Malformations
The patient who was the CTr index case (patient 2) had congenital malformation of her external and middle ears, a finding that hardly seems happenstance.

Differential Diagnosis

The main differential diagnosis is the Carney-Stratakis syndrome [16], a disorder that features 2 of the components of CTr, paraganglioma and gastric stromal sarcoma. The Carney-Stratakis syndrome is familial, transmitted by autosomal-dominant inheritance. The paraganglioma is usually the presenting tumor. In contrast, the gastric tumor is almost always the initial manifestation in CTr. Several other rare disorders feature multiple gastric GISTs [14]; none feature multiple pulmonary chondromas.

Genetics

CTr very likely results from genetic mutation. More than half of the patients known to have CTr and their tumors have been screened for mutations of the genes that are linked with sporadic or genetic forms of GIST and paraganglioma (*SDHB*, *SDHC*, SDHD, *KIT*, and *PDGFRA*). No mutations have been found [17].

References

1 Carney JA, Sheps SG, Go VLW, Gordon H: The triad of gastric leiomyosarcoma, functioning extra-adrenal paraganglioma and pulmonary chondroma. New Engl J Med 1977;296:1517–1518.

2 Grace MP, Batist G, Grace WR, Gillooley JF: Aorticopulmonary paraganglioma and gastric leiomyoblastoma in a young woman. Am J Med 1981;70: 1981.

3 Sawhney SA, Chapman AD, Carney JA, Gomersall LN, Dempsey OJ: Incomplete Carney triad – a review of two cases. Q J Med 2009;102:649–653.

4 Rutkowski P, Nowecki ZI, Debiec-Rychter M, Gerzesiakowska U, Michej W, Wozniak A, Siedlecki JA, Limon J, Jerzak vel Dobosz A, Kakol M, Osuch C, Ruka W: Predictive factors for long-term effects of imatinib therapy in patients with inoperable/metastatic CD117(+) gastrointestinal stromal tumors (GISTs). J Cancer Res Clin Oncol 2007;133:589–597.

5 Vio A, Abate L, Leogrande G: Considerazioni su un singolare caso di tumore gastrico a nodi multiplie (leiomioma bizzarro di Stout) associato ad amartochondroma pulmonare in una giovinetta di 12 anni. Ann Ital Chir 1969;45:750–768.

6 de Castro FJ, Olsen WR, Littler ER: Gastric leiomyoblastoma in an adolescent. Am J Surg 1972;123: 614–616.

7 Muller M, Ryncki PV, Saegesser F, Gardiol D: Hamartomes pulmonaires multiple bilatéraux. A propos d'une jeune femme préablement opérée d'une tumeur musculaire d'estomac. Schweiz med. Wschr 1974;104:511–514.

8 Hirota S, Isozaki K, Moriyama Y, Hashimoto K, Nishida T, Ishigure S, Kawano K, Hanada M, Kuratat A, Takeda M, Tunio GM, Matsduzawa Y, Kanakura Y, Shinomura Y, Kitamura Y: Gain-of-function mutations of *c-kit* in human gastrointestinal stromal tumors. Science 1998;279:577–580.

9 Appleman HD, Helwig EB: Gastric epithelioid leiomyoma and leiomyosarcoma (leiomyoblastomas). Cancer 1976;38:708–728.

10 Saul SH, Rast ML, Brooks JJ: The immunohistochemistry of gastrointestinal stromal tumors. Evidence supporting origin from smooth muscle. Am J Surg Pathol 1987;11:464–473.

11 Gjevre JA, Myers JL, Prakash UBS: Pulmonary hamartoma. Mayo Clin Proc 1996;71:14–20.

12 Carney JA: Gastric stromal sarcoma, pulmonary chondroma, and extra-adrenal paraganglioma (Carney triad): natural history, adrenocortical component, and possible familial occurrence. Mayo Clin Proc 1999;74:543–552.

13 Rodriguez F, Aubry MC, Tazelaar HD, Slezak J, Carney JA: Pulmonary chondroma: a tumor associated with Carney triad and different from pulmonary hamartoma. Am J Surg Pathol 2007;31:1844–1853.

14 Zhang L, Smyrk TC, Young WR Jr, Stratakis CA, Carney JA: Gastric stromal tumors in Carney triad are different clinically, pathologically, and behaviourly from sporadic gastric gastrointestinal stromal tumors: findings in 104 cases. Am J Surg Pathol 2010;34:53–64.

15 Gaal J, Stratakis CA, Carney JA, Ball ER, Korpershoek E, Lodish MB, Levy I, Xekoulki P, van Nederveen FH, den Bakker MA, O'Sullivan M, Dinjens WNM, de Krijger RR: SDHB immunohistochemistry: a useful tool in the diagnosis of Carney-Stratakis and Carney triad gastrointestinal stromal tumors. Mod Pathol 2011;24:147–151.

16 Carney JA, Stratakis CA: Familial paraganglioma and gastric stromal sarcoma: a new syndrome distinct from the Carney triad. Am J Med Genet 2002; 108:132–139.

17 Stratakis CA, Carney JA: The triad of paragangliomas, gastric stromal tumors and pulmonary chondromas (Carney triad), and the dyad of paragangliomas and gastric stromal sarcomas (Carney-Stratakis syndrome): molecular genetics and clinical implications. J Int Med 2009;266:43–52.

J. Aidan Carney, MD, PhD, FRCP
Plummer North 10, Mayo Clinic
200 Southwest First Street
Rochester, MN 55905 (USA)
E-Mail Carney.Aidan@mayo.edu

Stratakis CA (ed): Endocrine Tumor Syndromes and Their Genetics.
Front Horm Res. Basel, Karger, 2013, vol 41, pp 111–140 (DOI: 10.1159/000345673)

Genetics of Pituitary Adenomas

Monica R. Gadelha[a] · Giampaolo Trivellin[b] · Laura Cristina Hernández-Ramírez[b] · Márta Korbonits[b]

[a]Division of Endocrinology, Clementino Fraga Filho University Hospital, Federal University of Rio de Janeiro, Rio de Janeiro, Brazil; [b]Centre for Endocrinology, Barts and London School of Medicine, Queen Mary University of London, London, UK

Abstract

Pituitary adenomas are common tumors of the adenohypophysis which can cause considerable morbidity, due to excessive hormonal secretion or compression and local invasion of surrounding structures. The vast majority of pituitary adenomas occur sporadically. Altered gene expression is commonly detected but somatic mutations, epigenetic changes and abnormal microRNAs have also been described. Occurrence of *GNAS* mutations at a postzygotic stage lead to McCune-Albright syndrome (MAS), a disease causing endocrine hyperfunction and tumors in several organs, including the pituitary. Familial pituitary adenomas occur as part of a syndrome affecting other organs, such as in MEN1 or Carney complex, or occur with pituitary adenomas only as in familial isolated pituitary adenoma (FIPA). FIPA, an autosomal-dominant disease with variable penetrance, is explained in 20% of patients by germline mutations in the tumor suppressor *aryl hydrocarbon receptor interacting protein (AIP)*, while no gene abnormality has been identified to date in the majority of the FIPA families. AIP mutation-positive patients have a characteristic clinical phenotype with usually young- or childhood-onset growth hormone (GH) and/or prolactin (PRL)-secreting adenomas and can be seen in cases with no apparent family history as well. Understanding the tumorigenic process in *AIP*-positive and *AIP*-negative FIPA patients could result in better diagnostic and treatment options for both familial and sporadic cases.

Pituitary adenomas are common tumors of the adenohypophysis. They can cause considerable morbidity due to excessive hormonal secretion or lack of appropriate hormone release and due to compression and local invasion of important surrounding structures. The prevalence of pituitary adenomas is high (14–22%) in autopsy and MRI studies [1], but many of these lesions remain clinically silent and represent incidentalomas. Clinically relevant adenomas diagnosed due to symptoms are significantly less common, ~1:1,100 patients have been identified with pituitary adenomas in the general population in population-based studies [2, 3].

The vast majority of pituitary adenomas are sporadic tumors. Genetic alterations are commonly seen in the tumor tissue, such as *GNAS* gene mutations in 40% of somatotroph adenomas. On the other hand, increasing proportion of familial cases have been reported [4], and the recent establishment of a novel clinical entity, familial isolated pituitary adenoma (FIPA), is expected to increase awareness and lead to an improved recognition of familial cases.

Despite their relative rarity, familial pituitary tumors represent an important group of conditions as often they have a more aggressive course and show younger age of onset, such as in patients with mutations in the *multiple endocrine neoplasia 1 (MEN1,* MIM*613733*)* or *aryl hydrocarbon receptor interacting protein (AIP,* MIM*605555*)* genes. The genetic background of familial pituitary tumors is heterogeneous and the phenotype of the families varies quite widely. A better understanding of the causative genes and the pathogenic mechanisms of this particular group of tumors is needed to improve the diagnosis and management of these patients, which, hopefully, will lead to a better prognosis, and may help to understand the pathogenesis of sporadic adenomas as well.

The inherited conditions that, to date, are known to predispose to pituitary adenomas are multiple endocrine neoplasia type 1 (MEN1, MIM#131100, see chapter by Agarwal, this vol.) and type 4 (MEN4, MIM#610755, see chapter by Lee and Pellegata, this vol.), Carney complex (MIM#160980, see chapter by Espiard and Bertherat, this vol.) and FIPA (MIM#102200, this chapter). More recently case reports raised the possibility that mutations in the *DICER1* [5] and *succinate dehydrogenase (SDH)* genes [6–9] can also predispose to pituitary tumors. Genetic conditions associated with pituitary neoplasms have been summarized on figure 1. In the current chapter, we will discuss experimental and clinical data regarding FIPA and McCune-Albright syndrome. In addition, genes and microRNAs implicated in sporadic adenoma development will be discussed.

Familial Isolated Pituitary Adenomas

Clinical Characteristics

Approximately 5% of the pituitary adenomas occur with familial aggregation (MEN1, MEN4, Carney complex and FIPA). FIPA syndrome is defined as the occurrence of at least two cases of pituitary adenomas in a family that does not exhibit any other syndromic features, such as MEN1, MEN4 or Carney complex. Somatotroph, lactotroph and somatolactotroph adenomas are the most common subtypes, but other subtypes have also been reported. FIPA is an autosomal dominant disease with a variable penetrance. Germline *AIP* mutations are identified in 20% (range 15–40%) of patients with FIPA syndrome, while the causative gene in the majority of the families is unknown. The penetrance in *AIP*-positive FIPA families is usually 15–30% (range 10–80%) [12–14], while it is somewhat lower in *AIP*-negative families [13].

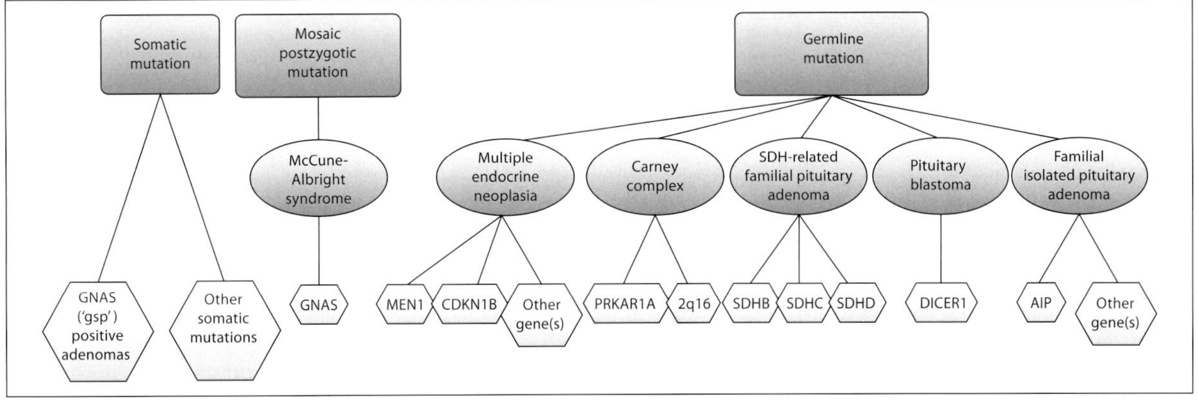

Fig. 1. Pituitary tumors due to genetic origin. A somatic activating mutation in the *GNAS* gene can be found in 30–40% of sporadic somatotroph adenomas. Theoretically, somatic mutations in other genes could also lead to pituitary adenoma development. Mosaic post-zygotic activating mutation of the *GNAS* gene leads to the McCune-Albright syndrome; some of these patients develop somatotroph hyperplasia or adenoma. Germline mutation in the *MEN1* gene or rarely in the *CDKN1B* (coding for cell cycle regulator protein p27) gene cause MEN1 or MEN4; in a small proportion other cell cycle regulators have been implicated (p18 (*CDKN2C*) and p21 (*CDKN1A*)) [11] or no gene abnormality can be found. A mutation in the type 1A regulatory subunit of the cAMP-dependent protein kinase A *(PRKAR1A)* is found in the majority (60%) of patients with Carney complex; in the remainder patients, data suggest a putative causative gene in the 2q16 chromosome region. Patients have been described with *SDH* mutation-related familial paraganglioma/pheochromocytoma and familial pituitary adenomas [6–9]. A mutation in the *DICER1* gene, a gene which regulates microRNAs, may cause an ACTH-secreting pituitary blastoma of infant onset [5]. A fifth of FIPA cases show a mutation in the *AIP* gene; in the majority of families the causative gene has not yet been identified. Adapted from Korbonits et al. [10].

There is a phenotypic difference between *AIP*-positive and *AIP*-negative families. The mean age at diagnosis (24 years) in *AIP*-positive families is approximately 13 years lower than in *AIP*-negative families and the majority of *AIP*-positive families harbor a childhood-onset case [15]. Two-thirds of *AIP*-positive patients are males, while there is no gender predominance in *AIP*-negative familial cases and in sporadic pituitary adenomas [16]. In addition, families with members harboring *AIP* mutations are mainly composed of patients with either pure somatotroph adenomas or with mixed somatotroph and lactotroph adenomas [12, 15]. Actually, *AIP* mutations are found in 50% of homogeneous somatotroph FIPA families [15, 17]. *AIP*-positive cases that presented clinically as nonfunctioning pituitary adenomas (NFPAs) can also exhibit positive growth hormone (GH)/prolactin (PRL) staining [15]. Rarely, ACTH-, LH/FSH- and TSH-secreting adenomas or true null cell adenomas were also identified. The *AIP*-negative families can have a more varied phenotype, with families composed of homologous prolactinoma, NFPA or rarely Cushing's disease or comprising heterogeneous families. *AIP*-positive acromegalic patients often exhibit sparsely granulated somatotroph adenomas [18]. Consistent with this, the tumors of *AIP*-positive patients usually have an aggressive clinical behavior, being large, with frequent invasion of nearby structures and, as a consequence, these patients are submitted to more surgical interventions [16]. Regarding the response to medical therapy, Leontiou et al. [18] observed that *AIP*-positive patients showed a poorer response to somatostatin analogues (SSAs). Indeed, Daly et al. [16] compared 38 *AIP*-positive acromegaly patients and 160 matched acromegaly controls (without *AIP* mutations). They observed that patients harboring *AIP* mutations presented less GH and insulin-like growth factor type 1 (IGF-1) reductions than controls with SSAs therapy (40.0 and 75.0% for GH and 47.4 and 56.0% for IGF-1, respectively). They also observed that the median magnitude of tumor shrinkage achieved with SSAs was significantly higher in the control group (median 41.1 vs. 0.0% in the *AIP*-mutated patients; $p < 0.001$). This poor response to SSAs therapy is not due to a different expression profile of somatostatin receptor (SSTR) in these tumors, as there is no significant reduction of the SSTR subtypes in *AIP*-positive samples compared to sporadic somatotroph adenomas; actually, SSTR5 staining was shown to be slightly higher in *AIP*-positive FIPA samples compared to sporadic adenoma samples [19].

Interestingly, AIP protein expression is reduced in a subset of acromegalic patients with sporadic disease without *AIP* mutation, especially in more invasive cases [20]. Indeed, low AIP expression has been shown to be a better predictor of tumor invasion in somatotrophinomas than Ki-67 or p53 [20]. The mechanism involved in this low AIP expression is currently under investigation. Kasuki et al. [21] reported that sporadic patients with acromegaly harboring somatotrophinomas with low AIP expression are more prone to exhibit resistance to SSAs therapy. The authors compared the AIP protein expression in somatotroph tumors from 35 sporadic patients with acromegaly treated with octreotide LAR after surgery. Of the 18 patients whose tumors exhibited low AIP expression, only 4 (22%) achieved disease control with octreotide therapy, in contrast with 11 of 17 patients (65%) whose tumors presented high AIP expression ($p = 0.013$). In the same study, the authors evaluated SSTR2 expression and observed that there was no difference in SSTR2 expression between patients with low or high AIP expression, in agreement with data on *AIP* mutant tissues [19, 21].

Assessment for FIPA

If a patient with pituitary adenoma has a relative presenting also with pituitary adenoma and no other known associated syndromes then we consider the diagnosis of FIPA. Genetic testing can be offered for *AIP*. According to our current practice, we screen all FIPA cases, all childhood-onset pituitary adenomas and all young-onset (<30 years) macroadenomas even without known family history. We summarized our current strategy in figure 2 [22].

If an *AIP* mutation is identified, genetic screening can be offered to family members. Based on the youngest known affected *AIP*-positive case, we currently suggest screening at age 4 years or earlier [12]. Unaffected carrier family members should undergo regular clinical assessment. For pediatric cases yearly measurements of height and weight with calculation of height velocity and documentation of development of puberty together with pituitary function tests are recommended. Baseline pituitary MRI is advised

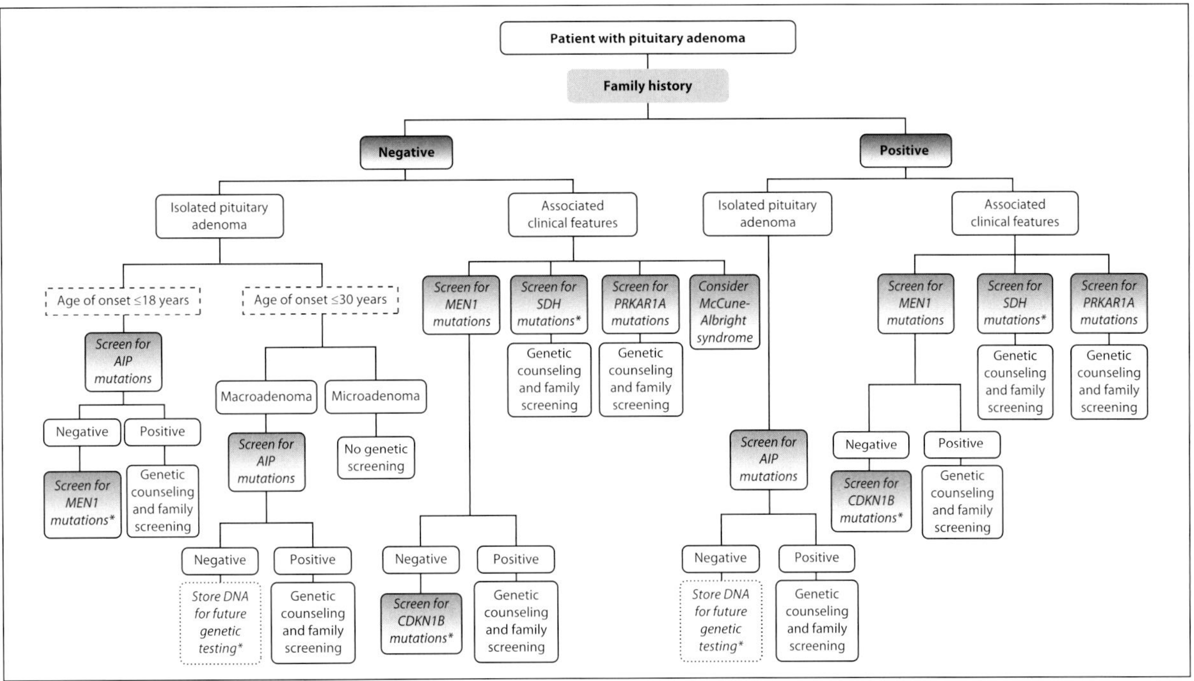

Fig. 2. Suggested approach for genetic testing in patients with pituitary adenomas. * Weak evidence for these suggestions. Adapted from Hernández-Ramírez and Korbonits [22].

around the age of 10 years and repeat MRI scanning of the pituitary every 5 years can be considered if clinical and pituitary function tests remain normal. Adult patients are suggested to have a baseline clinical assessment with pituitary function tests and MRI followed by yearly pituitary function tests. Although there is no long-term experience, repeat MRI of the pituitary every 5 years could be considered until the age of 30 years if clinical and pituitary function tests remain normal. Currently, we follow-up all patients, but in the future monitoring frequency may be reduced above the age of 30–50 years. Surveillance data from *AIP* mutation-positive families in the last few years have revealed a number of *AIP* mutation carrier patients with abnormal biochemical and MRI findings who either underwent treatment or are followed closely [12, 17, 23]. Clinical, laboratory and MRI screening for family members of *AIP*-negative FIPA patients could be performed upon patients request and/or under a research protocol.

AIP Function, Mutations and Animal Models

The human *AIP* gene is located at the 11q13 chromosome region, 2.7 Mb downstream of the *MEN1* gene. *AIP* consists of 6 exons, encoding a 330 amino acid (37 kDa) cytoplasmic co-chaperone phosphoprotein [24], also known as X-associated protein-2 (XAP2), Ah receptor-activated 9 (ARA9) or FK506-binding protein 37 (FKBP37). *AIP* is located on a conserved synthenic block in human, mouse and rat and the AIP protein sequence is evolutionarily conserved among species. The N-terminal AIP protein consists of a peptidyl-prolyl cis-trans isomerase (PPIase)-like domain, whose 3D structure has now been resolved [25]. The C-terminal protein consists of three tetratricopeptide repeat (TPR) motifs and a final α-7 helix and its structure has also been resolved [Prodromou and Korbonits, unpubl. data]. TPR domains are 34 amino acid sequences, often arranged in tandem repeats, formed by two α-helices forming an antiparallel structure that mediates intra- and intermolecular interactions [26]. Other TPR protein family members are aryl hydrocarbon receptor-interacting protein-like 1 (AIPL1), protein phosphatase 5 (PP5), FKBP51, FKBP52, cyclophilin 40 (Cyp40), carboxyl-terminus of hsc70-interacting protein (CHIP), and heat shock protein 70 (hsp70)/hsp90 organizing protein (Hop) [26].

Numerous proteins have been identified to interact with AIP directly (viral proteins (HBV X and EBNA-3), chaperone proteins (hsp90 and hsc70), phosphodiesterases (PDE4A5 and PDE2A3), nuclear receptors (AhR, PPARα and TRβ1), transmembrane receptors (RET and possibly EGFR), G proteins (Gα13 and Gαq), an inhibitor of apoptosis protein (survivin) and a mitochondrial import receptor (TOMM20)) or indirectly (glucocorticoid receptor and the co-chaperone protein p23) [26]. The potential for AIP to interact with several other steroid hormone receptors, such as the androgen and progesterone receptors, has recently been reported [27]. The multiplicity of AIP interactions suggests that AIP is involved in various cellular pathways; however, at the moment it is uncertain which of them play a role in pituitary tumorigenesis. The AhR-cAMP-PDE pathway seems to be a very attractive candidate as AhR activation has well-known tumorigenic effects and phosphodiesterases are involved in the tight control of cellular cAMP levels, which are known to be involved in Gsα mutation-related as well as Carney complex-related somatotroph tumorigenesis [26].

AIP is widely expressed in the human body, but its expression levels vary considerably among tissues. For instance, high expression levels have been observed in spleen and thymus, whereas low AIP expression was detected in liver, kidney and lung [28].

In the normal pituitary gland AIP is expressed only in somatotroph and lactotroph cells, where it associates with secretory vesicles, whereas in sporadic pituitary tumors AIP is expressed in all cell types and shows lack of colocalization with secretory vesicles in prolactinomas, corticotrophinomas and NFPAs [18]. High AIP expression levels are usually observed in NFPAs [18, 29], whereas a low expression was described in invasive GH-secreting adenomas [20]. These observations suggest that the regulation of AIP is different in somatotroph compared to other pituitary cell types.

Although AIP was originally identified in 1996, its clinical relevance was only established 10 years later when heterozygous germline mutations were found in pituitary adenomas [30]. No genotype-phenotype correlation for age of onset, tumor type or level of penetrance has been established to date.

The presence of somatic *AIP* mutations has been studied in both endocrine and nonendocrine tumors, but no mutations have been reported so far [10].

To date, 112 different *AIP* variants have been reported in the literature. In addition to single nucleotide polymorphisms, various missense, nonsense, splice-site and promoter mutations, as well as small deletions and insertions (in-frame or leading to frame-shift), and large genomic deletions have been described. The latter constitutes about 10% of mutations in *AIP*-positive FIPA families and can only be detected with specific techniques, such as MLPA (multiplex ligation-dependent probe amplification). About 65% of *AIP* mutations result in a truncated/lost protein, while missense variants and the in-frame changes mostly affect the TPR domain or the C-terminal α-helix. All known mutations are predicted to lead to loss of function of the protein. There are a few hotspot mutations described in *AIP*, mostly affecting CpG sites, such as codons 81, 271 and 304. Founder mutations have also been described in Finland, Northern Ireland and Italy [12, 14, 30].

The loss-of-function mutations, together with LOH and functional data, suggest that *AIP* functions as a tumor suppressor gene in the pituitary gland [13, 18, 30, 31]. Homozygous *Aip* loss in mice was shown to cause embryonic lethality due to congenital defects in heart development and inability to maintain productive erythropoiesis [32, 33], whereas heterozygous *Aip* (*Aip*+/–) mice were shown to be prone to develop pituitary adenomas, especially somatotrophinomas [34]. Interestingly, unlike in humans, Aip+/– mice display complete penetrance of pituitary tumors [34] possibly due to homogenous genetic background.

GNAS Mutations and McCune-Albright Syndrome

Definition and Epidemiology

Originally described in the 1930s (first by McCune [35] and then by Albright et al. [36]) as the triad of polyostotic fibrous dysplasia, *café-au-lait* spots and precocious puberty. McCune-Albright syndrome (MAS, MIM#174800) is a complex genetic syndrome encompassing other diseases due to endocrine hyperfunction. According to the current definition of MAS, this diagnosis is established in the presence of (1) monostotic or polyostotic fibrous dysplasia, and (2) at least one manifestation of endocrine hyperfunction and/or café-au-lait spots [37]. The original clinical triad is known as classic MAS, while the presence of only 2 manifestations is known as nonclassic MAS. Even though the presence of only one manifestation is not included in this definition, Lumbroso et al. [38] found that there is a subgroup of girls with isolated precocious puberty bearing GNAS mutations. This manifestation can appear isolated and remain like that, but it could also be the first manifestation in patients who will develop other components of the disease in the future. Café-au-lait spots are the commonest component of the syndrome (53–95% of patients) [39]. In the largest available series (113 patients with MAS-related abnormalities), the classic triad was present in only 24% of patients, one third had 2 components of the triad and the rest of them had only one (usually precocious puberty) [38].

MAS is a very rare disease with a prevalence around 1/100,000–1/1,000,000 in the general population, but fibrous dysplasia (especially the monostotic variant) is much more common [37]. There is a gender imbalance with a predominance of female patients [38]; the reason for this is unknown.

Genetic Issues

The genetic basis of MAS is a postzygotic (i.e. somatic) mutation in the *GNAS* (also known as *GNAS1*) gene; the patients are somatic mosaics for *GNAS* mutations [40]. The clinical manifestations are widely variable due to the variable mutation status of the various tissues [40, 41]. Germline *GNAS* mutations are never inherited, they are probably embryonically lethal [41, 42]. Theoretically, severe MAS cases are related to a mutational event at an early developmental stage [42]. In agreement with this hypothesis, in MAS patients with involvement of several tissues, the same *GNAS* mutation is found in all the tissues analyzed [38]. Apparently, somatic mosaicism is a sine qua non condition for the development of MAS: cells bearing the mutation can only survive if they are interspersed with normal cells in the affected tissues [41], as has been proved for fibrous dysplasia lesions [43].

The *GNAS* locus displays complex genomic imprinting, generating multiple alternative products from the paternal and maternal alleles, driven by the activation of alternative promoters (4 sense and 1 antisense), differently imprinted [44, 45].

Gsα is the best known product coded by *GNAS*. Gsα is transcribed from the exons 1–13, resulting in four alternatively spliced products (two long, Gsα-1 and Gsα-2, and two short, Gsα-3 and Gsα-4), that might have variable biological roles [46]. Exons 2–13 are common to the other *GNAS* gene products: NESP55 and XLαs.

Gsα constitutive activation at multiple tissues is the accepted pathogenic basis of MAS, whereas there is not a clear contribution of the other *GNAS* locus products to the clinical features [40]. A tissue-specific imprinting pattern in some organs has been proposed [47] and supported by data from inactivating *GNAS* mutations.

In humans, tissue-specific imprinting has been demonstrated in the pituitary, where Gsα is exclusively expressed from the maternal allele [48]. Somatotrophinomas (both those with and without *GNAS* mutations) often show a relaxation of Gsα monoallelic expression, but retain the normal imprinting of NESP55 and XLαs, implying a possible role for loss of Gsα imprinting in somatotroph cells tumorigenesis [48]. In *GNAS* mutation-positive somatotrophinomas, both sporadic and MAS-related, mutations are almost always located in the maternal allele, in agreement with the pituitary-specific imprinting of this gene [49]. In thyroid and gonads, the expression of Gsα is mainly dependent on the maternal allele, but the paternal contribution is not negligible, indicating that genetic imprinting is not necessarily an all-or-nothing phenomenon [50]. Therefore, acromegaly occurs only in those MAS patients with an affected maternal allele, but there is not an apparent relationship between the origin of the mutated allele and the rest of MAS components [49], each individual showing a particular distribution of abnormal cells in the affected tissues.

GNAS mutations in MAS patients always occur at codon 201 and usually result in the substitution of the residue arginine by a histidine or cysteine [46], or, infrequently, by a serine, glycine or leucine. On the other hand, in isolated endocrine tumors *GNAS* mutations can occur both at the 201 or 227 positions [51]. Indeed, 40% of sporadic somatotrophinomas bear a heterozygous activating *GNAS* mutation either at the position 201 or 227 (*gsp* oncogene) [52, 53]. Detection of *GNAS* mutations in affected tissues is high (90%), while peripheral blood lymphocytes show 21–27% positivity in MAS patients [38]. MAS is a clinical diagnosis but detection of *GNAS* mutations in affected tissues could be important in certain non-classical cases [38].

Pituitary Involvement

Pituitary disease in MAS is characterized by elevated GH and often (92%) accompanying high prolactin levels [54]. Excessive GH production is part of MAS in 21% of patients [54], but only 33–65% of these bear a pituitary adenoma detectable by imaging studies [54, 55]. The current concept is that pituitary involvement in MAS is widespread and diffuse, including areas of normal gland, somatotroph hyperplasia (most common), somatotroph neoplasia, lactotroph neoplasia and mammosomatotroph neoplasia [55]. Interestingly, *GNAS* mutation-related acromegaly patients (both MAS (100%) and sporadic acromegaly (78%)) respond positively to a TRH test while gsp negative cases only in 50% [54].

Surgical treatment in MAS-related acromegaly can be difficult due to the presence of craniofacial bone lesions, complicating surgical approaches [54, 55]. Visual and/or auditive compromise due to cranial nerve compression is more severe in patients with high GH and IGF-1 levels [54]. Medical treatment with cabergoline and octreotide can lead to disease control, although often partial. Combined treatment with pegvisomant and radiotherapy achieved total disease control in a series of 5 out of 6 acromegalic SSA-resistant MAS patients [56].

Other features of MAS include peripheral (primary) precocious puberty in girls (30–50% [57]), hyperthyroidism (50%), Cushing's syndrome (7%), renal phosphate wasting (50%) (explained by the production of the phosphaturic factor fibroblast growth factor 23 (FGF-23) by the fibrous dysplasia lesions [58]). Nonendocrine manifestations include fibrous dysplasia, irregular café-au-lait spots ('cost of Maine' pattern), rarely gastrointestinal reflux, gastrointestinal polyps, pancreatitis, neonatal cholestasis, sudden death, tachycardia, aortic root dilatation and platelet dysfunction [37, 38, 59]. Hyperparathyroidism in MAS is secondary to the abnormalities in mineral metabolism and not caused by *GNAS* mutations [37]. A few cases of thyroid and breast cancer have been reported in association with MAS; nevertheless, a causative association has not been established [59].

Table 1 . Genes potentially involved in the pathogenesis of sporadic pituitary adenomas

Gene name	MIM number	Location (Chr)	Function	TSG/ oncogene	Defect
AIP	605555	11q13.2	Co-chaperone protein	Tumor suppressor gene (TSG)	Decreased expression in invasive somatotrophinomas
AKT1	164730	14q32.33	Regulates many processes including metabolism, proliferation, cell survival, growth and angiogenesis	Oncogene	Increased expression, especially in NFPAs
AKT2	164731	19q13.2	Regulates many processes including metabolism, proliferation, cell survival, growth and angiogenesis	Oncogene	Increased expression, especially in NFPAs
BAG1	601497	9p13.3	Inhibits the chaperone activity of HSP70/HSC70 and the pro-apoptotic function of PPP1R15A	–	Increased expression
BMI1 (BMI-1)	164831	10p12.2	Component of the polycomb repressive complex 1, which is required to maintain the transcriptionally repressive state of many genes	Oncogene	Increased expression, genetic amplification in one adenoma
BMP4	112262	14q22.2	Plays a crucial role in the control of the differentiation and proliferation of the different cell types in the anterior pituitary	TSG	Increased expression
CCNA1 (cyclin A1)	604036	13q13.3	Involved in the control of the G1/S and G2/M phases of the cell cycle	Oncogene	Increased expression, especially in recurrent adenomas
CCNB1 (cyclin B1)	123836	5q13.2	Involved in G2-M transition	Oncogene	Increased expression
CCNB2 (cyclin B2)	602755	15q22.2	Involved in G2-M transition	Oncogene	Increased expression that correlates with HMGA1 and HMGA2 expression
CCND1 (cyclin D1)	168461	11q13.3	Promotes progression through the G1-S phase of the cell cycle	Oncogene	Increased expression, allelic imbalance
CCNE1 (cyclin E1)	123837	19q12	Promotes progression through the G1-S phase of the cell cycle	Oncogene	Increased expression
CDKN1A ($p21^{CIP1}$)	116899	6p21.2	Regulator of cell cycle progression at G1	TSG	Decreased expression in NFPAs, increased expression in hormone producing adenomas, especially somatotrophinomas
CDKN1B ($p27^{KIP1}$)	600778	12p13.1	Blocks the cell cycle in the G0/G1 phase. Also involved in cell migration, proliferation, neuronal differentiation and apoptosis	TSG or oncogene depending on cellular context	Decreased expression, especially in recurrent adenomas
CDKN2A ($p16^{INK4}$)	600160	9p21.3	Induces cell cycle arrest in G1 and G2 phases	TSG	Decreased expression mostly by promoter methylation

Tumor types	Animal models	References
Invasive somatotrophinomas	*Aip* +/– mice develop pituitary tumors with complete penetrance	Kasuki et al. [20], 2011; Kasuki et al. [21], 2012
Various tumor types	No pituitary tumors	Musat et al. [75], 2005
Various tumor types	No pituitary tumors	Musat et al. [75], 2005
Somatotrophinomas, prolactinomas, NFPAs	No pituitary tumors	Morris et al. [76], 2005
Various tumor types	Conditional, neural and glial-specific transgenic expression of *Bmi1* in mice lead to development of intermediate and anterior lobe ACTH-secreting pituitary adenomas	Sanchez-Beato et al. [77], 2006; Palumbo et al. [74], 2012; Westerman et al. [78], 2012
Prolactinomas	No pituitary tumors	Paez-Pereda et al. [79], 2003
Various tumor types	No pituitary tumors	Turner et al. [80] 2000; Nakabayashi et al. [81], 2001
Various tumor types	Homozygous *Ccnb1* KO is embryonic lethal in mice	Turner et al. [80], 2000; Wierinckx et al. [82], 2007
All tumor types	*Ccnb2*-KO mice, although develop normally, are smaller than normal mice and have reduced litter sizes	De Martino et al. [83], 2009
Aggressive and non-functioning adenomas, somatotrophinomas	No pituitary tumors	Hibberts et al. [84], 1999; Jordan et al. [85], 2000; Turner et al. [80] 2000; Simpson et al. [86], 2001; Elston et al. [87], 2008
Mainly corticotropinomas	No pituitary tumors	Jordan et al. [85], 2000; Turner et al. [80] 2000
All tumor types	*Cdkn1a* KO mice do not develop pituitary adenomas, but both double *Cdkn1a* and *Rb1*, and *Cdkn1a* and *Cdkn2c* KO mice develop pituitary adenomas with a shorter latency than single *Rb1* and *Cdkn2c* mutants, respectively. Double *Cdkn1a* and *Cdkn1b* KO mice show higher incidence of pituitary adenomas than *Cdkn1b* mutants	Neto et al. [88], 2005
All tumor types, especially corticotropinomas and pituitary carcinomas	*Cdkn1b* KO mice develop intermediate lobe hyperplasia leading to corticotropinomas	Qian et al. [89], 1996; Lloyd et al. [90], 1997; Bamberger et al. [91], 1999; Jin et al. [92], 1997; Lidhar et al. [93], 1999; Komatsubara et al. [94], 2001; Nakabayashi et al. [81], 2001; Korbonits et al. [95], 2002; Musat et al. [75], 2005
All tumor types, but especially NFPAs	*Cdkn2a* KO mice do not show pituitary adenomas, but double *Cdkn2a* and *Cdkn2c* KO mice develop intermediate lobe tumors with a shorter latency than single *Cdkn2c* mutants	Woloschak et al. [96], 1996; Jaffrain-Rea et al. [97], 1999; Simpson et al. [98], 1999; Ruebel et al. [99], 2001; Seemann et al. [100], 2001; Ogino et al. [101], 2005; Yoshino et al. [102], 2006; Machiavelli et al. [103], 2008; Kirsch et al. [104], 2009

Table 1 . Continued

Gene name	MIM number	Location (Chr)	Function	TSG/ oncogene	Defect
CDKN2B ($p15^{INK4B}$)	600431	9p21.3	Inhibits progression of cell cycle at G1	TSG	Decreased expression partly by promoter methylation, homozygous deletion
CDKN2C ($p18^{INK4C}$)	603369	1p32.3	Regulator of cell cycle progression at G1	TSG	Decreased expression mostly by promoter methylation
COPS5 (JAB1)	604850	8q13.1	Probable protease subunit of the COP9 signalosome complex, which is involved in various cellular and developmental processes	–	Increased expression
CREB1 (CREB)	123810	2q33.3	Phosphorylation-dependent transcriptional activator of cAMP response elements (CREs), that regulates mitogenesis, metabolism, differentiation, and proliferation	Oncogene	Constitutive activation by phosphorylation
DAPK1	600831	9q21.33	Positive mediator of the programmed cell death induced by gamma-interferon	TSG	Decreased expression either by promoter methylation or by homozygous deletion of the promoter CpG island
DKC1	300126	Xq28	Pseudouridine synthase that modifies rRNA and regulates telomerase activity	TSG	Loss-of-function somatic mutation
DRD2 (D2R)	126450	11q23.2	G protein-coupled receptor for dopamine	–	Decreased expression
EGFR	131550	7p11.2	Transmembrane glycoprotein required for normal cellular proliferation, survival, adhesion, migration and differentiation	Oncogene	Increased expression
FGF2 (bFGF)	134920	4q27-28	Plays an important role in the regulation of cell survival, cell division, angiogenesis, cell differentiation and cell migration	–	Increased expression, decreased mRNA expression in TSH-secreting adenomas
FGFR1	136350	8p11.23-p11.22	Receptor for fibroblast growth factor	Oncogene	Increased expression especially in NFPAs, decreased mRNA expression in TSH-secreting adenomas
FGFR2	176943	10q26.13	Receptor for fibroblast growth factor	Oncogene	Decreased expression by promoter methylation
FGFR4	134935	5q35.2	Membrane-anchored receptor for fibroblast growth factor (preferentially binds acidic fibroblast growth factors)	Oncogene	Increased expression of a N-terminally truncated cytoplasmic isoform (ptd-FGFR4) by alternative transcription initiation
FOLR1 (FR)	136430	11q13.4	Binds to folate and reduces folic acid derivatives and mediates delivery of 5-methyltetrahydrofolate to the interior of cells	Oncogene?	Increased expression in NFPAs, decreased expression in PRL- and GH-secreting adenomas
GADD45B (GADD45-β)	604948	19p13.3	Regulation of growth and apoptosis	TSG	Decreased expression

Tumor types	Animal models	References
Various tumor types	No pituitary tumors	Ogino et al. [101], 2005; Yoshino et al. [102], 2006
All tumor types	*Cdkn2c* KO mice display intermediated lobe and anterior pituitary adenomas	Morris et al. [76], 2005; Hossain et al. [105], 2009; Kirsch et al. [104], 2009
Pituitary carcinomas	No pituitary tumors	Korbonits et al. [95], 2002
Somatotrophinomas	A transcriptionally inactive *Creb* transgene in somatotrophs leads to dwarfism and somatotroph hypoplasia in mice	Bertherat et al. [106], 1995
Various tumor types, preferentially invasive adenomas	No pituitary tumors	Simpson et al. [107], 2002
1 NFPA	No pituitary tumors	Bellodi et al. [108], 2010
Resistant prolactinomas compared to non-resistant tumors	*Drd2* KO mice develop lactotroph hyperplasia which leads to PRL-secreting adenomas	Caccavelli et al. [109], 1994
NFPAs	No pituitary tumors	Chaidarun et al. [110], 1994
All tumor types	Transgenic *Fgfr2* mice show lactotroph hyperplasia	McCabe et al. [111], 2003
All tumor types	No pituitary tumors	McCabe et al. [111], 2003
Various tumor types	Transgenic *Fgfr2* mice die shortly after birth (no pituitary abnormalities)	Zhu et al. [112], 2007
ptd-FGFR4 in all tumor types	Transgenic *Fgfr4* mice develop lactotroph adenomas	Ezzat et al. [113], 2002
NFPAs, PRL- and GH-secreting adenomas	No pituitary tumors	Evans et al. [114], 2001
Gonadotroph adenomas	No pituitary tumors	Michaelis et al. [115], 2011

Table 1 . Continued

Gene name	MIM number	Location (Chr)	Function	TSG/ oncogene	Defect
GADD45G (GADD45-γ)	604949	9q22.2	Growth suppression and apoptosis	TSG	Decreased expression mainly due to promoter methylation
GHR	600946	5p13-p12	Transmembrane receptor that mediates GH action	–	Loss-of-function somatic mutation
GHRH	139190	20q11.23	Stimulates growth hormone secretion	–	Increased expression
GHRHR	139191	7p14.3	Transmembrane receptor that mediates GHRH action	–	Truncated alternatively spliced nonfunctioning receptor
GNAI2 (Gi2α)	139360	3p21.31	Inhibition of adenylate cyclase and calcium influx	Oncogene	Gain-of-function somatic mutations
GNAS (GNAS1)	139320	20q13.32	Alpha subunit of the stimulatory G protein that activates adenylate cyclase	Oncogene	Gain-of-function somatic mutations, loss of imprinting, increased expression in some somatotrophinomas
HDAC2	605164	6q21	Enzyme that deacetylates of lysine residues on the N-terminal region of the core histones	Oncogene	Decreased expression
HMGA1	600701	6p21.31	Variety of biological functions. Key role in growth and development	Oncogene	Overexpression
HMGA2	600698	12q14.3	Variety of biological functions. Key role in growth and development	Oncogene	Amplification and overexpression
HRAS (Ras)	190020	11p15.5	GDP/GTP binding protein that regulates cell division in response to growth factor stimulation	Oncogene	Gain-of-function somatic mutations
IKZF1	603023	7p12.2	DNA-binding protein with crucial functions in the hematopoietic system and in the development of the immune system	Oncogene	Dominant-negative truncated isoform (Ik6)
LAPTM4B	8q22.1	613296	Required for lysosome homeostasis, acidification and function	Oncogene	Increased expression
MAGEA3	300174	Xq28	Unknown function, but may play a role in embryonal development and tumor transformation or progression	Oncogene	Increased expression by promoter hypomethylation and histone acetylation in association with FGFR2 down-regulation
MEG3	605636	14q32.3	long non-coding RNA. Induces apoptosis and inhibits proliferation of tumor cells	TSG	Decreased expression
MEN1	613733	11q13.1	Transcriptional regulator	TSG	Loss-of-function somatic mutations and deletions, decreased expression

Tumor types	Animal models	References
NFPAs, somatotrophinomas, prolactinomas	No pituitary tumors	Zhang et al. [116], 2002; Bahar et al. [117], 2004
Somatotrophinomas	Homozygous *Ghr* KO mice exhibit retarded postnatal growth, proportionate dwarfism, decreased IGF1 levels, small pituitaries	Asa et al. [118], 2007
Somatotrophinomas	Transgenic *Ghrh*–expressing mice develop somatotroph hyperplasia which leads to GH-secreting adenomas	Thapar et al. [119], 1997
Somatotrophinomas	Homozygous mice for a spontaneous null mutation exhibit reduced growth, impaired GH synthesis and release	Hashimoto et al. [120], 1995
NFPAs, 1 corticotropinoma	*Gnai2* KO mice display growth retardation and die prematurely	Williamson et al. [121], 1994; Williamson et al. [122], 1995
Mainly somatotrophinomas (about 40%), some NFPAs, corticotropinomas	Cholera toxin-transgenic mice develop somatotroph hyperplasia	Vallar et al. [123], 1987; Landis et al. [52],1989; Tordjman et al. [124], 1993; Williamson et al. [121], 1994; Williamson et al. [122], 1995; Hamacher et al. [125], 1998; Hayward et al. [48], 2001; Riminucci et al. [126], 2002; Picard et al. [127], 2007
Corticotropinomas	*Hdac2* –/– mice show partially penetrant embryonic lethality	Bilodeau et al. [128], 2006
All tumor types	*Hmga1* transgenic mice develop pituitary adenomas secreting PRL and GH	De Martino et al. [83], 2009
Prolactinomas, NFPAs	*Hmga2* transgenic mice develop GH- and PRL-secreting adenomas	Finelli et al. [129], 2002; Pierantoni et al. [130], 2005
Pituitary carcinomas metastases, 1 aggressive prolactinoma, invasive adenomas	No pituitary tumors	Karga et al. [131], 1992; Cai et al. [132], 1994; Pei et al. [133], 1994; Lin et al. [134], 2009
Subset of adenomas	*Ikaros*-null mice had contraction of the pituitary corticomelanotroph population, reduced circulating adrenocorticotrophic hormone levels, and adrenal glucocorticoid insufficiency	Ezzat et al. [135], 2003
NFPAs and corticotropinomas	No animal models available	Morris et al. [76], 2005
Various tumor types	No animal models available	Zhu et al. [136], 2008
NFPAs	2 *Meg3* KO mouse models available. *Meg3* deletion results in perinatal death	Zhang et al. [116], 2002; Zhang et al. [137], 2003; Zhao et al. [138], 2005; Gejman et al. [139], 2008; Cheunsuchon et al. [140], 2011; Mezzomo et al. [141], 2012
All tumor types	Heterozygous *Men1* KO mice develop, among others, pituitary tumors	Zhuang et al. [142], 1997; Tanaka et al. [143], 1998; Wenbin et al. [144], 1999; Schmidt et al. [145],1999; McCabe et al. [146],1999

Table 1 . Continued

Gene name	MIM number	Location (Chr)	Function	TSG/ oncogene	Defect
MERTK (CMP-tk)	604705	2q13	Receptor tyrosine kinase that transduces signals from the extracellular matrix into the cytoplasm by binding to several ligands	Oncogene	Increased expression in corticotropinomas, decreased expression in prolactinomas
NR3C1 (GR, GCR)	138040	5q31.3	Nuclear receptor for glucocorticoids	–	Loss-of-function somatic mutation, LOH
ODC1 (ODC)	165640	2p25.1	Catalyzes the decarboxylation of ornithine to form putrescine	Oncogene	Increased expression in somatotrophinomas, decreased expression in corticotropinomas
PIK3CA	171834	3q26.32	Catalytic subunit of phosphatidylinositol 3-kinase, which coordinates a diverse range of cell functions such as proliferation, cell survival, degranulation, vesicular trafficking and cell migration	Oncogene	Gain-of-function somatic mutations and genetic amplification
PITX2	601542	4q25	Member of the bicoid-like homeobox transcription factor family, which is involved in the Wnt/ Dvl/β-catenin pathway	–	Increased expression
PLAGL1 (ZAC1)	603044	6q24.2	Zinc finger transcription factor that plays a role in pituitary development, differentiation, maturation and tumorigenesis	TSG	Decreased expression
POU1F1 (PIT1)	173110	3p11.2	Transcription factor with a key role in specification, expansion and survival of different pituitary cell types during anterior pituitary development	–	Increased expression
PRKCA (PKC α)	176960	17q24.2	Kinase that participates in growth factor- and hormone-mediated transmembrane signaling and cell proliferation	Oncogene	Increased expression, gain-of-function somatic mutations in invasive tumors
PTTG1 (PTTG, Securin)	604147	5q33.3	Cell cycle regulation and cell senescence	Oncogene	Increased expression, especially in corticotropinomas
PTTG1IP (PBF)	603784	21q22.3	Facilitates the nuclear translocation of PTTG1 and potentiates the transcriptional activation of FGF2 by PTTG1	Oncogene	Increased expression, especially in NFPAs
RB1 (pRB)	614041	13q14.2	Key regulator of entry into cell division	TSG	Decreased expression partly by promoter methylation
RHBDD3 (PTAG)	–	22q12.2	Pro-apoptotic mediator	TSG	Decreased expression partly due to promoter methylation
SMARCA4 (Brg1)	603254	19p13.2	Member of the SWI/SNF protein family with helicase and ATPase activities. Regulates gene transcription by altering chromatin structure	TSG	Decreased expression, altered subcellular localization
SSTR2	182452	17q25.1	G protein-coupled receptor for somatostatin	–	Decreased expression

Tumor types	Animal models	References
Corticotropinomas, prolactinomas	No pituitary tumors	Evans et al. [114], 2001
Corticotropinomas	Homozygous null mutants die at birth	Karl et al. [147], 1996; Huizenga et al. [148], 1998
Somatotrophinomas, corticotropinomas	Homozygous null embryos die prior to gastrulation	Evans et al. [114], 2001
Mutations in invasive corticotroph, lactotroph, plurihormonal and non-functioning adenomas, amplifications in all types of adenomas, both invasive and non-invasive	Homozygous KO or knock-in mutations of *Pik3ca* lead to embryonic death associated with growth retardation	Lin et al. [134], 2009
NFPAs	Transgenic overexpression of *Pitx2* in mouse pituitary increases gonadotroph population	Acunzo et al. [149], 2011
NFPAs	*Zac1* KO results in neonatal lethality in mice	Pagotto et al. [150], 2000; Noh et al. [151], 2009
GH-, PRL- and TSH-secreting adenomas	Homozygous *Pou1f1* KO mice for spontaneous mutations exhibit hypoplasia of the anterior pituitary cells resulting in deficiencies in GH, PRL, and TSH, dwarfism	Palmieri et al. [152], 2012
NFPAs	No pituitary tumors	Alvaro et al. [153], 1993
All tumor types	Targeted *Pttg* overexpression in mice results in focal pituitary hyperplasia with hormone hypersecretion; transgenic zebrafish overexpressing *zPttg* targeted to POMC cells show hypercortisolism and pituitary corticotroph expansion	Zhang et al. [154], 1999; McCabe et al. [111], 2003; Morris et al. [76], 2005; Salehi et al. [155], 2010
All tumor types	No animal models available	McCabe et al. [111], 2003
Aggressive adenomas	pRB+/- mice develop intermediate lobe hyperplasia which leads to ACTH-secreting adenomas	Simpson et al. [156], 2000; Ogino et al. [101], 2005; Yoshino et al. [102], 2006
Various tumor types	No animal models available	Bahar et al. [157], 2004
Corticotropinomas	*Brg1* -/- mice died during the periimplantation stage. Brg1 +/- mice are predisposed to exencephaly and various tumors (no pituitary)	Bilodeau et al. [128], 2006
Resistant somatotrophinomas compared to non-resistant tumors	No pituitary tumors	Corbella et al. [158], 2001

Table 1 . Continued

Gene name	MIM number	Location (Chr)	Function	TSG/ oncogene	Defect
THRB (TRβ)	190160	3p24.2	Nuclear receptor that mediates gene regulation by thyroid hormone	TSG	Loss-of-function somatic mutation and aberrant alternatively spliced variant
TP53 (P53)	191170	17p13.1	Involved in cell cycle regulation as a trans-activator that acts to negatively regulate cell division by controlling a set of genes required for this process	TSG	Loss-of-function somatic mutations
WIF1	605186	12q14.3	Secreted protein that binds WNT proteins and inhibits their activities	TSG	Decreased expression by promoter methylation

White background = Abnormal gene expression; light grey background = genetic defects; dark grey background = both genetic defects and abnormal expression. Gene names are shown accordingly to the HGNC (HUGO Gene Nomenclature Committee) approved gene symbol. Commonly used alternative symbols are shown in brackets. Data from nonvalidated microarray experiments are not reported in the table. MIM = Mendelian inheritance in man database; Chr = chromosome; TSG = tumor suppressor gene; SNP = single nucleotide polymorphism; KO = knock-out; LOH = loss of heterozygosity; NFPAs = nonfunctioning pituitary adenomas.

Somatic Alterations in Pituitary Adenomas

Pituitary adenomas are monoclonal in origin, expanding from molecular abnormalities in a single somatic cell [60]. These alterations, which include activation of proto-oncogenes, inactivation of tumor suppressor genes, and epimutations, confer the cell a growth advantage. The resulting genomic instability facilitates subsequent mutation accumulation [61].

The majority (about 95%) of pituitary adenomas occur sporadically. The most common somatic mutation is in the *GNAS* gene (gsp mutation), which occurs in around 40% of GH-secreting adenomas. Alterations in classical tumor suppressor genes such as *TP53* and *RB1* or oncogenes such as *HRAS* and *MYC* are only rarely identified, and exclusively in aggressive tumors or pituitary carcinomas [62] (table 1).

Numerous genes show altered expression in pituitary tumors (table 1), but it is still unknown whether they initiate the tumorigenic process or if they represent a later event. A number of alterations have been found to alter the expression of genes implicated in the regulation of the cell cycle, apoptosis, growth factors and their receptors, signal transduction pathways (in particular, the cAMP, MAPK and PI3K/Akt pathways [63]), specific hormonal factors, or other molecules with still unclear

Tumor types	Animal models	References
Thyrotropinomas	No pituitary tumors	Ando et al. [159], 2001; Ando et al. [160], 2001
1 atypical ACTH-secreting adenoma, 1 aggressive ACTH-secreting adenoma after radiotherapy, 1 atypical PRL-secreting adenoma and 1 pituitary carcinoma from the same patient, 2 ACTH-secreting carcinomas	*Tp53* KO mice are predisposed to develop pituitary adenomas, double *Tp53* and *Rb1* KO mice develop pituitary adenomas with a shorter latency than single *Tp53* and *Rb1* mutants	Tanizaki et al. [161], 2007; Kawashima et al. [162], 2009; Pinto et al. [163], 2011; Murakami et al. [164], 2011
Reduction of mRNA common to all tumor subtypes, reduction of protein levels predominantly limited to NFPAs	No pituitary tumors	Elston et al. [87], 2008

functions. Different mechanisms leading to abnormal gene expression have been described, such as allelic loss, gene amplification, and epigenetic changes [64]. Several tumor suppressor genes, in particular the inhibitors of cyclin-dependent kinase complexes, were shown to be frequently downregulated in pituitary tumors without presenting somatic mutations but as a consequence of epigenetic alterations like promoter hypermethylation or histone modifications [65, 66]. Moreover, abnormal miRNA expression profiles have been reported in recent years in pituitary adenomas [67] (table 2). Several animal models have been generated, which usually confirmed the functional role of these genes in the pathogenesis of pituitary tumors [62, 66].

To explain the predominance of benign versus malignant pituitary tumors, the occurrence of cellular senescence has been proposed [68]. Cellular senescence is an antiproliferative response triggered by DNA damage, chromosomal instability and aneuploidy, loss of tumor-suppressive signaling or oncogene activation, which leads to irreversible cell cycle arrest via activation of inhibitors of cell cycle progression, such as $p16^{INK4}$, $p19^{ARF}$, and $p21^{CIP1}$. Pituitary adenoma cells may undergo premature senescence in order to escape from the deleterious consequences that proliferative pressure of oncogenes, hormones and transformation factors could exert on their crucial physiological function on homeostasis control. More than 70% of GH-secreting adenomas overexpress the *PTTG* gene, which leads to aneuploidy and induction of senescence markers, including $p21^{CIP1}$ and senescence-associated β-galactosidase. In contrast, $p21^{CIP1}$ is weakly expressed in normal pituitary tissue and undetectable in pituitary carcinomas [69].

MicroRNAs in Pituitary Adenomas

MicroRNAs (miRNAs) are small (approximately 22 nucleotides) noncoding RNA molecules involved in posttranscriptional regulation of gene expression [70]. They regulate about 30% of human genes, constituting a major class of molecular regulators. The mature miRNA, as part of a complex called RNA-induced silencing complex (RISC), either binds to a perfectly complementary sequence in the mRNA strand resulting in degradation of the mRNA by RISC, or binds to a partially complementary mRNA sequence and this induces translational repression of the target mRNA [71].

miRNAs have been implicated in the regulation of many cellular processes, including cell proliferation, apoptosis, cell adhesion and metabolism. Thus, alterations in miRNA expression can potentially be involved in the development of many diseases, including human neoplasias. miRNAs can act either as activators or inhibitors of carcinogenesis, being called oncomiRs and tumor suppressor miRNAs, respectively.

miRNA expression has been associated with pituitary tumor type, characteristics (size, invasion) and response to therapy. miRNAs have also been involved in the regulation of some genes associated with the pathogenesis of pituitary adenomas (table 2) [67].

Several different miRNAs have been shown to be differently expressed in the various subtypes of pituitary adenomas in comparison with normal pituitary and also in adenomas in comparison with carcinomas (table 2) [67, 72]. Degli Uberti's group observed that miR-15a and miR-16–1 were downregulated in GH- and PRL-producing adenomas in comparison with normal pituitary and the expression of these miRNAs was inversely correlated with tumor size [72]. Moreover, some miRNAs targets were evaluated individually in different studies:

- miR-16–1 predicted target arginyl-tRNA synthetase (RARS) mRNA levels inversely correlated with miR-16-1 expression and tumor size in both somatotrophinomas and prolactinomas [67, 72].
- The expression of miR let-7 inversely correlated with mRNA levels of *high-mobility group A protein 2 (HMGA2)*, a gene known to cause pituitary adenomas in transgenic mice, suggesting that the reduction of this miRNA may be responsible for the higher expression of HMGA2 in more invasive tumors [67]. Moreover, functional studies showed that transfection of this miRNA reduced the proliferation of GH3 cells, indicating that it might act as a tumor suppressor miRNA.

Table 2. Studies addressing microRNAs expression in pituitary adenomas

Study	Tumor type	Aberrant microRNAs expression	Affected gene(s)	Clinical correlation
Bottoni et al. [165], 2005	10 GH and 10 PRL	Underexpression of miR-15a and miR-16-1 in adenomas × NP	*RARS*	Inverse correlation with tumor size
Bottoni et al. [166], 2007	17 NFPA, 5 PRL, 4 ACTH and 6 GH	30 miRNAs differently expressed between adenomas and NP. 29 miRNAs predict tumor type	–	6 miRNAs correlated with tumor size in NFPA. 3 miRNAs up- and 3 down-regulated in NFPA treated with DA in comparison with non-treated ones
Qian et al. [167], 2009	98 adenomas of all types	Let-7 overexpression in tumors with low HMGA2 expression	*HMGA2*	
Amaral et al. [168], 2009	14 ACTH	Underexpression of miR-145, miR-21, miR-141, miR-150, miR-15a, miR-16, miR-143 and let-7a in adenomas × NP	–	miR-141 levels directly correlated with chance of disease recurrence
Stilling et al. [169], 2010	8 ACTH 2 ACTH carcinomas	188 miRNAs over- and 160 under-expressed in ACTH × NP 98 miRNAs differently expressed in adenoma × carcinoma	–	–
Butz et al. [170], 2010*	27 NFPA and 15 GH	miR-20a, miR-128a and miR-516-3p overexpressed in NFPA. miR-93 and miR-155 overexpressed in GH and NFPA	*WEE1*	–
Mao et al. [171], 2010	21 GH	23 miRNAs over- and 29 under-expressed in GH × NP	–	9 miRNAs differently expressed in micro × macroadenomas 13 differently expressed in lanreotide treated × surgery alone 7 differently expressed in lanreotide responders × non responders
Butz et al. [172], 2011	8 NFPA	70 miRNAs over- and 92 under-expressed in NFPA × NP	–	18 miRNAs inversely correlated with tumor size
Palmieri et al. [173], 2011*	14 PRL, 9 GH and 18 NFPA	miR-15, miR-16, miR26a, miR-196ab and Let-7a underexpressed in adenomas × NP	*HMGA1* and *HMGA2*	–
D'Ángelo et al. [174], 2012*	18 GH	miR34b, miR-326, miR-374b, miR-432, miR-548c-3p, miR-570, miR-603 and miR-633 under-expressed, and miR-320 over-expressed in adenomas × NP	*HMGA1*, *HMGA2* and *E2F1*	–
Palumbo et al. [74], 2012*	12 GH	5 miRNAs over- and 12 underexpressed in GH × NP	*PTEN* and *BMI1*	–
Trivellin et al. [73], 2012*	10 GH and 7 NFPA	miR-107 overexpressed in tumors × NP AIP expression inhibited by miR-107	*AIP*	–

GH = Somatotrophinoma; PRL = prolactinoma; NFPA = nonfunctioning pituitary adenoma; ACTH = corticotropinoma; NP = normal pituitary tissue; DA = dopamine agonist; × = versus. * Studies where functional validation was done.

- Several miRNAs (miR-135a, miR-140–5p, miR-582–3p, miR-582–2p and miR-938), known to inhibit Smad3, a protein underexpressed in NFPAs, were shown to be significantly overexpressed in NFPAs [67].
- Another group of miRNAs were suggested to influence the expression of cell cycle inhibitor *Wee1*. miR-155, miR-20a, miR-93, miR-128a and miR-516–3p were significantly overexpressed in NFPAs and GH-secreting adenomas compared to NP.

Functional studies proved that overexpression of miR-128a, miR-516–3p and miR-155 was associated with the reduced expression of Wee1 kinase, thereby indicating a role of these miRNAs in pituitary tumorigenesis [67].

- miR-107 is an interesting miRNA as it has been shown to have both tumor suppressor miR and oncomiR properties, depending on the tissue type. In pituitary adenomas it is upregulated in comparison with normal pituitary [73], however, it inhibits cell proliferation in human neuroblastoma SH-SY5Y and rat pituitary GH3 cell lines. *AIP* is a functional target of miR-107 as miR-107 inhibits human AIP expression [73]; therefore, miR-107 unlikely exerts its tumor suppressor role via *AIP*.
- A recent study using somatotroph hyperplasia samples showed that miR-26b was overexpressed and miR-128 was underexpressed compared to normal pituitary [74]. Molecular analysis revealed that these miRNAs regulate the expression levels of *PTEN* and *BMI1*, genes known to be involved in the regulation of cell proliferation.

Conclusion

Tumorigenesis is influenced by inherited and acquired mutations as well as epigenetic changes. An important feature of pituitary adenomas is that they are relatively common but rarely cause clinically relevant disease and exceedingly rarely develop into a metastatic carcinoma. One of the suggested mechanisms of lack of malignant transformation is the development of cellular senescence. However, the regulating factors influencing these processes in the vast majority of sporadic adenoma cases are unknown. On the other hand, understanding the tumorigenic process in the rare familial adenomas could result in better diagnostic and treatment options for both familial and sporadic cases.

References

1 Ezzat S, Asa SL, Couldwell WT, Barr CE, Dodge WE, Vance ML, McCutcheon IE: The prevalence of pituitary adenomas: a systematic review. Cancer 2004;101:613–619.

2 Daly AF, Rixhon M, Adam C, Dempegioti A, Tichomirowa MA, Beckers A: High prevalence of pituitary adenomas: a cross-sectional study in the province of Liege, Belgium. J Clin Endocrinol Metab 2006;91:4769–4775.

3 Fernandez A, Karavitaki N, Wass JA: Prevalence of pituitary adenomas: a community-based, cross-sectional study in Banbury (Oxfordshire, UK). Clin Endocrinol (Oxf) 2010;72:377–382.

4 Couldwell WT, Cannon-Albright L: A heritable predisposition to pituitary tumors. Pituitary 2010; 13:130–137.

5 Wildi-Runge S, Bahubeshi A, Carret A, Crevier L, Robitaille Y, Kovacs K, Horvath E, Schenck S, Foulkes WD, Deal C: New phenotype in the familial DICER1 tumor syndrome: pituitary blastoma presenting at age 9 months. Endocrine Rev 2011;32:P1–P777.

6 Denes J, Swords FM, Xekouki P, Kumar AV, Maher ER, Ferscht N, Grieve J, Baldeweg SE, Stratakis CA, Korbonits M: Familial pituitary adenoma and paraganglioma syndrome – a novel type of multiple endocrine neoplasia. Endocrine Rev 2012;33:OR41–OR42.

7 Brahma A, Heyburn P, Swords F: Familial prolactinoma occurring in association with SDHB mutation positive paraganglioma. Endocrine Abstr 2009;19:239.
8 Xekouki P, Pacak K, Almeida M, Wassif CA, Rustin P, Nesterova M, de la Luz SM, Matro J, Ball E, Azevedo M, Horvath A, Lyssikatos C, Quezado M, Patronas N, Ferrando B, Pasini B, Lytras A, Tolis G, Stratakis CA: Succinate dehydrogenase (SDH) D subunit (SDHD) inactivation in a growth-hormone-producing pituitary tumor: a new association for SDH? J Clin Endocrinol Metab 2012; 97:E357–E366.
9 Varsavsky M, Sebastian-Ochoa A, Torres VE: Coexistence of a pituitary macroadenoma and multicentric paraganglioma: a strange coincidence. Endocrinol Nutr 2012, epub ahead of print.
10 Korbonits M, Storr H, Kumar AV: Familial pituitary adenomas. Who should be tested for AIP mutations? Clin Endocrinol (Oxf) 2012;77:3513–3556.
11 Agarwal SK, Mateo CM, Marx SJ: Rare germline mutations in cyclin-dependent kinase inhibitor genes in multiple endocrine neoplasia type 1 and related states. J Clin Endocrinol Metab 2009;94: 1826–1834.
12 Chahal HS, Stals K, Unterlander M, Balding DJ, Thomas MG, Kumar AV, Besser GM, Atkinson AB, Morrison PJ, Howlett TA, Levy MJ, Orme SM, Akker SA, Abel RL, Grossman AB, Burger J, Ellard S, Korbonits M: AIP mutation in pituitary adenomas in the 18th century and today. N Eng J Med 2011; 364:43–50.
13 Igreja S, Chahal HS, King P, Bolger GB, Srirangalingam U, Guasti L, Chapple JP, Trivellin G, Gueorguiev M, Guegan K, Stals K, Khoo B, Kumar AV, Ellard S, Grossman AB, Korbonits M: Characterization of aryl hydrocarbon receptor interacting protein (AIP) mutations in familial isolated pituitary adenoma families. Hum Mutat 2010;31:950–960.
14 Occhi G, Jaffrain Rea ML, Trivellin G, Albiger N, Ceccato F, De ME, Angelini M, Ferasin S, Beckers A, Mantero F, Scaroni C: The R304X mutation of the aryl hydrocarbon receptor interacting protein gene in familial isolated pituitary adenomas: mutational hot-spot or founder effect? J Endocrinol Invest 2010;33:800–805.
15 Chahal HS, Chapple JP, Frohman LA, Grossman AB, Korbonits M: Clinical, genetic and molecular characterization of patients with familial isolated pituitary adenomas (FIPA). Trends Endocrinol Metab 2010;21:419–427.
16 Daly AF, Tichomirowa MA, Petrossians P, et al: Clinical characteristics and therapeutic responses in patients with germ-line AIP mutations and pituitary adenomas: an international collaborative study. J Clin Endocrinol Metab 2010;95:E373–E383.
17 Tichomirowa MA, Barlier A, Daly AF, et al: High prevalence of AIP gene mutations following focused screening in young patients with sporadic pituitary macroadenomas. Eur J Endocrinol 2011; 165:509–515.
18 Leontiou CA, Gueorguiev M, van der SJ, et al: The role of the aryl hydrocarbon receptor-interacting protein gene in familial and sporadic pituitary adenomas. J Clin Endocrinol Metab 2008;93:2390–2401.
19 Chahal HS, Trivellin G, Leontiou CA, Alband N, Fowkes RC, Tahir A, Igreja SC, Chapple JP, Jordan S, Lupp A, Schulz S, Ansorge O, Karavitaki N, Carlsen E, Wass JAH, Grossman AB, Korbonits M: Somatostatin analogues modulate AIP in somatotroph adenomas – the role of the ZAC1 pathway. J Clin Endocrinol Metab 2012;97:E14111–E14420.
20 Kasuki Jomori de PL, Vieira NL, Armondi Wildemberg LE, Gasparetto EL, Marcondes J, de Almeida NB, Takiya CM, Gadelha MR: Low aryl hydrocarbon receptor-interacting protein expression is a better marker of invasiveness in somatotropinomas than ki-67 and p53. Neuroendocrinology 2011;94: 39–48.
21 Kasuki L, Vieira NL, Wildemberg LE, Colli LM, de CM, Takiya CM, Gadelha MR: AIP expression in sporadic somatotropinomas is a predictor of the response to octreotide LAR therapy independent of SSTR2 expression. Endocr Relat Cancer 2012; 19:L25–L29.
22 Hernández-Ramírez LC, Korbonits M: Familial pituitary adenomas; in Laws ER, Ezzat S, Asa SL, Rio LM, Michel L, Knutzen R: Pituitary Disorders: Diagnosis and Management. John Wiley & Sons, Ltd., 2013, pp 87–110.
23 Korbonits M: Tracing back a gene's influence. Endocrine Abstr 2012;29:S22.2.
24 Dull AB, Carlson DB, Petrulis JR, Perdew GH: Characterization of the phosphorylation status of the hepatitis B virus X-associated protein 2. Arch Biochem Biophys 2002;406:209–221.
25 Linnert M, Haupt K, Lin YJ, Kissing S, Paschke AK, Fischer G, Weiwad M, Lucke C: NMR assignments of the FKBP-type PPIase domain of the human aryl-hydrocarbon receptor-interacting protein (AIP). Biomol NMR Assign 2012;6:209–212.
26 Trivellin G, Korbonits M: AIP and its interacting partners. J Endocrinol 2011;210:137–155.

27 Schulke JP, Wochnik GM, Lang-Rollin I, Gassen NC, Knapp RT, Berning B, Yassouridis A, Rein T: Differential impact of tetratricopeptide repeat proteins on the steroid hormone receptors. PLoS One 2010;5:e11717.
28 Petrulis JR, Perdew GH: The role of chaperone proteins in the aryl hydrocarbon receptor core complex. Chem Biol Interact 2002;141:25–40.
29 Jaffrain-Rea ML, Angelini M, Gargano D, et al: Expression of aryl hydrocarbon receptor (AHR) and AHR-interacting protein in pituitary adenomas: pathological and clinical implications. Endocr Relat Cancer 2009;16:1029–1043.
30 Vierimaa O, Georgitsi M, Lehtonen R, Vahteristo P, Kokko A, Raitila A, Tuppurainen K, Ebeling TM, Salmela PI, Paschke R, Gundogdu S, De ME, Makinen MJ, Launonen V, Karhu A, Aaltonen LA: Pituitary adenoma predisposition caused by germline mutations in the AIP gene. Science 2006;312:1228–1230.
31 Heliovaara E, Raitila A, Launonen V, Paetau A, Arola J, Lehtonen H, Sane T, Weil RJ, Vierimaa O, Salmela P, Tuppurainen K, Makinen M, Aaltonen LA, Karhu A: The expression of AIP-related molecules in elucidation of cellular pathways in pituitary adenomas. Am J Pathol 2009;175:2501–2507.
32 Lin BC, Sullivan R, Lee Y, Moran S, Glover E, Bradfield CA: Deletion of the aryl hydrocarbon receptor-associated protein 9 leads to cardiac malformation and embryonic lethality. J Biol Chem 2007;282: 35924–35932.
33 Kang BH, Xia F, Pop R, Dohi T, Socolovsky M, Altieri DC: Developmental control of apoptosis by the immunophilin aryl hydrocarbon receptor-interacting protein (AIP) involves mitochondrial import of survivin. J Biol Chem 2011;286:16758–16767.
34 Raitila A, Lehtonen HJ, Arola J, Heliovaara E, Ahlsten M, Georgitsi M, Jalanko A, Paetau A, Aaltonen LA, Karhu A: Mice with inactivation of aryl hydrocarbon receptor-interacting protein (AIP) display complete penetrance of pituitary adenomas with aberrant ARNT expression. Am J Pathol 2010;177: 1969–1976.
35 McCune DJ: Osteitis fibrosa cystica: the case of a nine year old girl who also exhibits precocious puberty, multiple pigmentation of the skin and hyperthyroidism. Am J Dis Child 1936;52:743–744.
36 Albright F, Butler AM, Hampton AO, Smith P: Syndrome characterized by osteitis fibrosa disseminata, areas of pigmentation and endocrine dysfunction, with precocious puberty in females – report of five cases. N Eng J Med 1937;216:727–746.
37 Dumitrescu CE, Collins MT: McCune-Albright syndrome. Orphanet J Rare Dis 2008;3:12.
38 Lumbroso S, Paris F, Sultan C: Activating Gsalpha mutations: analysis of 113 patients with signs of McCune-Albright syndrome – a European Collaborative Study. J Clin Endocrinol Metab 2004;89:2107–2113.
39 Shah KN: The diagnostic and clinical significance of cafe-au-lait macules. Pediatr Clin N Am 2010;57: 1131–1153.
40 Weinstein LS, Shenker A, Gejman PV, Merino MJ, Friedman E, Spiegel AM: Activating mutations of the stimulatory G protein in the McCune-Albright syndrome. N Eng J Med 1991;325:1688–1695.
41 Happle R: The McCune-Albright syndrome: a lethal gene surviving by mosaicism. Clin Genet 1986; 29:321–324.
42 Weinstein LS, Liu J, Sakamoto A, Xie T, Chen M: GNAS: normal and abnormal functions. Endocrinology 2004;145:5459–5464.
43 Bianco P, Kuznetsov SA, Riminucci M, Fisher LW, Spiegel AM, Robey PG: Reproduction of human fibrous dysplasia of bone in immunocompromised mice by transplanted mosaics of normal and Gsalpha-mutated skeletal progenitor cells. J Clin Invest 1998;101:1737–1744.
44 Hayward BE, Moran V, Strain L, Bonthron DT: Bidirectional imprinting of a single gene: GNAS1 encodes maternally, paternally, and biallelically derived proteins. Proc Natl Acad Sci USA 1998;95: 15475–15480.
45 Hayward BE, Bonthron DT: An imprinted antisense transcript at the human GNAS1 locus. Hum Mol Genet 2000;9:835–841.
46 Weinstein LS, Yu S, Warner DR, Liu J: Endocrine manifestations of stimulatory G protein alpha-subunit mutations and the role of genomic imprinting. Endocrine Rev 2001;22:675–705.
47 Weinstein LS: The stimulatory G protein alpha-subunit gene: mutations and imprinting lead to complex phenotypes. J Clin Endocrinol Metab 2001;86:4622–4626.
48 Hayward BE, Barlier A, Korbonits M, Grossman AB, Jacquet P, Enjalbert A, Bonthron DT: Imprinting of the G(s)alpha gene GNAS1 in the pathogenesis of acromegaly. J Clin Invest 2001;107:R31–R36.
49 Mantovani G, Bondioni S, Lania AG, Corbetta S, de SL, Cappa M, Di BE, Chanson P, Beck-Peccoz P, Spada A: Parental origin of Gsalpha mutations in the McCune-Albright syndrome and in isolated endocrine tumors. J Clin Endocrinol Metab 2004;89: 3007–3009.
50 Mantovani G, Ballare E, Giammona E, Beck-Peccoz P, Spada A: The gsalpha gene: predominant maternal origin of transcription in human thyroid gland and gonads. J Clin Endocrinol Metab 2002;87: 4736–4740.

51 Lyons J, Landis CA, Harsh G, Vallar L, Grunewald K, Feichtinger H, Duh QY, Clark OH, Kawasaki E, Bourne HR: Two G protein oncogenes in human endocrine tumors. Science 1990;249:655–659.

52 Landis CA, Masters SB, Spada A, Pace AM, Bourne HR, Vallar L: GTPase inhibiting mutations activate the alpha chain of Gs and stimulate adenylyl cyclase in human pituitary tumours. Nature 1989;340: 692–696.

53 Freda PU, Chung WK, Matsuoka N, Walsh JE, Kanibir MN, Kleinman G, Wang Y, Bruce JN, Post KD: Analysis of GNAS mutations in 60 growth hormone secreting pituitary tumors: correlation with clinical and pathological characteristics and surgical outcome based on highly sensitive GH and IGF-I criteria for remission. Pituitary 2007;10:275–282.

54 Akintoye SO, Chebli C, Booher S, Feuillan P, Kushner H, Leroith D, Cherman N, Bianco P, Wientroub S, Robey PG, Collins MT: Characterization of gsp-mediated growth hormone excess in the context of McCune-Albright syndrome. J Clin Endocrinol Metab 2002;87:5104–5112.

55 Vortmeyer AO, Glasker S, Mehta GU, Abu-Asab MS, Smith JH, Zhuang Z, Collins MT, Oldfield EH: Somatic GNAS mutation causes widespread and diffuse pituitary disease in acromegalic patients with McCune-Albright syndrome. J Clin Endocrinol Metab 2012;97:2404–2413.

56 Galland F, Kamenicky P, Affres H, Reznik Y, Pontvert D, Le BY, Young J, Chanson P: McCune-Albright syndrome and acromegaly: effects of hypothalamopituitary radiotherapy and/or pegvisomant in somatostatin analog-resistant patients. J Clin Endocrinol Metab 2006;91:4957–4961.

57 De SC, Lala R, Matarazzo P, Balsamo A, Bergamaschi R, Cappa M, Cisternino M, de SV, Lucci M, Franzese A, Ghizzoni L, Pasquino AM, Segni M, Rigon F, Saggese G, Bertelloni S, Buzi F: McCune-Albright syndrome: a longitudinal clinical study of 32 patients. J Pediatr Endocrinol Metab 1999;12: 817–826.

58 Riminucci M, Collins MT, Fedarko NS, Cherman N, Corsi A, White KE, Waguespack S, Gupta A, Hannon T, Econs MJ, Bianco P, Gehron RP: FGF-23 in fibrous dysplasia of bone and its relationship to renal phosphate wasting. J Clin Invest 2003;112: 683–692.

59 Collins MT, Singer FR, Eugster E: McCune-Albright syndrome and the extraskeletal manifestations of fibrous dysplasia. Orphanet J Rare Dis 2012;7(suppl 1):S4.

60 Herman V, Fagin J, Gonsky R, Kovacs K, Melmed S: Clonal origin of pituitary adenomas. J Clin Endocrinol Metab 1990;71:1427–1433.

61 Peltomaki P: Mutations and epimutations in the origin of cancer. Exp Cell Res 2012;318:299–310.

62 Lania A, Mantovani G, Spada A: Genetics of pituitary tumors: Focus on G-protein mutations. Exp Biol Med (Maywood) 2003;228:1004–1017.

63 Cuny T, Gerard C, Saveanu A, Barlier A, Enjalbert A: Physiopathology of somatolactotroph cells: from transduction mechanisms to cotargeting therapy. Ann NY Acad Sci 2011;1220:60–70.

64 Vandeva S, Jaffrain-Rea ML, Daly AF, Tichomirowa M, Zacharieva S, Beckers A: The genetics of pituitary adenomas. Best Pract Res Clin Endocrinol Metab 2010;24:461–476.

65 Musat M, Vax VV, Borboli N, Gueorguiev M, Bonner S, Korbonits M, Grossman AB: Cell cycle dysregulation in pituitary oncogenesis. Front Horm Res 2004;32:34–62.

66 Quereda V, Malumbres M: Cell cycle control of pituitary development and disease. J Mol Endocrinol 2009;42:75–86.

67 Sivapragasam M, Rotondo F, Lloyd RV, Scheithauer BW, Cusimano M, Syro LV, Kovacs K: MicroRNAs in the human pituitary. Endocr Pathol 2011;22:134–143.

68 Chesnokova V, Zonis S, Ben-Shlomo A, Wawrowsky K, Melmed S: Molecular mechanisms of pituitary adenoma senescence. Front Horm Res 2010; 38:7–14.

69 Chesnokova V, Melmed S: Pituitary senescence: the evolving role of PTTG. Mol Cell Endocrinol 2010; 326:55–59.

70 Taft RJ, Pang KC, Mercer TR, Dinger M, Mattick JS: Non-coding RNAs: regulators of disease. J Pathol 2010;220:126–139.

71 Lee RC, Feinbaum RL, Ambros V: The *C. elegans* heterochronic gene lin-4 encodes small RNAs with antisense complementarity to lin-14. Cell 1993;75: 843–854.

72 Zatelli MC, Degli Uberti EC: MicroRNAs and possible role in pituitary adenoma. Semin Reprod Med 2008;26:453–460.

73 Trivellin G, Butz H, Delhove J, Igreja S, Chahal HS, Zivkovic V, McKay TR, Patocs A, Grossman AB, Korbonits M: MicroRNA miR-107 is overexpressed in pituitary adenomas and in vitro inhibits the expression of aryl hydrocarbon receptor-interacting protein (AIP). Am J Physiol Endocrinol Metab 2012;303:E708–E719.

74 Palumbo T, Faucz FR, Azevedo M, Xekouki P, Iliopoulos D, Stratakis CA: Functional screen analysis reveals miR-26b and miR-128 as central regulators of pituitary somatomammotrophic tumor growth through activation of the PTEN-AKT pathway. Oncogene 2012, epub ahead of print.

75 Musat M, Korbonits M, Kola B, Borboli N, Hanson MR, Nanzer AM, Grigson J, Jordan S, Morris DG, Gueorguiev M, Coculescu M, Basu S, Grossman AB: Enhanced protein kinase B/Akt signalling in pituitary tumours. Endocr Relat Cancer 2005;12:423–433.

76 Morris DG, Musat M, Czirjak S, Hanzely Z, Lillington DM, Korbonits M, Grossman AB: Differential gene expression in pituitary adenomas by oligonucleotide array analysis. Eur J Endocrinol 2005;153: 143–151.
77 Sanchez-Beato M, Sanchez E, Gonzalez-Carrero J, Morente M, Diez A, Sanchez-Verde L, Martin MC, Cigudosa JC, Vidal M, Piris MA: Variability in the expression of polycomb proteins in different normal and tumoral tissues. A pilot study using tissue microarrays. Mod Pathol 2006;19:684–694.
78 Westerman BA, Blom M, Tanger E, van DV, Song JY, van SM, Gadiot J, Cornelissen-Steijger P, Zevenhoven J, Prosser HM, Uren A, Aronica E, van LM: GFAP-Cre-mediated transgenic activation of Bmi1 results in pituitary tumors. PLoS One 2012; 7:e35943.
79 Paez-Pereda M, Giacomini D, Refojo D, Nagashima AC, Hopfner U, Grubler Y, Chervin A, Goldberg V, Goya R, Hentges ST, Low MJ, Holsboer F, Stalla GK, Arzt E: Involvement of bone morphogenetic protein 4 (BMP-4) in pituitary prolactinoma pathogenesis through a Smad/estrogen receptor crosstalk. Proc Natl Acad Sci USA 2003;100:1034–1039.
80 Turner HE, Nagy Z, Sullivan N, Esiri MM, Wass JA: Expression analysis of cyclins in pituitary adenomas and the normal pituitary gland. Clin Endocrinol (Oxf) 2000;53:337–344.
81 Nakabayashi H, Sunada I, Hara M: Immunohistochemical analyses of cell cycle-related proteins, apoptosis, and proliferation in pituitary adenomas. J Histochem Cytochem 2001;49:1193–1194.
82 Wierinckx A, Auger C, Devauchelle P, Reynaud A, Chevallier P, Jan M, Perrin G, Fevre-Montange M, Rey C, Figarella-Branger D, Raverot G, Belin MF, Lachuer J, Trouillas J: A diagnostic marker set for invasion, proliferation, and aggressiveness of prolactin pituitary tumors. Endocr Relat Cancer 2007; 14:887–900.
83 De MI, Visone R, Wierinckx A, Palmieri D, Ferraro A, Cappabianca P, Chiappetta G, Forzati F, Lombardi G, Colao A, Trouillas J, Fedele M, Fusco A: HMGA proteins up-regulate CCNB2 gene in mouse and human pituitary adenomas. Cancer Res 2009; 69:1844–1850.
84 Hibberts NA, Simpson DJ, Bicknell JE, Broome JC, Hoban PR, Clayton RN, Farrell WE: Analysis of cyclin D1 (CCND1) allelic imbalance and overexpression in sporadic human pituitary tumors. Clin Cancer Res 1999;5:2133–2139.
85 Jordan S, Lidhar K, Korbonits M, Lowe DG, Grossman AB: Cyclin D and cyclin E expression in normal and adenomatous pituitary. Eur J Endocrinol 2000;143:R1–R6.
86 Simpson DJ, Frost SJ, Bicknell JE, Broome JC, McNicol AM, Clayton RN, Farrell WE: Aberrant expression of G(1)/S regulators is a frequent event in sporadic pituitary adenomas. Carcinogenesis 2001; 22:1149–1154.
87 Elston MS, Gill AJ, Conaglen JV, Clarkson A, Shaw JM, Law AJ, Cook RJ, Little NS, Clifton-Bligh RJ, Robinson BG, McDonald KL: Wnt pathway inhibitors are strongly down-regulated in pituitary tumors. Endocrinology 2008;149:1235–1242.
88 Neto AG, McCutcheon IE, Vang R, Spencer ML, Zhang W, Fuller GN: Elevated expression of p21 (WAF1/Cip1) in hormonally active pituitary adenomas. Ann Diagn Pathol 2005;9:6–10.
89 Qian X, Jin L, Grande JP, Lloyd RV: Transforming growth factor-beta and p27 expression in pituitary cells. Endocrinology 1996;137:3051–3060.
90 Lloyd RV, Jin L, Qian X, Kulig E: Aberrant p27kip1 expression in endocrine and other tumors. Am J Pathol 1997;150:401–407.
91 Bamberger CM, Fehn M, Bamberger AM, Ludecke DK, Beil FU, Saeger W, Schulte HM: Reduced expression levels of the cell-cycle inhibitor p27Kip1 in human pituitary adenomas. Eur J Endocrinol 1999; 140:250–255.
92 Jin L, Qian X, Kulig E, Sanno N, Scheithauer BW, Kovacs K, Young WF Jr, Lloyd RV: Transforming growth factor-beta, transforming growth factor-beta receptor II, and p27Kip1 expression in nontumorous and neoplastic human pituitaries. Am J Pathol 1997;151:509–519.
93 Lidhar K, Korbonits M, Jordan S, Khalimova Z, Kaltsas G, Lu X, Clayton RN, Jenkins PJ, Monson JP, Besser GM, Lowe DG, Grossman AB: Low expression of the cell cycle inhibitor p27Kip1 in normal corticotroph cells, corticotroph tumors, and malignant pituitary tumors. J Clin Endocrinol Metab 1999;84:3823–3830.
94 Komatsubara K, Tahara S, Umeoka K, Sanno N, Teramoto A, Osamura RY: Immunohistochemical analysis of p27 (Kip1) in human pituitary glands and in various types of pituitary adenomas. Endocr Pathol 2001;12:181–188.
95 Korbonits M, Chahal HS, Kaltsas G, Jordan S, Urmanova Y, Khalimova Z, Harris PE, Farrell WE, Claret FX, Grossman AB: Expression of phosphorylated p27(Kip1) protein and Jun activation domain-binding protein 1 in human pituitary tumors. J Clin Endocrinol Metab 2002;87:2635–2643.
96 Woloschak M, Yu A, Xiao J, Post KD: Frequent loss of the P16INK4a gene product in human pituitary tumors. Cancer Res 1996;56:2493–2496.

97 Jaffrain-Rea ML, Ferretti E, Toniato E, Cannita K, Santoro A, Di SD, Ricevuto E, Maroder M, Tamburrano G, Cantore G, Gulino A, Martinotti S: p16 (INK4a, MTS-1) gene polymorphism and methylation status in human pituitary tumours. Clin Endocrinol (Oxf) 1999;51:317–325.
98 Simpson DJ, Bicknell JE, McNicol AM, Clayton RN, Farrell WE: Hypermethylation of the p16/CDKN2A/MTSI gene and loss of protein expression is associated with nonfunctional pituitary adenomas but not somatotrophinomas. Genes Chromosomes Cancer 1999;24:328–336.
99 Ruebel KH, Jin L, Zhang S, Scheithauer BW, Lloyd RV: Inactivation of the p16 gene in human pituitary nonfunctioning tumors by hypermethylation is more common in null cell adenomas. Endocr Pathol 2001;12:281–289.
100 Seemann N, Kuhn D, Wrocklage C, Keyvani K, Hackl W, Buchfelder M, Fahlbusch R, Paulus W: CDKN2A/p16 inactivation is related to pituitary adenoma type and size. J Pathol 2001;193:491–497.
101 Ogino A, Yoshino A, Katayama Y, Watanabe T, Ota T, Komine C, Yokoyama T, Fukushima T: The p15(INK4b)/p16(INK4a)/RB1 pathway is frequently deregulated in human pituitary adenomas. J Neuropathol Exp Neurol 2005;64:398–403.
102 Yoshino A, Katayama Y, Ogino A, Watanabe T, Yachi K, Ohta T, Komine C, Yokoyama T, Fukushima T: Promoter hypermethylation profile of cell cycle regulator genes in pituitary adenomas. J Neurooncol 2007;83:153–162.
103 Machiavelli G, Cotignola J, Danilowicz K, Carbonara C, Paes de LA, Basso A, Bruno OD, Szijan I: Expression of p16(INK4A) gene in human pituitary tumours. Pituitary 2008;11:71–75.
104 Kirsch M, Morz M, Pinzer T, Schackert HK, Schackert G: Frequent loss of the CDKN2C (p18INK4c) gene product in pituitary adenomas. Genes Chromosomes Cancer 2009;48:143–154.
105 Hossain MG, Iwata T, Mizusawa N, Qian ZR, Shima SW, Okutsu T, Yamada S, Sano T, Yoshimoto K: Expression of p18(INK4C) is down-regulated in human pituitary adenomas. Endocr Pathol 2009; 20:114–121.
106 Bertherat J, Chanson P, Montminy M: The cyclic adenosine 3′,5′-monophosphate-responsive factor CREB is constitutively activated in human somatotroph adenomas. Mol Endocrinol 1995;9:777–783.
107 Simpson DJ, Clayton RN, Farrell WE: Preferential loss of death associated protein kinase expression in invasive pituitary tumours is associated with either CpG island methylation or homozygous deletion. Oncogene 2002;21:1217–1224.
108 Bellodi C, Krasnykh O, Haynes N, Theodoropoulou M, Peng G, Montanaro L, Ruggero D: Loss of function of the tumor suppressor DKC1 perturbs p27 translation control and contributes to pituitary tumorigenesis. Cancer Res 2010;70:6026–6035.
109 Caccavelli L, Feron F, Morange I, Rouer E, Benarous R, Dewailly D, Jaquet P, Kordon C, Enjalbert A: Decreased expression of the two D2 dopamine receptor isoforms in bromocriptine-resistant prolactinomas. Neuroendocrinology 1994;60:314–322.
110 Chaidarun SS, Eggo MC, Sheppard MC, Stewart PM: Expression of epidermal growth factor (EGF), its receptor, and related oncoprotein (erbB-2) in human pituitary tumors and response to EGF in vitro. Endocrinology 1994;135:2012–2021.
111 McCabe CJ, Khaira JS, Boelaert K, Heaney AP, Tannahill LA, Hussain S, Mitchell R, Olliff J, Sheppard MC, Franklyn JA, Gittoes NJ: Expression of pituitary tumour transforming gene (PTTG) and fibroblast growth factor-2 (FGF-2) in human pituitary adenomas: relationships to clinical tumour behaviour. Clin Endocrinol (Oxf) 2003;58:141–150.
112 Zhu X, Lee K, Asa SL, Ezzat S: Epigenetic silencing through DNA and histone methylation of fibroblast growth factor receptor 2 in neoplastic pituitary cells. Am J Pathol 2007;170:1618–1628.
113 Ezzat S, Zheng L, Zhu XF, Wu GE, Asa SL: Targeted expression of a human pituitary tumor-derived isoform of FGF receptor-4 recapitulates pituitary tumorigenesis. J Clin Invest 2002;109:69–78.
114 Evans CO, Young AN, Brown MR, Brat DJ, Parks JS, Neish AS, Oyesiku NM: Novel patterns of gene expression in pituitary adenomas identified by complementary deoxyribonucleic acid microarrays and quantitative reverse transcription-polymerase chain reaction. J Clin Endocrinol Metab 2001;86:3097–3107.
115 Michaelis KA, Knox AJ, Xu M, Kiseljak-Vassiliades K, Edwards MG, Geraci M, Kleinschmidt DeMasters BK, Lillehei KO, Wierman ME: Identification of growth arrest and DNA-damage-inducible gene beta (GADD45beta) as a novel tumor suppressor in pituitary gonadotrope tumors. Endocrinology 2011;152:3603–3613.
116 Zhang X, Sun H, Danila DC, Johnson SR, Zhou Y, Swearingen B, Klibanski A: Loss of expression of GADD45 gamma, a growth inhibitory gene, in human pituitary adenomas: implications for tumorigenesis. J Clin Endocrinol Metab 2002;87:1262–1267.
117 Bahar A, Bicknell JE, Simpson DJ, Clayton RN, Farrell WE: Loss of expression of the growth inhibitory gene GADD45gamma, in human pituitary adenomas, is associated with CpG island methylation. Oncogene 2004;23:936–944.

118 Asa SL, DiGiovanni R, Jiang J, Ward ML, Loesch K, Yamada S, Sano T, Yoshimoto K, Frank SJ, Ezzat S: A growth hormone receptor mutation impairs growth hormone autofeedback signaling in pituitary tumors. Cancer Res 2007;67:7505–7511.
119 Thapar K, Kovacs K, Stefaneanu L, Scheithauer B, Killinger DW, Lioyd RV, Smyth HS, Barr A, Thorner MO, Gaylinn B, Laws ER Jr: Overexpression of the growth-hormone-releasing hormone gene in acromegaly-associated pituitary tumors. An event associated with neoplastic progression and aggressive behavior. Am J Pathol 1997;151:769–784.
120 Hashimoto K, Koga M, Motomura T, Kasayama S, Kouhara H, Ohnishi T, Arita N, Hayakawa T, Sato B, Kishimoto T: Identification of alternatively spliced messenger ribonucleic acid encoding truncated growth hormone-releasing hormone receptor in human pituitary adenomas. J Clin Endocrinol Metab 1995;80:2933–2939.
121 Williamson EA, Daniels M, Foster S, Kelly WF, Kendall-Taylor P, Harris PE: Gs alpha and Gi2 alpha mutations in clinically non-functioning pituitary tumours. Clin Endocrinol (Oxf) 1994;41:815–820.
122 Williamson EA, Ince PG, Harrison D, Kendall-Taylor P, Harris PE: G-protein mutations in human pituitary adrenocorticotrophic hormone-secreting adenomas. Eur J Clin Invest 1995;25:128–131.
123 Vallar L, Spada A, Giannattasio G: Altered Gs and adenylate cyclase activity in human GH-secreting pituitary adenomas. Nature 1987;330:566–568.
124 Tordjman K, Stern N, Ouaknine G, Yossiphov Y, Razon N, Nordenskjold M, Friedman E: Activating mutations of the Gs alpha-gene in nonfunctioning pituitary tumors. J Clin Endocrinol Metab 1993;77: 765–769.
125 Hamacher C, Brocker M, Adams EF, Lei T, Fahlbusch R, Buchfelder M, Derwahl M: Overexpression of stimulatory G protein alpha-subunit is a hallmark of most human somatotrophic pituitary tumours and is associated with resistance to GH-releasing hormone. Pituitary 1998;1:13–23.
126 Riminucci M, Collins MT, Lala R, Corsi A, Matarazzo P, Gehron RP, Bianco P: An R201H activating mutation of the GNAS1 (Gsalpha) gene in a corticotroph pituitary adenoma. Mol Pathol 2002;55:58–60.
127 Picard C, Silvy M, Gerard C, Buffat C, Lavaque E, Figarella-Branger D, Dufour H, Gabert J, Beckers A, Brue T, Enjalbert A, Barlier A: Gs alpha overexpression and loss of Gs alpha imprinting in human somatotroph adenomas: association with tumor size and response to pharmacologic treatment. Int J Cancer 2007;121:1245–1252.
128 Bilodeau S, Vallette-Kasic S, Gauthier Y, Figarella-Branger D, Brue T, Berthelet F, LaCroix A, Batista D, Stratakis C, Hanson J, Meij B, Drouin J: Role of Brg1 and HDAC2 in GR trans-repression of the pituitary POMC gene and misexpression in Cushing disease. Genes Dev 2006;20:2871–2886.
129 Finelli P, Pierantoni GM, Giardino D, Losa M, Rodeschini O, Fedele M, Valtorta E, Mortini P, Croce CM, Larizza L, Fusco A: The High Mobility Group A2 gene is amplified and overexpressed in human prolactinomas. Cancer Res 2002;62:2398–2405.
130 Pierantoni GM, Finelli P, Valtorta E, Giardino D, Rodeschini O, Esposito F, Losa M, Fusco A, Larizza L: High-mobility group A2 gene expression is frequently induced in non-functioning pituitary adenomas (NFPAs), even in the absence of chromosome 12 polysomy. Endocr Relat Cancer 2005;12: 867–874.
131 Karga HJ, Alexander JM, Hedley-Whyte ET, Klibanski A, Jameson JL: Ras mutations in human pituitary tumors. J Clin Endocrinol Metab 1992;74: 914–919.
132 Cai WY, Alexander JM, Hedley-Whyte ET, Scheithauer BW, Jameson JL, Zervas NT, Klibanski A: ras mutations in human prolactinomas and pituitary carcinomas. J Clin Endocrinol Metab 1994;78: 89–93.
133 Pei L, Melmed S, Scheithauer B, Kovacs K, Prager D: H-ras mutations in human pituitary carcinoma metastases. J Clin Endocrinol Metab 1994;78:842–846.
134 Lin Y, Jiang X, Shen Y, Li M, Ma H, Xing M, Lu Y: Frequent mutations and amplifications of the PIK3CA gene in pituitary tumors. Endocr Relat Cancer 2009;16:301–310.
135 Ezzat S, Yu S, Asa SL: Ikaros isoforms in human pituitary tumors: distinct localization, histone acetylation, and activation of the 5′ fibroblast growth factor receptor-4 promoter. Am J Pathol 2003;163: 1177–1184.
136 Zhu X, Asa SL, Ezzat S: Fibroblast growth factor 2 and estrogen control the balance of histone 3 modifications targeting MAGE-A3 in pituitary neoplasia. Clin Cancer Res 2008;14:1984–1996.
137 Zhang X, Zhou Y, Mehta KR, Danila DC, Scolavino S, Johnson SR, Klibanski A: A pituitary-derived MEG3 isoform functions as a growth suppressor in tumor cells. J Clin Endocrinol Metab 2003;88: 5119–5126.
138 Zhao J, Dahle D, Zhou Y, Zhang X, Klibanski A: Hypermethylation of the promoter region is associated with the loss of MEG3 gene expression in human pituitary tumors. J Clin Endocrinol Metab 2005;90:2179–2186.

139 Gejman R, Batista DL, Zhong Y, Zhou Y, Zhang X, Swearingen B, Stratakis CA, Hedley-Whyte ET, Klibanski A: Selective loss of MEG3 expression and intergenic differentially methylated region hypermethylation in the MEG3/DLK1 locus in human clinically nonfunctioning pituitary adenomas. J Clin Endocrinol Metab 2008;93:4119–4125.
140 Cheunsuchon P, Zhou Y, Zhang X, Lee H, Chen W, Nakayama Y, Rice KA, Tessa Hedley-Whyte E, Swearingen B, Klibanski A: Silencing of the imprinted DLK1-MEG3 locus in human clinically nonfunctioning pituitary adenomas. Am J Pathol 2011;179:2120–2130.
141 Mezzomo LC, Gonzales PH, Pesce FG, Kretzmann FN, Ferreira NP, Oliveira MC, Kohek MB: Expression of cell growth negative regulators MEG3 and GADD45gamma is lost in most sporadic human pituitary adenomas. Pituitary 2012;15:420–427.
142 Zhuang Z, Ezzat SZ, Vortmeyer AO, Weil R, Oldfield EH, Park WS, Pack S, Huang S, Agarwal SK, Guru SC, Manickam P, Debelenko LV, Kester MB, Olufemi SE, Heppner C, Crabtree JS, Burns AL, Spiegel AM, Marx SJ, Chandrasekharappa SC, Collins FS, Emmert-Buck MR, Liotta LA, Asa SL, Lubensky IA: Mutations of the MEN1 tumor suppressor gene in pituitary tumors. Cancer Res 1997; 57:5446–5451.
143 Tanaka C, Yoshimoto K, Yamada S, Nishioka H, Ii S, Moritani M, Yamaoka T, Itakura M: Absence of germ-line mutations of the multiple endocrine neoplasia type 1 (MEN1) gene in familial pituitary adenoma in contrast to MEN1 in Japanese. J Clin Endocrinol Metab 1998;83:960–965.
144 Wenbin C, Asai A, Teramoto A, Sanno N, Kirino T: Mutations of the MEN1 tumor suppressor gene in sporadic pituitary tumors. Cancer Lett 1999;142: 43–47.
145 Schmidt MC, Henke RT, Stangl AP, Meyer-Puttlitz B, Stoffel Wagner B, Schramm J, von DA: Analysis of the MEN1 gene in sporadic pituitary adenomas. J Pathol 1999;188:168–173.
146 McCabe CJ, Gittoes NJ, Sheppard MC, Franklyn JA: Increased MEN1 mRNA expression in sporadic pituitary tumours. Clin Endocrinol (Oxf) 1999;50: 727–733.
147 Karl M, Von WG, Kempter E, Katz DA, Reincke M, Monig H, Ali IU, Stratakis CA, Oldfield EH, Chrousos GP, Schulte HM: Nelson's syndrome associated with a somatic frame shift mutation in the glucocorticoid receptor gene. J Clin Endocrinol Metab 1996;81:124–129.
148 Huizenga NA, de LP, Koper JW, Clayton RN, Farrell WE, van der Lely AJ, Brinkmann AO, de Jong FH, Lamberts SW: Human adrenocorticotropin-secreting pituitary adenomas show frequent loss of heterozygosity at the glucocorticoid receptor gene locus. J Clin Endocrinol Metab 1998;83:917–921.
149 Acunzo J, Roche C, Defilles C, Thirion S, Quentien MH, Figarella-Branger D, Graillon T, Dufour H, Brue T, Pellegrini I, Enjalbert A, Barlier A: Inactivation of PITX2 transcription factor induced apoptosis of gonadotroph tumoral cells. Endocrinology 2011;152:3884–3892.
150 Pagotto U, Arzberger T, Theodoropoulou M, Grubler Y, Pantaloni C, Saeger W, Losa M, Journot L, Stalla GK, Spengler D: The expression of the antiproliferative gene ZAC is lost or highly reduced in nonfunctioning pituitary adenomas. Cancer Res 2000;60:6794–6799.
151 Noh TW, Jeong HJ, Lee MK, Kim TS, Kim SH, Lee EJ: Predicting recurrence of nonfunctioning pituitary adenomas. J Clin Endocrinol Metab 2009;94: 4406–4413.
152 Palmieri D, Valentino T, De MI, Esposito F, Cappabianca P, Wierinckx A, Vitiello M, Lombardi G, Colao A, Trouillas J, Pierantoni GM, Fusco A, Fedele M: PIT1 upregulation by HMGA proteins has a role in pituitary tumorigenesis. Endocr Relat Cancer 2012;19:123–135.
153 Alvaro V, Levy L, Dubray C, Roche A, Peillon F, Querat B, Joubert D: Invasive human pituitary tumors express a point-mutated alpha-protein kinase-C. J Clin Endocrinol Metab 1993;77:1125–1129.
154 Zhang X, Horwitz GA, Heaney AP, Nakashima M, Prezant TR, Bronstein MD, Melmed S: Pituitary tumor transforming gene (PTTG) expression in pituitary adenomas. J Clin Endocrinol Metab 1999;84: 761–767.
155 Salehi F, Kovacs K, Scheithauer BW, Cantelmi D, Horvath E, Lloyd RV, Cusimano M: Immunohistochemical expression of pituitary tumor transforming gene (PTTG) in pituitary adenomas: a correlative study of tumor subtypes. Int J Surg Pathol 2010; 18:5–13.
156 Simpson DJ, Hibberts NA, McNicol AM, Clayton RN, Farrell WE: Loss of pRb expression in pituitary adenomas is associated with methylation of the RB1 CpG island. Cancer Res 2000;60:1211–1216.
157 Bahar A, Simpson DJ, Cutty SJ, Bicknell JE, Hoban PR, Holley S, Mourtada-Maarabouni M, Williams GT, Clayton RN, Farrell WE: Isolation and characterization of a novel pituitary tumor apoptosis gene. Mol Endocrinol 2004;18:1827–1839.
158 Corbetta S, Ballare E, Mantovani G, Lania A, Losa M, Di Blasio AM, Spada A: Somatostatin receptor subtype 2 and 5 in human GH-secreting pituitary adenomas: analysis of gene sequence and mRNA expression. Eur J Clin Invest 2001;31:208–214.
159 Ando S, Sarlis NJ, Oldfield EH, Yen PM: Somatic mutation of TRbeta can cause a defect in negative regulation of TSH in a TSH-secreting pituitary tumor. J Clin Endocrinol Metab 2001;86:5572–5576.

160 Ando S, Sarlis NJ, Krishnan J, Feng X, Refetoff S, Zhang MQ, Oldfield EH, Yen PM: Aberrant alternative splicing of thyroid hormone receptor in a TSH-secreting pituitary tumor is a mechanism for hormone resistance. Mol Endocrinol 2001;15:1529–1538.
161 Tanizaki Y, Jin L, Scheithauer BW, Kovacs K, Roncaroli F, Lloyd RV: P53 gene mutations in pituitary carcinomas. Endocr Pathol 2007;18:217–222.
162 Kawashima ST, Usui T, Sano T, Iogawa H, Hagiwara H, Tamanaha T, Tagami T, Naruse M, Hojo M, Takahashi JA, Shimatsu A: P53 gene mutation in an atypical corticotroph adenoma with Cushing's disease. Clin Endocrinol (Oxf) 2009;70:656–657.
163 Pinto EM, Siqueira SA, Cukier P, Fragoso MC, Lin CJ, de Mendonca BB: Possible role of a radiation-induced p53 mutation in a Nelson's syndrome patient with a fatal outcome. Pituitary 2011;14:400–404.
164 Murakami M, Mizutani A, Asano S, Katakami H, Ozawa Y, Yamazaki K, Ishida Y, Takano K, Okinaga H, Matsuno A: A mechanism of acquiring temozolomide resistance during transformation of atypical prolactinoma into prolactin-producing pituitary carcinoma: case report. Neurosurgery 2011; 68:E1761–E1767.
165 Bottoni A, Piccin D, Tagliati F, Luchin A, Zatelli MC, Degli Uberti EC: miR-15a and miR-16-1 down-regulation in pituitary adenomas. J Cell Physiol 2005;204:280–285.
166 Bottoni A, Zatelli MC, Ferracin M, Tagliati F, Piccin D, Vignali C, Calin GA, Negrini M, Croce CM, Degli Uberti EC: Identification of differentially expressed microRNAs by microarray: a possible role for microRNA genes in pituitary adenomas. J Cell Physiol 2007;210:370–377.
167 Qian ZR, Asa SL, Siomi H, Siomi MC, Yoshimoto K, Yamada S, Wang EL, Rahman MM, Inoue H, Itakura M, Kudo E, Sano T: Overexpression of HMGA2 relates to reduction of the let-7 and its relationship to clinicopathological features in pituitary adenomas. Mod Pathol 2009;22:431–441.
168 Amaral FC, Torres N, Saggioro F, Neder L, Machado HR, Silva WA Jr, Moreira AC, Castro M: MicroRNAs differentially expressed in ACTH-secreting pituitary tumors. J Clin Endocrinol Metab 2009;94:320–323.
169 Stilling G, Sun Z, Zhang S, Jin L, Righi A, Kovacs G, Korbonits M, Scheithauer BW, Kovacs K, Lloyd RV: MicroRNA expression in ACTH-producing pituitary tumors: up-regulation of microRNA-122 and -493 in pituitary carcinomas. Endocrine 2010;38: 67–75.
170 Butz H, Liko I, Czirjak S, Igaz P, Munayem KM, Zivkovic V, Balint K, Korbonits M, Racz K, Patocs A: Down-regulation of Wee1 kinase by a specific subset of microRNA in human sporadic pituitary adenomas. J Clin Endocrinol Metab 2010;95:E181–E191.
171 Mao ZG, He DS, Zhou J, Yao B, Xiao WW, Chen CH, Zhu YH, Wang HJ: Differential expression of microRNAs in GH-secreting pituitary adenomas. Diagn Pathol 2010;5:79.
172 Butz H, Liko I, Czirjak S, Igaz P, Korbonits M, Racz K, Patocs A: MicroRNA profile indicates downregulation of the TGFbeta pathway in sporadic nonfunctioning pituitary adenomas. Pituitary 2011;14: 112–124.
173 Palmieri D, D'Angelo D, Valentino T, De Martino I, Ferraro A, Wierinckx A, Fedele M, Trouillas J, Fusco A: Downregulation of HMGA-targeting microRNAs has a critical role in human pituitary tumorigenesis. Oncogene 2012;31:3857–3865.
174 D'Angelo D, Palmieri D, Mussnich P, Roche M, Wierinckx A, Raverot G, Fedele M, Maria CC, Trouillas J, Fusco A: Altered MicroRNA expression profile in human pituitary GH adenomas: down-regulation of miRNA targeting HMGA1, HMGA2, and E2F1. J Clin Endocrinol Metab 2012; 97:E1128–E1138.

Márta Korbonits, MD, PhD
Department of Endocrinology, Barts and London
School of Medicine and Dentistry, Charterhouse Square
London EC1M 6BQ (UK)
E-Mail m.korbonits@qmul.ac.uk

Stratakis CA (ed): Endocrine Tumor Syndromes and Their Genetics.
Front Horm Res. Basel, Karger, 2013, vol 41, pp 141–148 (DOI: 10.1159/000345674)

Clinical Behavior and Genetics of Nonsyndromic, Familial Nonmedullary Thyroid Cancer

Andrew J. Bauer

Thyroid Center, Division of Endocrinology and Diabetes, Children's Hospital of Philadelphia, Philadelphia, Pa., USA

Abstract

Nonmedullary thyroid cancer (NMTC) is one of the most inheritable forms of all cancers with an 8- to 10-fold risk of a first-degree relative developing disease. Familial nonmedullary thyroid cancer (FNMTC) describes this familial aggregation and is comprised of two distinct subgroups; syndromic and nonsyndromic. Greater than 85% of thyroid tumors in nonsyndromic FNMTC are papillary thyroid cancer, followed by FTC (~10%), poorly differentiated, and anaplastic thyroid cancer (~5%). Compared to sporadic NMTC, FNMTC presents at a younger age and is associated with a higher incidence of multifocal disease and metastasis. The transmission pattern most frequently follows an autosomal dominant mode of inheritance. While there has been extensive investigation to find a high-penetrant, single locus as the causative genetic factor, more recent data suggest that FNMTC is a polygenic disorder with variable penetrance likely associated with a low-to-moderate number of low-penetrant alleles. A number of case-controlled, familial and population-based studies using genomewide association single-nucleotide polymorphism arrays have begun to unravel the complex genetic environment of FNMTC. These studies highlight the significant challenges in identifying markers predictive of disease onset and progression. Continued efforts will hopefully lead to identification of a panel of genetic markers used to identify family members at risk. Until this time, clinical factors appear to be the most efficient and accurate method for surveillance and diagnosis.

Familial nonmedullary thyroid carcinoma (FNMTC) describes follicular-cell-derived tumors, either papillary thyroid cancer (PTC) or follicular thyroid cancer (FTC), that occur with increased frequency within a family. This classification may be further divided into two subgroups; syndromic and nonsyndromic. This chapter will focus on nonsyndromic FNMTC, follicular-cell-derived tumors that occur in isolation from other endocrine tumors or disorders but carry an increased incidence of presentation within an extended family. Syndromic forms of FNMTC, such as

PTEN hamartoma syndrome, Peutz-Jeghers syndrome and others, are discussed in the chapter by Kalkan and Waguespack [this vol.].

The first evidence of an inheritable predisposition to develop NMTC was reported in 1955 by Robinson and Orr [1]. In this sentinel paper, two 24-year-old monozygotic twin sisters were diagnosed with multifocal, bilateral papillary adenocarcinoma with regional metastasis. Since this initial report there have been increased efforts to more accurately define both the clinical behavior and the molecular etiology of FNMTC. Unfortunately, because of the high incidence of sporadic disease, and significant inconsistencies in study design, most notably a variation in inclusion criteria used to define how many family members constitute a FNMTC kindred, the pattern of inheritance, clinical phenotype and identification of susceptibility loci remain elusive.

What is clear, however, is that FNMTC is a clinically identifiable syndrome showing a higher degree of familial predisposition when compared to many other well-characterized cancers. Data from large, case-controlled population studies show that the familial relative risk, a ratio describing the age-adjusted risk for a first-degree relative developing a cancer compared to the general population, for thyroid cancer is as high as 8- to 10-fold compared to 2–4 for breast, colon and prostate cancer, cancers with well-described Mendelian patterns of inheritance [2–5]. While environmental factors also contribute to the development of thyroid cancer, most notably ionizing radiation for PTC, the strong heritability of thyroid cancer suggests that the genetic component may provide the highest attributable risk for the majority of patients [4]. While great strides have been made in identifying genetic markers of thyroid tumorigenesis, consensus on a strict definition of FNMTC, as well as study designs that include multiplex families, segregate data based on precise tumor phenotype, and the use of appropriate control groups, are critical to unraveling the clinical behavior and genetic etiology of FNMTC [6].

Clinical Behavior and Definition of FNMTC

Based on family history, it is estimated that FNMTC accounts for approximately 3.5–6% of all thyroid carcinomas of follicular cell origin [5, 7]. On a cellular level, there does not appear to be any distinguishing histologic features between FNMTC and sporadic tumors [8]; however, in regard to clinical behavior, there are mixed data on whether FNMTC follows a more or less aggressive pattern of disease compared to sporadic NMTC.

Studies supporting a more aggressive pattern suggest that FNMTC presents at an earlier age of onset, is more frequently multifocal and bilateral, is associated with a higher incidence of locoregional (LR) lymph node metastasis, and, subsequently, a higher incidence of LR recurrence and shorter disease-free survival [9–12]. In addition to these findings in the individual patient, there is also evidence to suggest clinical anticipation between generations, where second-generation family members present with disease at an earlier age and with larger and more invasive tumors at the time of diagnosis [9, 13].

These data have led clinicians to suggest early screening of family members in order to monitor for the development of benign and malignant thyroid disease. In addition, due to concern for an increased risk of invasive disease, a more aggressive treatment plan for FNMTC family members may be pursued, to include total thyroidectomy with prophylactic central neck dissection and radioiodine remnant ablation for all [9]. Similar to sporadic NMTC, lateral neck dissection is only recommended if pre-operative staging identifies malignant disease in the lateral-cervical compartments [9].

Results from early US surveillance of apparently unaffected family members have been favorable [14, 15]. A recent report by Rosario et al. [14] showed an increased incidence of multicentricity, extrathyroidal extension, and LR lymph node and distant metastasis in siblings of PTC patients (n = 723) compared to matched controls (n = 241). In addition, in siblings found to harbor PTC, US surveillance was associated with earlier detection of clinically significant disease, as reflected by smaller tumor size (0.8 vs. 2.85 cm; p = <0.001), a lower incidence of lymph node metastasis (23.2 vs. 65.6%; p = <0.001) as well as a lower incidence of extrathyroidal extension (20.9 vs. 56.2%; p = 0.002) when compared to the proband [14].

In contrast to these results there are several additional studies suggesting that FNMTC follows a similar pattern of behavior compared to sporadic disease [16, 17] and that treatment should be based solely on consensus guidelines for sporadic disease [18, 19]. Robenshtok et al. [17] reported that FNMTC patients (n = 67) present with a similar stage of disease at diagnosis, experience a similar incidence of persistent and recurrent disease and show no difference in disease-free survival after a mean follow-up period of 8.6 ±10 years when compared to controls (n = 375). In addition, there was no evidence to support the presence of more aggressive disease in subsequent generations [17].

Whether FNMTC follows a similar clinical course compared to sporadic thyroid cancers of follicular origin has been complicated by the lack of consensus over defining how many affected family members are required to define the familial form of disease. The relative high incidence of disease in the general population predicts that clustering of sporadic disease within a family may be common and that using a minimum standard of 2 affected family members to define FNMTC may lead to inclusion of sporadic cases [17]. This risk is exaggerated by inclusion of benign thyroid disease, such as multinodular goiter, as well as the current rising incidence of disease in both the United States and Europe, estimated to be approximately 2% annually since 2004 [20]. The risk of including sporadic cases into the clinical and/or genetic evaluation of FNMTC has been mathematically defined by Charkes [21] who predicted that using a 2-family-member definition model to define FNMTC carries a 62–69% risk of including sporadic disease while using a 3 or more affected family member model reduces the risk to less than 6%.

In reviewing the clinical studies to date, the majority have used a minimum definition model of 2 or more family members to define FNMTC [9–13, 16]. There are two studies that have segregated the data based on a minimum affected model (2 or more) and compared their findings against the more mathematically stringent model or 3 or more affected family members. Triponez et al. [22] reported decreased survival for families with 3 or more affected family members; however, the subgroup of tumor types was broad and all 3 of the anaplastic thyroid cancer patients were in the 3 or more family member group. In contrast, Robenshtok et al. [17] found no statistical difference in clinical behavior when comparing families based on 2 or more compared to a 3 or more definition model.

Overall, the features that appear to be most frequently reported across studies are that FNMTC most closely follows an autosomal-dominant mode of inheritance and that earlier onset of disease, and a more invasive phenotype, are common. US surveillance appears to be warranted; however, the age at which to start surveillance, and the frequency of repeat US, has not been defined. A reasonable approach may be to initiate US surveillance approximately 5 years prior to the youngest adult family member diagnosed with FNMTC. These limitations should be discussed with the family prior to initiation of a screening program. In addition, families should be counseled over the potential of identifying benign disease that may subsequently require FNA biopsy and long-term follow-up. Large, prospective studies with clearly defined inclusion criteria, to include the number of patients that define FNMTC, subgrouping of specific tumor subtypes, and inclusion of matched controls are needed to more accurately characterize the pattern of inheritance and the clinical behavior of disease. This is particularly relevant for patients that present with NMTC prior to 18 years of age.

Genetics

Approximately 85% of thyroid tumors included in FNMTC are PTC (85%), followed by follicular thyroid carcinoma (10–15%) and, finally, a very small number of poorly differentiated and anaplastic tumors (~5%) [23]. In general, NMTC are associated with activation of the mitogen-activated protein kinase and PI3K/AKT pathways [24], most frequently associated with somatic rearrangement of *RET/PTC* or mutations in *BRAF* in PTC, and rearrangements in *PAX8/PPARγ* or mutations in *PTEN* or *RAS* in FTC [25]. The incidence of these well-described, somatic mutations does not appear to be different between sporadic or FNMTC [7].

In general, the molecular etiology of a familial cancer syndrome may be the result of altered expression of a single gene or secondary to the cumulative concurrence of multiple, lower penetrance susceptibility genes. Initial efforts to define the predisposing genetic etiology of FNMTC focused on examining large kindreds for high-penetrance, single-locus candidate genes and often included the presence of common, benign conditions as a component of the inheritable trait [26]. More recently, with the realization that linkage studies may not have sufficient power or resolution to define complex, multifactorial disease, genomewide association studies (GWAS) have been explored [6].

Several groups have attempted to use linkage analysis based on a selected number of microsatellite markers, or single-nucleotide polymorphisms (SNP) evenly distributed across the genome, in an effort to identify mutations in high penetrance genes. Khan et al. [27] provided a concise review on the majority of these studies. Six potential regions for FNMTC were identified from this collective group of studies, and included; multinodular goiter with PTC – *MNG1* (14q32), thyroid tumors with cell oxyphilia – *TCO* (19p13.2), PTC with papillary renal neoplasm – *fPTC/PRN* (1q21), PTC with increased risk of follicular variant of PTC (fvPTC) – *NMTC* (2q21), benign thyroid disease with an increased risk of PTC – *FTEN* (8p23.1-p22), and the telomere-telomerase complex [27]. Many of these loci achieved a lod score sufficient to confirm linkage with a range from +2.85 to a maximum score of +235 [27]. Unfortunately, many of these loci could not be validated in subsequent studies [27]. In addition, several other genes associated with benign thyroid disease (thyroid-stimulating hormone receptor), sporadic PTC *(RET/PTC1, RET/PTC3, NRAS, KRAS*, hepatocyte growth factor – *MET* and *JUNB)*, and syndromic PTC (adenomatous polyposis coli – *APC* and the phosphate and tenisin homolog gene – *PTEN*) have also been excluded as a potential causative factor in FNMTC [7, 27]. Last, while germline mutations in *BRAF* do not appear to be a causative factor in FNMTC there is some evidence to suggest an association between mutations in *BRAF* and FNMTC tumor progression [7, 27].

Two additional SNP array-based linkage analysis have been published subsequent to Khan's review. In the first, SNP array-based linkage analysis was performed on 38 FNMTC families, with 49 members consenting to pooled analysis after histologic confirmation of NMTC; 41 were from families with 2 or more affected members [28]. In keeping with previous studies, exclusion criteria included known exposure to ionizing radiation. Significant linkage was found for markers rs990033 at locus 1q21.1 and for rs12183572 at locus 6q22.31, with lod scores of 3.04 and 3.30, respectively. No known genes are located at these markers; however, the locus at 1q21 had been previously identified as PRN1 by Malchoff et al. [29]. Unfortunately, this study did not examine the presence or absence of these markers in nonaffected family members and to date these markers have not been validated by independent examination.

In the second study, GWAS, using a 50K or 500K SNP array platform, was used to examine a kindred with 8 individuals diagnosed with PTC, of which 2 had both PTC and melanoma, and compared the results against 14 other family members without PTC; 2 with melanoma, 2 with chronic lymphocytic leukemia, 1 with breast cancer, goiter, and both cutaneous and ocular melanoma and 9 others with benign thyroid disease [30]. Linkage analysis identified a locus at 8q24. This locus was subsequently confirmed by examination of an additional 25 families with at least 2 confirmed cases of NMTC (22 of 25 with 3 or more affected family members). The overall maximum non-parametric linkage score of all cases combined for the 8q24 locus was 3.2 ($p = 0.007$). Resequencing of the thyroglobulin and Src-like adaptor genes located at 8q24 did not lead to discovery of an associated mutation. However, downregulation of a noncoding

RNA gene (*AK023948*) was found in 24 of 26 examined PTC samples leading the authors to conclude that *AK023948* is a candidate susceptibility gene for FNMTC [30].

A number of additional SNP variants associated with the development of NMTC from well-powered studies, validated by independent groups, and including patients from non-Caucasian ancestry populations, have also been reported (for review see Landa and Robledo [26]). However, many of these variants have not been validated in case-control studies and few have been examined in FNMTC kindred.

Lastly, four well-powered, case-control studies have been reported, three using GWAS [31–33] and one using a candidate gene approach [34]. Three of the four studies examined tumors for low penetrance genes in sporadic PTC [31, 32, 34] with the study by Takahashi et al. [33] examining 660 cases of radiation-induced PTC from the Chernobyl accident. Variants rs965513 located at 9q22.33 and rs944289 located at 14q13.3 have emerged as strong predictors of PTC tumorigenesis and are located in close proximity to the well-described thyroid transcription factors FOXE1 (thyroid transcription factor-1), located in close proximity to 9q22.33, and NKX2–1 (TTF-2), located in close proximity to 14q13.3 [31, 33, 34]. The most recent of the four studies has identified a new polymorphism, rs944289, located 3.2 kb downstream from rs944289 in a region with no previously recognized genes [32]. Subsequent studies of this region have identified a new candidate gene, designated papillary thyroid carcinoma susceptibility candidate 3, *PTCSC3*, with expression and function analysis suggesting that *PTCSC3* may be a newly discovered, thyroid specific tumor suppressor gene [32]. None of these most recent markers have been explored in a case-controlled FNMTC study.

Conclusion

Familial aggregation is a necessary but insufficient criteria to predict the heritability of a complex disease process. For NMTC, most notably PTC, there are clear epidemiologic and clinical data suggesting a high degree of heritability, with first-degree relatives of patients diagnosed with NMTC showing the greatest risk for developing disease compared to all other cancers [2–4]. While there is a lack of consensus on when to initiate, and with what frequency to conduct, clinical surveillance, the data support that annual clinical surveillance of first-degree relatives with physical exam and/or thyroid US is reasonable and associated with identification of NMTC at an earlier stage of progression. The lack of prospective, case-controlled studies, with defined subgrouping of NMTC tumor types, limits any conclusion in regard to recommending a more aggressive treatment strategy. As such, once diagnosed, treatment of FNMTC should follow general guidelines for treatment and management of sporadic disease.

On a genetic level, the data are still limited in regard to identifying markers that predict the risk of developing disease in apparently unaffected family members or afford an ability to predict clinical behavior in patients with FNMTC. Similar to sporadic forms of NMTC, the likelihood of identifying a single, highly penetrant genetic marker appears to be quite low. More recent data suggest that similar to many other cancers, FNMTC is likely a polygenic disorder that segregates in an autosomal-dominant pattern of inheritance, but with multiple low-penetrant susceptibility loci. Interaction of these loci with an individual person's genetic landscape, endogenous endocrine and immune factors, as well as the external environment, likely further influence the expression and behavior of disease. The use of GWAS may afford an increased ability to discover susceptibility alleles; however, the greatest challenge in the post-GWAS era is to understand the functional consequences and causality of finding these low penetrance alleles [35].

Large, prospective, case-controlled studies, with defined subtypes of NMTC, validated across multiple ancestral genetic landscapes, will be needed in order to identify a group of low-penetrant polymorphisms that predict the risk for developing disease, as well as define a strategy to stratify and individualize therapy [6]. In the meantime, as recently shown by Jendrzejewski et al. [32], identification and functional analysis of these polymorphisms provides novel and important insight into the genetic predisposition and molecular mechanisms involved in PTC tumorigenesis, and, hopefully, a greater understanding of the heritability of NMTC.

While disease-specific mortality for FNMTC is low, a large percentage of patients are exposed to unnecessary risks during evaluation, treatment and surveillance secondary to our inability to accurately predict the invasive potential for the individual patient and their family members.

References

1 Robinson DW, Orr TG: Carcinoma of the thyroid and other diseases of the thyroid in identical twins. AMA Arch Surg 1955;70:923–928.

2 Dong C, Hemminki K: Modification of cancer risks in offspring by sibling and parental cancers from 2,112,616 nuclear families. Int J Cancer 2001;92: 144–150.

3 Goldgar DE, et al: Systematic population-based assessment of cancer risk in first-degree relatives of cancer probands. J Natl Cancer Inst 1994;86:1600–1608.

4 Risch N: The genetic epidemiology of cancer: interpreting family and twin studies and their implications for molecular genetic approaches. Cancer Epidemiol Biomarkers Prev 2001;10:733–741.

5 Pal T, et al: Increased risk for nonmedullary thyroid cancer in the first degree relatives of prevalent cases of nonmedullary thyroid cancer: a hospital-based study. J Clin Endocrinol Metab 2001;86:5307–5312.

6 Manolio TA, et al: Finding the missing heritability of complex diseases. Nature 2009;461:747–753.

7 Moses W, Weng J, Kebebew E: Prevalence, clinicopathologic features, and somatic genetic mutation profile in familial versus sporadic nonmedullary thyroid cancer. Thyroid 2011;21:367–371.

8 Nose V: Familial thyroid cancer: a review. Mod Pathol 2011;24(suppl 2):S19–S33.

9 Hillenbrand A, et al: Familial nonmedullary thyroid carcinoma-clinical relevance and prognosis. A European multicenter study. ESES Vienna presentation. Langenbecks Arch Surg 2010;395:851–858.

10 Ito Y, et al: Biological behavior and prognosis of familial papillary thyroid carcinoma. Surgery 2009; 145:100–105.

11 Mazeh H, et al: In patients with thyroid cancer of follicular cell origin, a family history of nonmedullary thyroid cancer in one first-degree relative is associated with more aggressive disease. Thyroid 2012;22:3–8.

12 Sippel RS, Caron NR, Clark OH: An evidence-based approach to familial nonmedullary thyroid cancer: screening, clinical management, and follow-up. World J Surg 2007;31:924–933.

13 Capezzone M, et al: Familial non-medullary thyroid carcinoma displays the features of clinical anticipation suggestive of a distinct biological entity. Endocr Relat Cancer 2008;15:1075–1081.
14 Rosario PW, et al: Ultrasonographic screening for thyroid cancer in siblings of patients with apparently sporadic papillary carcinoma. Thyroid 2012; 22:805–808.
15 Uchino S, et al: Detection of asymptomatic differentiated thyroid carcinoma by neck ultrasonographic screening for familial nonmedullary thyroid carcinoma. World J Surg 2004;28:1099–1102.
16 Maxwell EL, Hall FT, Freeman JL: Familial nonmedullary thyroid cancer: a matched-case control study. Laryngoscope 2004;114:2182–2186.
17 Robenshtok E, et al: Clinical characteristics and outcome of familial nonmedullary thyroid cancer: a retrospective controlled study. Thyroid 2011;21: 43–48.
18 Cooper DS, et al: Revised American Thyroid Association management guidelines for patients with thyroid nodules and differentiated thyroid cancer. Thyroid 2009;19:1167–1214.
19 Pacini F, et al: European consensus for the management of patients with differentiated thyroid carcinoma of the follicular epithelium. Eur J Endocrinol 2006;154:787–803.
20 Howlader N, et al: SEER Cancer Statistics Review, 1975–2009. Available from: http://seer.cancer.gov/statfacts/html/thyro.html.
21 Charkes ND: On the prevalence of familial nonmedullary thyroid cancer in multiply affected kindreds. Thyroid 2006;16:181–186.
22 Triponez F, et al: Does familial non-medullary thyroid cancer adversely affect survival? World J Surg 2006;30:787–793.
23 Bonora E, Tallini G, Romeo G: Genetic predisposition to familial nonmedullary thyroid cancer: an update of molecular findings and state-of-the-art studies. J Oncol 2010;2010:385206.
24 Liu Z, et al: Highly prevalent genetic alterations in receptor tyrosine kinases and phosphatidylinositol 3-kinase/akt and mitogen-activated protein kinase pathways in anaplastic and follicular thyroid cancers. J Clin Endocrinol Metab 2008;93:3106–3116.
25 Bauer AJ, Francis GL: Update on the molecular signature of differentiated thyroid cancer: clinical implications and potential opportunities. Expert Rev Endocrinol Metab 2011;6:819–834.
26 Landa I, Robledo M: Association studies in thyroid cancer susceptibility: are we on the right track? J Mol Endocrinol 2011;47:R43–R58.
27 Khan A, et al: Familial nonmedullary thyroid cancer: a review of the genetics. Thyroid 2010;20:795–801.
28 Suh I, et al: Distinct loci on chromosome 1q21 and 6q22 predispose to familial nonmedullary thyroid cancer: a SNP array-based linkage analysis of 38 families. Surgery 2009;146:1073–1080.
29 Malchoff CD, Malchoff DM: Familial nonmedullary thyroid carcinoma. Semin Surg Oncol 1999;16: 16–18.
30 He H, et al: A susceptibility locus for papillary thyroid carcinoma on chromosome 8q24. Cancer Res 2009;69:625–631.
31 Gudmundsson J, et al: Common variants on 9q22.33 and 14q13.3 predispose to thyroid cancer in European populations. Nat Genet 2009;41:460–464.
32 Jendrzejewski J, et al: The polymorphism rs944289 predisposes to papillary thyroid carcinoma through a large intergenic noncoding RNA gene of tumor suppressor type. Proc Natl Acad Sci USA 2012;109: 8646–8651.
33 Takahashi M, et al: The FOXE1 locus is a major genetic determinant for radiation-related thyroid carcinoma in Chernobyl. Hum Mol Genet 2010;19: 2516–2523.
34 Landa I, et al: The variant rs1867277 in FOXE1 gene confers thyroid cancer susceptibility through the recruitment of USF1/USF2 transcription factors. PLoS Genet 2009;5:e1000637.
35 Freedman ML, et al: Principles for the post-GWAS functional characterization of cancer risk loci. Nat Genet 2011;43:513–518.

Andrew J. Bauer, MD, FAAP
Thyroid Center, Division of Endocrinology and Diabetes, Children's Hospital of Philadelphia
34th Street and Civic Center Boulevard, Suite 11NW30
Philadelphia, PA 19104–4399 (USA)
E-Mail bauera@chop.edu

Stratakis CA (ed): Endocrine Tumor Syndromes and Their Genetics.
Front Horm Res. Basel, Karger, 2013, vol 41, pp 149–165 (DOI: 10.1159/000345675)

Genetic Defects Associated with Familial and Sporadic Hyperparathyroidism

Geoffrey N. Hendy[a] · David E.C. Cole[b]

[a]Departments of Medicine, Physiology and Human Genetics, McGill University, and Calcium Research Laboratory and Hormones and Cancer Research Unit, Royal Victoria Hospital, Montreal, Que., and [b]Departments of Laboratory Medicine and Pathobiology, Medicine, and Genetics, University of Toronto, Toronto, Ont., Canada

Abstract

Primary hyperparathyroidism (PHPT) occurs sporadically, but occasionally it may be a feature of a familial condition, such as multiple endocrine neoplasia type 1 (MEN1), MEN2A, or the HPT-jaw tumor syndrome (HPT-JT), and familial hypocalciuric hypercalcemia/neonatal severe hyperparathyroidism (FHH/NSHPT). PHPT may also occur as familial isolated hyperparathyroidism (FIHP), and has been observed as a consequence of mutations in the *CDKN1B* gene (MEN4). Tumorigenesis in these conditions may be the result of protooncogene activation (e.g. *RET* in MEN2) or two-hit losses of a tumor suppressor (e.g. MEN1, HPT-JT). In patients with MEN1, HPT-JT or FHH/NSHPT, the hyperparathyroidism manifests at a younger age and affects both sexes equally. In MEN1, mutations of the *MEN1* gene also cause enteropancreatic and anterior pituitary tumors. In MEN2, activating mutations in the *RET* protooncogene also cause medullary thyroid carcinoma and pheochromocytoma. In HPT-JT, mutations of *CDC73/HRPT2* are associated with parathyroid carcinoma, but tumors of the kidneys and uterus are additional features. In some FIHP families, a *CASR* mutation may be identified. In parathyroid carcinoma, even if sporadic, molecular diagnostics for *CDC73/HRPT2* should be considered, as it should be for younger patients. Further exploration of these hereditary syndromes may shed light on the molecular mechanisms giving rise to nonhereditary PHPT.

Primary Hyperparathyroidism

Clinical Features

Primary hyperparathyroidism is a common cause of hypercalcemia in adults, with an incidence of about 1 per 1,000. Laboratory features are elevated serum calcium, decreased fasting serum phosphate, increased serum parathyroid hormone (PTH), and hypercalciuria. The disorder can present at any age, but occurs most frequently in the sixth decade. More women than men are affected, the ratio being about three to one.

When found in children, primary hyperparathyroidism is likely to be a component of a familial endocrinopathy and a sex bias is not observed [1]. Approximately 85% of cases involve a single benign adenoma, while hyperplasia (multiple hypercellular glands) is present in 15%. Parathyroid carcinoma is seen in less than 1% of cases, and ectopic secretion of PTH by nonparathyroid tumors is rare.

In primary hyperparathyroidism, the other organ systems involved include the kidneys, skeleton, gastrointestinal tract and central nervous system. Nephrolithiasis is the most important manifestation clinically, with kidney stones occurring in 20% of patients. Formally, a classic sign, overt bone disease (osteitis fibrosa cystica, brown tumors, or pathological fractures), is uncommon. Gastrointestinal manifestations (nausea, vomiting, or constipation) are common but often mild and nonspecific; pancreatitis and peptic ulcer disease are now rare. In contrast, decreased bone mineral density (BMD) is an increasingly common mode of presentation. Even mild elevations of calcium can be accompanied with weakness and a feeling of lassitude. Major mood disturbances and psychotic behavior are associated with more severe hypercalcemia. Hypercalcemia and hypercalciuria lead to increased urinary frequency, and in more severe cases, dehydration and secondary electrolyte disturbances may be present.

Genetics

About 1 in 10 cases of primary hyperparathyroidism is hereditary, occurring as an isolated form or associated with other abnormalities. If sporadic, individuals should be advised that there is a nonnegligible recurrence risk, since there is a small but significant genetic component to this multifactorial disease but it can be difficult to exclude a hereditary syndrome.

Genetic linkage studies confirmed the hereditary nature of the known syndromes and in some cases identified mutations in specific genes responsible for parathyroid hyperfunction [2]. Thus, individuals with idiopathic primary hyperparathyroidism should be carefully investigated for a hereditary syndrome if they are young (<45 years of age) or there is any suggestion of a positive family history.

Known disorders with associated hyperparathyroidism include: multiple endocrine neoplasia, type 1 (MEN1), type 2 (MEN2) and type 4 (MEN4), the hyperparathyroidism-jaw tumor syndrome (HPT-JT), familial hypocalciuric hypercalcemia/neonatal severe hyperparathyroidism (FHH/NSHPT), and familial isolated hyperparathyroidism (FIHP) (table 1).

Multiple Endocrine Neoplasia Type 1

Clinical Features

The most common of the hereditary hyperparathyroidism syndromes is MEN1. Primary hyperparathyroidism occurs in 95% of MEN1 cases and is the first endocrinopathy to be detected in 90% of affected patients [3]. The hypercalcemia is generally

Table 1. Familial hyperparathyroid syndromes

	MEN1	MEN2A	MEN4	HPT-JT	FHH	NSHPT	FIHP[1]
OMIM#	131100	171400	610755	145001	145980	239200	145000
Mode of inheritance	AD	AD	AD	AD	AD	AR	AD
Genetic locus	11q13	10q11.2	12p13.1	1q31.2	3q13.3–21	3q13.3–21	2p130.3–14
Mutated gene	*MEN1*	*RET*	*CDKN1B*	*CDC73/HRPT2*	*CASR*	*CASR*	not known
Gene product	MENIN	RET	p27(Kip1)	parafibromin/CDC73	CASR	CASR	–
Associated conditions	pancreatic islet and pituitary tumors; other neuroendocrine and nonendocrine tumors	medullary thyroid carcinoma and pheochromocytoma	pituitary tumors and carcinoid; lipomas	jaw fibromas; renal and uterine tumors	chondrocalcinosis and pancreatitis	–	–
Defect in sporadic parathyroid tumors	inactivation in 25–35% of benign tumors; mutation extremely rare in carcinoma	mutation not found in benign tumors	mutations found in some sporadic adenomas	inactivation in ~70% of carcinomas; mutation extremely rare in sporadic adenomas	mutation extremely rare in benign tumors	–	–

AD = Autosomal dominant; AR = autosomal recessive.
[1] In some FIHP cases, mutations in *MEN1, CASR* or *CDC73/HRPT*2 genes were identified.

mild. The mean age of onset is 20 years in the familial disorder versus 55 years in sporadic primary hyperparathyroidism, and there is no sex bias [4]. MEN1 patients should be followed carefully for the onset of symptoms and complications, at which time total parathyroidectomy should be considered.

Pancreatic islet cell tumors are frequently seen. The most common are gastrinomas, giving rise to the marked gastric acid production and recurrent peptic ulceration of the Zollinger-Ellison syndrome. This is the major cause of morbidity and mortality in MEN1 patients. Insulinomas and asymptomatic pancreatic polypeptidomas are also frequent, while glucagonomas and VIPomas are less common. Anterior pituitary tumors occur in one third of MEN1 patients and, of these, most are prolactinomas. However, somatotropinomas, corticotropinomas, and nonfunctioning pituitary tumors are also common. Other associated tumors include carcinoid, adrenalcortical carcinoma, thyroid follicular carcinoma, facial angiofibromas, collagenomas and lipomas.

Genetics

The *MEN1* locus was mapped to chromosome 11q13 by linkage analysis in families and loss of heterozygosity (LOH) studies in MEN1-associated tumors. These studies indicate that *MEN1* encodes a tumor suppressor, consistent with the Knudson two-hit model of tumorigenesis. The *MEN1* gene was identified by positional cloning, and now more than 1,000 independent germline and somatic mutations have been found

[5]. Somatic mutations occur to a variable extent in parathyroid adenoma, gastrinoma, insulinoma, lung carcinoid, and anterior pituitary tumors. Many of the mutations are predicted to lead to a truncated inactive form of menin, the *MEN1* gene product. The lack of menin, caused by the loss of both alleles, leads to tumor development. Ten percent of the *MEN1* mutations occur de novo and 25% of MEN1 patients do not have mutations in the coding region of the *MEN1* gene. There is no apparent correlation between genotype and phenotype, and there is a wide diversity of mutations throughout the 1,830-bp coding region.

Somatic *MEN1* mutations occur in sporadic parathyroid adenomas with frequencies up to 40%. When examined, LOH at 11q13 has been found in ~40% of cases. In a few reports, germline *MEN1* mutations have also been noted in sporadic parathyroid adenomas. *MEN1* mutations contribute to some of the FIHP cases. Association of *MEN1* mutations with parathyroid carcinoma in MEN1 patients occurs but it is rare.

Menin

Human menin is a 610-amino acid protein without homology to known proteins [6]. Two novel nuclear localization signals reside in the carboxy-terminal portion and menin is localized predominantly to the nucleus. How loss of menin leads to tumorigenesis in only certain tissues, given its ubiquitous expression, is unclear. Some menin mutant proteins are selectively trafficked to and rapidly degraded by the ubiquitin-proteasome pathway. The chaperone, heat shock protein 70, and the ubiquitin ligase, COOH-terminus of Hsp70 interacting protein, are important for this [7, 8]. Menin functions as a scaffold protein and is a component of complexes important for chromatin remodeling, such as the mixed lineage leukemia (MLL) complex. MLL has histone methyltransferase activity that controls Hox gene expression important for early development, as well as cyclin-dependent kinase inhibitors (CDKIs) such as p18(Ink4c) and p27(Kip1) important for cell cycle control. Menin may be involved in telomere biology and DNA replication and repair. Menin also interacts with several transcription factors including Smads, JunD, and NF-κB and modulates their activities. Menin is a Smad3-interacting protein and inactivation blocks transforming growth factor-β (TGF-β) and activin signaling, antagonizing their growth inhibitory properties in anterior pituitary cells [9]. In cultured parathyroid cells, menin inactivation achieved by menin antisense oligonucleotides leads to loss of TGF-β inhibition of cell proliferation and PTH secretion. Moreover, TGF-β does not block the proliferation and PTH production of parathyroid cells from MEN1 patients [10]. Loss of various TGF-β signaling pathway components by genetic or epigenetic means is common in cancer and is likely to be important in MEN1 tumorigenesis.

In contrast to its role as a tumor suppressor, menin also acts as an essential oncogenic cofactor in the action of MLL fusion proteins in acute leukemias. Recently, the crystal structures for menin from sea anemone *(Nematostella vectensis)* and humans have been reported [11, 12]. The protein core of menin comprises three tetratricopeptide motifs that are flanked by two α-helical bundles and covered by a β-sheet motif. There is a large central cavity and this pocket constitutes the binding site for MLL or JunD leading to up- or downregulation of gene transcription, respectively. Menin-MLL inhibitors that reverse the oncogenic activity of MLL fusion proteins in leukemia have been developed using this new structural knowledge [13]. In addition, results obtained with a stable in-frame MEN1 mutant and a homology model of human menin protein show that the Smad3 interacting region (important for TGF-β action) is distant from the central cavity and located on the exposed surface adjacent to the β-sheet motif [14].

Menin is widely expressed from an early developmental stage and found in both nonendocrine and endocrine tissues. Mice heterozygous for the ablation of the *Men1* gene develop endocrine tumors during their lifetime similar to MEN1 patients [15]. Reduced TGF-β signaling has been noted in the mouse model tumors. Homozygous deletion of *Men1* is an embryonic lethal with fetuses dying at mid-gestation with defects in multiple organs [16]. Menin is necessary for the proper functioning of the signaling pathways activated by the TGF-β ligand family members that are critical for development and maintenance of many organ systems [17]. Therefore, the importance of menin in this particular pathway extends beyond control of endocrine and nonendocrine cells that when dysregulated lead to tumorigenesis.

Multiple Endocrine Neoplasia Type 2A

Clinical Features

The most common form of MEN2 is MEN2A (MIM #171400). Medullary thyroid carcinoma is seen in 95% of cases, pheochromocytoma in 50% and hyperparathyroidism in 20%. The primary hyperparathyroidism is due to parathyroid hyperplasia or multiple parathyroid adenomas. The incomplete suppression of PTH in response to a calcium infusion test and the observation of parathyroid hyperplasia at the time of thyroidectomy in MEN2A patients without clear-cut hypercalcemia both suggest that parathyroid abnormalities are probably present in most cases.

Genetics

The *MEN2* gene maps to chromosome 10cen-10q11.2. This region contains the REarranged during Transfection (*RET*) protooncogene encoding a tyrosine kinase receptor with cadherin-like, cysteine-rich extracellular domains and a tyrosine kinase intracellular domain. *RET* point mutations have been identified in all variants of MEN2 [18] (www.arup.utah.edu/database/MEN2/MEN2_welcome.php). In MEN2A, missense mutations recur most often in one of five cysteine codons (609, 611, 618 and 620 in exon 10 and 634 in exon 11) affecting the tyrosine kinase function. In 85% of MEN2A kindreds, it is the *RET* codon 634 (p.Cys634Arg) which is mutated.

The *RET* gene is a candidate for involvement in nonfamilial hyperparathyroidism. Although MEN2-type RET mutations – predominantly the M918T mutation of MEN2B – have been implicated in the pathogenesis of some sporadic medullary thyroid carcinomas and pheochromocytomas, no mutations have been found in sporadic parathyroid tumors. In addition, mutations of the RET receptor ligand, glial cell-derived neurotrophic factor, do not appear to play a role in the genesis of MEN2 neoplasms, nor in parathyroid adenomas.

Multiple Endocrine Neoplasia Type 4

Ten percent of MEN1 patients do not have detectable mutations of the *MEN1* gene and thus may have mutations in other genes. Attention has been directed towards the *CDNK1B* gene that encodes the 196 amino acid CDKI, p27(Kip1), because of the finding that a naturally occurring rat model (MENX) expressing a recessive MEN-like trait had a homozygous 8-bp frameshifting insertion at codon 177 of p27 with a missense peptide terminating at codon 218 [19]. The p27 protein was absent in rat tumor cells. In one family with MEN1, affected members were heterozygous for a germline *CDNK1B* W76X mutation. Other cases of mutations of p27 as well as other CDKIs, p15, p18 and p21 have been identified [20]. It should be noted that such mutations are uncommon (~2%) in mutation-negative MEN1 cases. MEN due to the *CDKN1B* mutation has been designated as MEN4 (MIM #610755) to distinguish it from MEN1, MEN2A or MEN2B (previously known as MEN3) (table 1). Although parathyroid involvement is present in all MEN4 cases described to date, presentation of other MEN1-type tumors varies widely and the full clinical phenotype has not been established.

Functionally impaired *CDKN1B* mutations have been identified in a few percent of typical sporadic adenomas. In addition, germline *CDKN1B* variants have been found in some hyperparathyroid patients presenting sporadically, providing further evidence of *CDKN1B* as a susceptibility gene for typical parathyroid adenomas [21]. Modest and marked reduced levels of expression of p27 protein have been noted in parathyroid adenomas and carcinomas, respectively.

Hyperparathyroidism-Jaw Tumor Syndrome

Clinical Spectrum

The hyperparathyroidism-jaw tumor (HPT-JT) syndrome is a multisystem disorder characterized by early onset of recurrent parathyroid tumors, fibrous ossifying tumors of the mandible and maxilla, and tumors of kidney, uterus, and other organs (table 1). Inherited in an autosomal-dominant fashion, this condition shows a considerable range of expression [22]. In childhood and adolescence, patients may be markedly hypercalcemic, and there is a greater risk of hypercalcemic crisis and severe bone disease than in other forms of familial hyperparathyroidism. The condition may be associated with crippling skeletal disease and death.

In contrast to the glandular hyperplasia found in other inherited hyperparathyroid conditions, there is usually a solitary, enlarged cystic gland. After removal of the tumor, the patient usually becomes normocalcemic, but double adenomas have been reported and recurrence is well documented. The incidence of parathyroid carcinoma is much higher than in sporadic hyperparathyroidism or MEN syndromes, potentially affecting more than 15% of hyperparathyroid carriers.

Fibro-osseous jaw tumors are frequent, appearing as cystic lesions on radiographs. They are restricted to maxilla and mandible and their natural history is independent of the hyperparathyroidism. The tumors may be small and asymptomatic or they may be large, destructive, and recurrent. They consist of woven trabecular bone on a stromal background but the aberrant cell type has not been identified. Importantly, the tumors lack osteoclasts and are quite different histopathologically from the brown tumors of longstanding untreated hyperparathyroidism.

Associated renal lesions include Wilms' tumor, hamartomas, and polycystic kidneys. Uterine tumors include adenosarcoma, but benign adenofibromas and leiomyomas are more commonly reported. However, the population frequency of uterine leiomyomas is high, and it is difficult to distinguish such tumors clinically. Given that uterine tumors may have a significant impact on reproductive fitness, careful gynecologic assessment is warranted. Renal and uterine anomalies tend to occur in familial clusters, and are more common in patients who have jaw fibromas.

Genetics

In a large group of families, this condition was linked to 1q21–31 and mutation analysis led to the identification of the responsible gene, *CDC73/HRPT2*, which encodes a novel transcription factor, parafibromin/CDC73 [23]. Subsequently, studies of familial and sporadic parathyroid carcinoma suggest that the two-hit hypothesis of Knudson applies to the *CDC73* gene and parathyroid carcinogenesis. HPT-JT and its variant forms are transmitted in an autosomal dominant manner with incomplete, age-dependent penetrance. Although the variability of the phenotype is reduced within families that share a common mutation and similar genetic background, genotype-phenotype correlations have not yet emerged. In a small number of kindreds, only hyperparathyroidism is observed, adding to the genetic heterogeneity characteristic of familial isolated hyperparathyroidism (FIHP or HRPT1; MIM #145000).

Parafibromin/CDC73

The single-copy *CDC73/HRPT2* gene at 1q31.2 with 17 exons produces a mature transcript of 2.7 kb and predicts a protein of 531 amino acids, originally named parafibromin [24]. The carboxy-terminal half of parafibromin has strong homology with the yeast cell division cycle protein 73 (Cdc73); hence, the dual designations of the gene (*CDC73/HRPT2* – MIM #607393) and the protein (parafibromin/CDC73). Parafibromin is ubiquitously expressed and found predominantly in the nucleus: a nuclear localization signal is found at amino acids 125–139 [25] and a nucleolar localization signal at amino acids 76–92 [26]. Parafibromin is a component of the polymerase-associated factor 1 (PAF1) complex that interacts with RNA polymerase II and is involved in transcript elongation and mRNA 3′ end processing. Like menin, parafibromin can function as a tumor suppressor or an oncogene in a cell context-dependent manner. For both, their binding proteins determine the particular functional roles in transcription that, in turn, can direct opposing responses, either promitogenic or antiproliferative. For example, the protein tyrosine phosphatase, SHP2, encoded by the *PTPN11* gene, dephosphorylates parafibromin converting it from a transrepressor of c-myc and cyclin D1 into an activator of promitogenic Wnt signaling through direct interactions with β-catenin [27].

Most of the more than 110 mutations identified to date (two-thirds, germline; one-third somatic) involve truncation or premature stops [28]. Nearly half of the mutations are found in exon 1, while most of the remainder are found in exons 2 and 7. Exons 3–6, 8, and 14 are also mutation sites, but mutations in the 3′ half of the cDNA sequence occur much less frequently. Mutations are only detected in half of HPT-JT families, even when there is evidence linking the family disorder to chromosome 1q31.2. Moreover, de novo mutations have been identified and parental mosaicism is known [28].

Parafibromin/CDC73 in Parathyroid Carcinoma

Somatic *CDC73* mutations are not found in sporadic typical benign parathyroid adenomas. In parathyroid carcinomas, LOH at chromosome 1q, particularly in tumors from HPT-JT kindreds, has been well characterized, supporting a tumor suppressor function for parafibromin. Studies of sporadic parathyroid carcinomas show somatic mutations of the *CDC73* gene in tissue, while carcinomas in HPT-JT kindreds show tissue LOH in affected carriers. Of particular note is the finding that patients with apparently sporadic parathyroid carcinomas harbor germline mutations [29, 30]. Parathyroid carcinoma is potentially resectable when contained within the gland, but difficult to control when it has metastasized. Accordingly, all patients with newly diagnosed parathyroid carcinoma should have a careful review of family history, and should be offered *CDC73* mutation screening [31]. Parafibromin immunostaining (see below) may serve as a clinical screen for tumors resulting from a germline *CDC73* mutation that will help direct molecular testing for patients and families most at risk. Guidelines have been proposed and monitoring of asymptomatic carriers is now recommended [32].

Distinction between parathyroid carcinoma and adenoma is difficult using histopathologic criteria. Features of parathyroid cancers, including parenchymal mitoses, trabeculated parenchyma, thick fibrous bands, and even partial capsular and vascular invasion, may also be found in atypical adenomas. Capsular breach and lymphovascular invasion are the most specific histopathologic features of parathyroid carcinoma, and predictive of metastases. Therefore, identification of useful immunohistochemical tumor markers has become of primary importance. To date, parafibromin, either alone or in combination with other markers, is one of the most promising. An initial report found that loss of nuclear parafibromin expression identified parathyroid malignancies with near complete sensitivity and specificity [33], but others have subsequently observed incomplete specificity and sensitivity, but even then acknowledging it to be a useful marker [34]. Staining for multiple markers has been suggested to be advantageous in comparison to staining for parafibromin alone, two examples being loss of *RB1* and overexpression of galectin-3. The combined loss of parafibromin staining and downregulation of calcium-sensing receptor (CASR) expression indicates increased malignant potential in parathyroid carcinoma patients.

Familial Hypocalciuric Hypercalcemia

In autosomal-dominant familial hypocalciuric hypercalcemia (FHH; MIM# 145980) or familial benign hypercalcemia (FBH) syndrome, lifelong hypercalcemia (similar to that of mild primary hyperparathyroidism) is often asymptomatic but there is abnormal renal calcium handling [35, 36]. In FHH, serum PTH levels are inappropriately normal, given the degree of hypercalcemia. Diagnostic difficulties arise in differentiating FHH from the 10% of primary hyperparathyroid patients with PTH levels at the upper limit of normal [37]. FHH patients who undergo parathyroidectomy most often remain hypercalcemic, and the consensus is that surgery is to be avoided. The enhanced renal tubular reabsorption of calcium may persist following induction of hypoparathyroidism by total parathyroidectomy, emphasizing that the abnormal renal handling of calcium in FHH can be independent of PTH.

Neonatal Severe Hyperparathyroidism

Primary hyperparathyroidism occurs very rarely in infancy and childhood. Neonatal severe hyperparathyroidism or NSHPT (MIM #239200) involves multiglandular parathyroid hyperplasia rather than a single adenoma. Affected infants develop severe, symptomatic hypercalcemia with florid rickets and other bony changes of hyperparathyroidism. Delay in effective treatment can lead to a devastating neurodevelopmental disorder, if it is not fatal. Some forms of neonatal hyperparathyroidism present with milder, less symptomatic disease that can be transient [36].

Genetics

FHH is inherited in an autosomal-dominant manner with almost 100% penetrance. The population prevalence of FHH is not well defined but this may reflect the infrequency of recognition rather than rarity of the disorder itself. The trait in most FHH families maps to chromosome 3q13–21 (FHH1, MIM# 145980) where the *CASR* gene is located, but in one kindred the trait was mapped to 19p13 (FHH2, MIM# 145981). In a family from Oklahoma with atypical features (osteomalacia and increasing circulating PTH with age) and one other family, the condition mapped to 19q13.3 (FHH3, MIM# 600740). Thus, FHH is genetically heterogeneous.

Calcium-Sensing Receptor

The human *CASR* gene that maps to 3q13.3–21 spans about 103 kb and has eight exons. Exons 2–7 encode a CASR protein of 1,078 amino acids. Exons 1A and 1B encode alternative 5′-untranslated regions that splice to exon 2. CASR is a member of family C of the superfamily of G-coupled plasma membrane proteins, a family that includes the metabotropic glutamate, taste and odorant, and γ-aminobutyric B receptors [36]. The large extracellular domain of the mature protein has ~600 amino acids comprised of a bilobed Venus flytrap-like domain (VFT) that connects to the seven-transmembrane domain with a ~200 amino acid intracellular tail. The CASR functions as a dimer with both covalent and noncovalent interaction between the VFTs of each monomer. Ca^{2+} and other orthosteric agonists bind in the cleft of each VFT causing the lobes to close in on each other and rotate, thereby causing movement of transmembrane α-helices that allows coupling to G-proteins and initiation of cell signaling. Small orally-active compounds, allosteric modulators, bind within the transmembrane region and either sensitize (calcimimetics) or desensitize (calcilytics) the CASR to changing Ca^{2+} concentrations. Calcimimetics are approved for use in patients with chronic kidney disease on dialysis and in severe hypercalcemia due to parathyroid carcinoma. Clinical trials with mild primary hyperparathyroidism patients show that calcimimetics reduce serum calcium and PTH levels and increase serum phosphate but do not significantly affect bone turnover or bone mineral density. Successful off-label applications for other indications have been reported, one example being infants with neonatal hyperparathyroidism [38].

About 300 unique mutations in the CASR have been identified: two-thirds are inactivating, causing FHH/NSHPT, while one-third are activating, and result in autosomal dominant hypocalcemia (CASRdb; www.casrdb.mcgill.ca). The majority of inactivating mutations are missense, but insertion, deletion, frame-shift, truncation, and splice-site mutations are also found. The spread of mutations across the coding exons is consistent with the evidence for multiple functional components that collectively contribute to signaling activity of the CASR dimer, so that a critical mutation in any one of them may result in substantial functional impairment.

Overt hyperparathyroidism is usually not part of the FHH syndrome and histologically the parathyroid glands removed from FHH patients are only occasionally hyperplastic. This is in contrast with the marked hypercellularity of the glands removed from NSHPT patients and the *Casr* knockout mouse model. However, some FHH families (and FIHP kindreds with *CASR* mutations) have affected members with elevated PTH levels and parathyroid tumors and parathyroidectomy can be curative. Thus, it may be that particular mutant CASRs, even in the heterozygous state, have deleterious effects specifically with respect to parathyroid cell proliferation. At one point, the link between parathyroid calcium sensing and proliferative pathways suggested that somatic mutations of *CASR* might be tumorigenic. However, all the evidence to date suggests that somatic mutations rarely if ever contribute to the pathogenesis of sporadic parathyroid tumors. On the other hand, the majority of the parathyroid glands of patients with primary hyperparathyroidism have reduced CASR expression. Thus, the calcium set-point is shifted to the right, parathyroid enlargement occurs, and serum calcium and PTH levels are increased. In addition, the regulator of G protein signaling 5 (RGS5) that inhibits signaling by the CASR is overexpressed in neoplastic parathyroid tissues [39]. Thus, reduced RGS5 expression and/or activity may contribute to altered CASR signaling in parathyroid tumors. Mutations in other genes regulating the calcium-sensing pathway may play a role in the initiation or progression of parathyroid tumorigenesis.

Vitamin D insufficiency is common among patients with PHPT and vitamin D deficiency is associated with more severe progressive disease. The active metabolite, 1,25$(OH)_2$D, regulates parathyroid cell proliferation, and expression of the *PTH* and *CASR* genes [40]. Humans or mice in which there is homozygous inactivation of the VDR or its ligand manifest marked parathyroid hyperplasia and elevated circulating PTH levels. Like the *CASR*, somatic mutation of the *VDR* does not contribute to parathyroid tumorigenesis, but *VDR* expression is reduced in PHPT. The reduced *CASR* expression may, in part, be secondary to decreased *VDR* expression. In FHH-affected individuals, the clinical severity can be exacerbated by vitamin D deficiency, promoting frank hyperparathyroidism, and with vitamin D supplementation can revert to an FHH phenotype with modestly elevated serum calcium with normal PTH levels [41].

Both exonic and intronic polymorphisms (SNPs) at the *CASR* locus have been studied. The most common missense SNP is A986S. Both ionized and total serum calcium concentrations are increased (within the normal range) in individuals carrying at least one 986S allele. There is a small but significant overall association between the PHPT phenotype and both A986S and R990G SNPs [42]. The minor 986S allele appears to act as a mild inactivating variant, promoting increases in serum calcium and relative decreases in calcium excretion. While 986S is more common in PHPT patients overall, it is less frequent, while 990G is more common, in patients with renal stones.

Familial Isolated Hyperparathyroidism

Familial isolated hyperparathyroidism (FIHP or HRPT1; MIM #145000) has been defined as hereditary primary hyperparathyroidism without the association of other disease or tumors (table 1). A small proportion of these cases are variants of the other monogenic diseases – MEN1, HPT-JT or FHH – but additional genes as yet unknown may be involved in the other cases. In some families, FIHP has been linked to a 1.7-Mb region on chromosome 2p13.3–14 but the causative gene has yet to be identified.

Cyclin D1 Oncogene and Parathyroid Neoplasia

To date the only oncogene implicated in parathyroid neoplasia is *CCND1* encoding cyclin D1, originally known as parathyroid adenomatosis 1 (PRAD1) [43]. A few sporadic parathyroid adenomas contain a tumor-specific DNA rearrangement involving a pericentromeric inversion of chromosome 11. This mutation brings the *CCND1* gene under the control of the 5′ regulatory region of the *PTH* gene and causes overexpression of cyclin D1. The tumor cells still possess one intact copy of the *PTH* gene that accounts for expression of PTH by the tumor. The protein cyclin D1 is overexpressed in up to 40% of sporadic parathyroid adenomas and an even higher percentage of carcinomas. The mechanism of the overexpression in the majority of cases remains unclear but likely involves a trans-acting regulatory disturbance rather than a clonal mutation in one gene allele.

Cyclin D1 is a 295-amino acid protein homologous to other members of the cyclin family. Cyclins play important roles in regulation of cell cycle progression, and human cyclins have been grouped into several types based upon sequence similarities. Each cyclin regulates the cell cycle at a specific time point by binding to and activating cyclin-dependent kinases (CDKs). Expression of the cyclins is cell cycle phase-dependent and controlled by both transcriptional and posttranscriptional mechanisms. Cyclin D1 is a key regulator of the critical G1-S phase transition in the cell cycle and its major CDK partners are CDK4 or CDK6, depending upon the tissue type examined.

Animal modeling has provided direct experimental evidence that cyclin D1 overexpression is capable of driving parathyroid tumorigenesis. A transgenic mouse model for parathyroid neoplasia has been generated in which the *CCND1* gene is under the control of the regulatory region of the *PTH* gene, mimicking the rearrangement and resultant overexpression observed in human tumors. These mice develop parathyroid enlargement and increased serum calcium and PTH levels. It had been suggested that mutation of a gene involved in the parathyroid gland calcium set point control might be an initial stimulus for cell proliferation. However, calcium regulatory abnormalities occur at a relative late stage in the transgenic mice with cyclin D1-driven hyperparathyroidism, suggesting that mutations in 'set-point' genes need not be the primary instigators in this disease.

Other Aspects of Parathyroid Tumorigenesis

A single case report documented an R83X mutation in the *PTH* gene predicting a truncation after amino acid 52 of the PTH polypeptide [44]. The patient exhibited hypercalcemia, skeletal changes of primary hyperparathyroidism but undetectable circulating intact PTH. While the patient leukocyte DNA was heterozygous for the mutation, the wild-type allele *PTH* allele had been deleted in the tumor. Hence, the truncated mutant PTH that retained the biological active amino-terminal part was secreted from the gland and was active at PTH target tissues.

Primary hyperparathyroidism occurs with increasing frequency in individuals exposed to neck irradiation. Irrespective of the actual involvement of irradiation, mutations in genes important for DNA repair and recombination may contribute to the tumorigenesis. However, no somatic mutations in the *RAD51* and *RAD54* genes on chromosomes 15q and 1p have been identified even though they are within regions that demonstrate allelic loss in parathyroid adenomas using techniques such as comparative genomic hybridization (CGH). Other regions of chromosomal loss are 6q, 9p and 13q, suggesting tumor suppressor genes, and chromosomal gains at 9q, 16p and 19p hint at the possible loci of still unidentified oncogenes.

Are genes that play an important role in the pathogenesis of other tumor types involved in the pathogenesis of benign parathyroid adenomas? Candidate genes, such as *H-ras, K-ras, N-ras, p53* and *RB,* contribute rarely, or not at all. β-Catenin, a target of the Wnt pathway, and encoded by the *CTNNB1* gene, is implicated in a variety of tumor types. Data from several studies indicate that activating mutations of the regulatory GSK-3β phosphorylation sites at serines 33 and 37 can be seen but are extremely infrequent in parathyroid adenomas [45]. Recently, some studies have suggested altered expression and cellular location of β-catenin may be brought about by other means, including epigenetic modifications.

The tumor suppressor gene, hypermethylated in cancer 1 (*HIC1*), is epigenetically deregulated in hyperparathyroid tumors by histone H3 lysine 27 methylation status modification [46]. A growth-regulatory role of HIC1 in parathyroid glands is suggested and altered expression of *HIC1* may represent an early event in tumor development. While the methylation status of *HIC1* is not consistently abnormal in parathyroid adenomas, it is clearly hypermethylated in parathyroid carcinomas, consistent with its underexpression.

In parathyroid tumors, promoter hypermethylation at CpG sites has been reported in the following tumor suppressor genes: (1) retinoblastoma protein-interacting zinc finger gene (*RIZ1*), a member of the nuclear protein-methyltransferase superfamily; (2) the Ras association (RalGDS/AF6) domain family member gene, *RASSF1A*; (3) the *CDC73* gene, and (4) the adenomatosis polyposis coli gene *(APC)* whose encoded protein acts as an antagonist of the Wnt signaling pathway, Indeed, aberrant WNT/β-catenin signaling in parathyroid carcinoma due to hypermethylation of the *APC* gene has been reported [47].

Recently, an unbiased microchip platform analysis was applied to benign and malignant parathyroid tumors revealing tumor suppressor hypermethylation with associated reduced expression of: (1) *CDKN2A* and *CDKN2B*, encoding CDKIs p15 and p16, respectively; (2) *WT1*, encoding the Wilms' tumor zinc finger transcription factor that can act as a tumor suppressor, and (3) *SFRP1*, *SFRP2* and *SFRP4*, encoding secreted frizzled related proteins that directly interact with Wnts thereby reducing β-catenin levels and regulating cell growth and differentiation [48].

MicroRNAs (miRs) are small noncoding RNAs that function as negative regulators of gene expression through mRNA degradation, translation inhibition, or a chromatin-based silencing mechanism. There are about 800 miRs in humans and some miRs may act as either tumor suppressors or oncogenes that control growth and apoptosis. One study has reported differential expression of a few miRs in human parathyroid carcinomas compared with normal parathyroid tissue [49]. Levels of miR-296 and miR-222 negatively correlated with the mRNA levels of hepatocyte growth factor receptor-regulated tyrosine kinase substrate and p27/Kip1 levels, respectively.

Expression profiling of familial and sporadic parathyroid tumors using a microarray class discovery approach identified three distinct groups: (1) a hyperplastic cluster, (2) a *CDC73* carcinoma cluster, and (3) an adenoma/*MEN1* cluster. The findings largely preclude an adenoma-to-carcinogenesis progression model except in the case of a germline or somatic *CDC73* mutation [50]. A proteomic approach using two-dimensional electrophoresis and mass spectrometry comparing parathyroid adenomas with normal parathyroid tissues identified 20 proteins that were differentially expressed and could be classified into functional categories encompassing biotic stimuli, cell organization, and signal transduction [51].

Most recently, whole exome sequencing was applied to matched tumor-constitutional DNA pairs from patients with sporadic parathyroid adenomas [52]. Selected identified genes were examined further in a large panel of parathyroid adenomas. This revealed a high rate (35%) of *MEN1* mutations and a low frequency of mutations in other genes, one of which was the histone methyltransferase *EZH2* gene.

Conclusions

The study of familial hyperparathyroid syndromes has provided insights into the molecular pathogenesis of the much more common sporadic hyperparathyroidsm. This is most pertinent to the role of *CDC73* mutation in parathyroid carcinoma. Evidence is accumulating that molecular testing for mutations in genes responsible for familial forms of hyperparathyroidism leads to more accurate diagnosis and assessment, and improves patient management and carrier surveillance. Future analysis of epigenetic as well as microRNA changes in sporadic parathyroid tumorigenesis may shed light on cases for which no genetic changes have been identified thus far.

References

1 Starker LF, Akerström T, Long WD, Delgado-Verdugo A, Donovan P, Udelsman R, Lifton RP, Carling T: Frequent germ-line mutations of the MEN1, CASR and HRPT2/CDC73 genes in young patients with clinically non-familial primary hyperparathyroidism. Horm Cancer 2012;3:44–51.

2 Marx SJ: Hyperparathyroid genes: sequences reveal answers and questions. Endocr Pract 2011;17Suppl7:18–27.

3 Thakker RV: Multiple endocrine neoplasia type 1 (MEN1). Best Pract Res Clin Endocrinol Metab 2010;24:355–370.

4 Eller-Vainicher C, Chiodini I, Battista C, Viti R, Mascia ML, Massironi S, Peracchi M, D'Agruma L, Minisola S, Corbetta S, Cole DEC, Spada A, Scillitani A: Sporadic and MEN1-related primary hyperparathyroidism: differences in clinical expression and severity. J Bone Miner Res 2009;24:1404–1410.

5 Lemos MC, Thakker RV: Multiple endocrine neoplasia type 1 (MEN1): analysis of 1336 mutations reported in the first decade following identification of the gene. Hum Mutat 2008;29:22–32.

6 Hendy GN, Kaji H, Canaff L: Cellular functions of menin. Adv Exp Med Biol 2009;668:37–50.

7 Yaguchi H, Ohkura N, Takahashi M, Nagamura Y, Kitabayashi I, Tsukada T: Menin missense mutants associated with multiple endocrine neoplasia type 1 are rapidly degraded via the ubiquitin-proteasome pathway. Mol Cell Biol 2004;24:6569–6580.

8 Canaff L, Vanbellinghen J-F, Kanazawa I, Kwak H, Garfield N, Vautour L, Hendy GN: Menin missense mutants encoded by the *MEN1*gene that are targeted to the proteasome: restoration of expression and activity by CHIP siRNA. J Clin Endocrinol Metab 2012;97:E282–E291.

9 Kaji H, Canaff L, Lebrun J-J, Goltzman D, Hendy GN: Inactivation of menin, a Smad3-interacting protein, blocks transforming growth factor type β signaling. Proc Natl Acad Sci USA 2001;98:3837–3842.

10 Sowa H, Kaji H, Kitazawa R, Kitazawa S, Tsukamoto T, Yano S, Tsukada T, Canaff L, Hendy GN, Sugimoto T, Chihara K: Menin inactivation leads to loss of transforming growth factor beta inhibition of parathyroid cell proliferation and parathyroid hormone secretion. Cancer Res 2004;64:2222–2228.

11 Murai MJ, Chruszcz M, Reddy G, Grembecka J, Cierpicki T: Crystal structure of menin reveals binding site for mixed lineage leukemia (MLL) protein. J Biol Chem 2011;286:31742–31748.

12 Huang J, Gurung B, Wan B, Matkar S, Veniaminova NA, Wan K, Merchant JL, Hua X, Lei M: The same pocket in menin binds both MLL and JUND but has opposite effects on transcription. Nature 2012;482:542–546.

13 Grembecka J, He S, Shi A, Purohit T, Muntean AG, Sorenson RJ, Showalter HD, Murai MJ, Belcher AM, Hartley T, Hess JL, Cierpicki T: Menin-MLL inhibitors reverse oncogenic activity of MLL fusion proteins in leukemia. Nat Chem Biol 2012;8:277–284.

14 Canaff L, Vanbellinghen J-F, Kaji H, Goltzman D, Hendy GN: Impaired transforming growth factor-β (TGF-β) transcriptional activity and cell proliferation control of a menin in-frame deletion mutant associated with multiple endocrine neoplasia type 1 (MEN1). J Biol Chem 2012;287:8584–8597.

15 Crabtree JS, Scacheri PC, Ward JM, Garrett-Beal L, Emmert-Buck MR, Edgemon KA, Lorang D, Libutti SK, Chandrasekharappa SC, Marx SJ, Spiegel AM, Collins FS: A mouse model of multiple endocrine neoplasia, type 1 develops multiple endocrine tumors. Proc Natl Acad Sci USA 2001;98:1118–1123.

16 Bertolino P, Radovanovic I, Casse H, Aguzzi A, Wang ZQ, Zhang CX: Genetic ablation of the tumor suppressor menin causes lethality at mid-gestation with defects in multiple organs. Mech Dev 2003;120:549–560.

17 Engleka KA, Wu M, Zhang M, Antonucci NB, Epstein JA: Menin is required in cranial neural crest for palatogenesis and perinatal viability. Dev Biol 2007;311:524–537.

18 Margraf RL, Crockett DK, Krautscheid PM, Seamons R, Calderon FR, Wittwer CT, Mao R: Multiple endocrine neoplasia type 2 RET protooncogene database: repository of MEN2-associated RET sequence variation and reference for genotype/phenotype correlations. Hum Mutat 2009;30:548–556.

19 Pellegata NS, Quintanilla-Martinez L, Siggelkow H, Samson E, Bink K, Höfler H, Fend F, Graw J, Atkinson MJ : Germ-line mutations in p27Kip1 cause a multiple endocrine neoplasia syndrome in rats and humans. Proc Natl Acad Sci USA 2006;103:15558–15563.

20 Agarwal SK, Mateo CM, Marx SJ: Rare germline mutations in cyclin-dependent kinase inhibitor genes in multiple endocrine neoplasia type 1 and related states. J Clin Endocr Metab 2009;94:1826–1834.

21 Costa-Guda J, Marinoni I, Molatore S, Pellegata NS, Arnold A: Somatic mutation and germline sequence abnormalities in *CDKN1B*, encoding p27Kip1, in sporadic parathyroid adenomas. J Clin Endocrinol Metab 2011;96:E701–E706.

22 Chen JD, Morrison C, Zhang C, Kahnoski K, Carpten JD, Teh BT: Hyperparathyroidism-jaw tumour syndrome. J Intern Med 2003;253:634–642.

23 Carpten JD, Robbins CM, Villablanca A, et al: HRPT2, encoding parafibromin, is mutated in hyperparathyroidism-jaw tumor syndrome. Nat Genet 2002;32:676–680.

24 Newey PJ, Bowl MR, Thakker RV: Parafibromin – functional insights. J Intern Med 2009;266:84–98.
25 Lin L, Czapiga M, Nini L, Zhang J-H, Simonds WF: Nuclear localization of the parafibromin tumor suppressor protein implicated in the hyperparathyroidism-jaw tumor syndrome enhances its proapoptotic function. Mol Cancer Res 2007;5:183–193.
26 Panicker LM, Zhang J-H, Dagur PK, Gastinger MJ, Simonds WF: Defective nucleolar localization and dominant interfering properties of a parafibromin L95P missense mutant causing the hyperparathyroidism-jaw tumor syndrome. Endocr Relat Cancer 2010;17:513–524.
27 Takahashi A, Tsutsumi R, Kikuchi I, Obuse C, Saito Y, Seidi A, Karisch R, Fernandez M, Cho T, Ohnishi N, Rozenblatt-Rosen O, Meyerson M, Neel BG, Hatakeyama M: SHP2 tyrosine phosphatase converts parafibromin/Cdc73 from a tumor suppressor to an oncogenic driver. Molec Cell 2011;43:45–56.
28 Newey PJ, Bowl MR, Cranston T, Thakker RV: Cell division cycle protein 73 homolog (CDC73) mutations in the hyperparathyroidism-jaw tumor syndrome (HPT-JT) and parathyroid tumors. Hum Mutat 2010;31:295–307.
29 Howell VM, Haven CJ, Kahnoski K, et al: HRPT2 mutations are associated with malignancy in sporadic parathyroid tumours. J Med Genet 2003;40: 657–663.
30 Shattuck TM, Valionaki S, Obara T, Gaz RD, Clark OH, Shoback D, Wierman ME, Tojo K, Robbins CM, Carpten JD, Farnebo LO, Larsson C, Arnold A: Somatic and germ-line mutations of the HRPT2 gene in sporadic parathyroid carcinoma. N Engl J Med 2003;349:1722–1729.
31 Guarnieri V, Scillitani A, Muscarella LA, Battista C, Bonfitto N, Bisceglia M, Minisola S, Mascia ML, D'Agruma L, Cole DEC: Diagnosis of parathyroid tumors in familial isolated hyperparathyroidism with *HRPT2* mutation: implications for cancer surveillance. J Clin Endocrinol Metab 2006;91:2827–2832.
32 Frank-Raue K, Haag C, Schulze E, Keuser R, Raue F, Dralle H, Lorenz K: CDC73-related hereditary hyperparathyroidism: five new mutations and the clinical spectrum. Eur J Endocrinol 2011;165:477–483.
33 Tan MH, Morrison C, Wang P, Yang X, Haven CJ, Zhang C, Zhao P, Tretiakova MS, Korpi-Hyovalti E, Burgess JR, Soo KC, Cheah WK, Cao B, Resau J, Morreau H, Teh BT: Loss of parafibromin immunoreactivity is a distinguishing feature of parathyroid carcinoma. Clin Cancer Res 2004;10:6629–6637.
34 Cetani F, Ambrogini E, Viacava P, Pardi E, Fanelli G, Naccarato AG, Borsari S, Lemmi M, Berti P, Miccoli P, Pinchera A, Marcocci C: Should parafibromin staining replace HRPT2 gene analysis as an additional tool for histologic diagnosis of parathyroid carcinoma? Eur J Endocrinol 2007;156:547–554.
35 Brown EM: Clinical lessons from the calcium-sensing receptor. Nat Clin Pract Endocrinol Metab 2007;3:122–133.
36 Hendy GN, Guarnieri V, Canaff L: Calcium-sensing receptor and associated diseases. Prog Mol Biol Transl Sci 2009;89C:31–95.
37 Christensen SE, Nissen PH, Vestergaard P, Mosekilde L: Familial hypocalciuric hypercalcemia: a review. Curr Opin Endocrinol Diabetes Obes 2011;18: 359–370.
38 Reh CM, Hendy GN, Cole DEC, Jeandron DD: Neonatal hyperparathyroidism with a heterozygous calcium-sensing receptor (CASR) R185Q mutation: clinical benefit from cinacalcet, J Clin Endocrinol Metab 2011;96:E707–E712.
39 Koh J, Dar M, Untch BR, Dixit D, Shi Y, Yang Z, Adam MA, Dressman H, Wang X, Gesty-Palmer D, Marks JR, Spurney R, Druey KM, Olson JA Jr: Regulator of G protein signaling 5 is highly expressed in parathyroid tumors and inhibits signaling by the calcium-sensing receptor. Molec Endocrinol 2011; 25:867–876.
40 Canaff L, Hendy GN: Human calcium-sensing receptor gene. Vitamin D response elements in promoters P1 and P2 confer transcriptional responsiveness to 1,25-dihydroxyvitamin D. J Biol Chem 2002;277:30337–30350.
41 Zajickova K, Vrbikova J, Canaff L, Pawelek PD, Goltzman D, Hendy GN: Identification and functional characterization of a novel mutation in the calcium-sensing receptor gene in familial hypocalciuric hypercalcemia: modulation of clinical severity by vitamin D status. J Clin Endocrinol Metab 2007;92:2616–2623.
42 Scillitani A, Guarnieri V, Battista C, De Gerinimo S, Muscarella LA, Chiodini I, Cignarelli M, Minisola S, Bertoldo F, Francucci CM, Malavolta N, Piovesan A, Mascia ML, Muscarella S, Hendy GN, D'Agruma L, Cole DEC: Primary hyperparathyroidism and the presence of kidney stones are associated with different haplotypes of the calcium-sensing receptor. J Clin Endocrinol Metab 2007;92:277–283.
43 Hendy GN, Arnold A: Molecular basis of PTH overexpression; in Bilezikian JP, Martin TJ, Raisz LG (eds): Principles of Bone Biology, ed 3. San Diego, Academic Press, 2008, pp 1311–1326.
44 Au AYM, McDonald K, Gill A, Sywak M, Diamond T, Conigrave AD, Clifton-Bligh RJ: *PTH* mutation with primary hyperparathyroidism and undetectable intact PTH. N Engl J Med 2008;359:1184–1186.
45 Guarnieri V, Baorda F, Battista C, Bisceglia M, Balsamo T, Gruppioni E, Florentino M, Muscarella LA, Coco M, Barbano R, Corbetta S, Spada A, Cole DEC, Canaff L, Hendy GN, Carella, M, Scillitani A: A rare S33C mutation of *CTNNB1* encoding β-catenin in a parathyroid adenoma found in an Italian primary hyperparathyroid cohort. Endocr 2012;41:152–155.

46 Svedlund J, Edblom SK, Marquez VE, Åkerström G, Björklund P, Westin G: Hypermethylated in cancer *(HIC1)*, a tumor suppressor gene epigenetically deregulated in hyperparathyroid tumors by histone H3 lysine modification. J Clin Endocrinol Metab 2012;97:E1307–E1315.

47 Svedlund J, Aurén M, Sundström M, Dralle H, Åkerström G, Björklund P, Westin G: Aberrant WNT/β-catenin signaling in parathyroid carcinoma. Molec Cancer 2010;9:294.

48 Starker LF, Svedlund J, Udelsman R, Dralle H, Åkerström G, Westin G, Lifton RP, Björklund P, Carling T: The DNA methylome of benign and malignant parathyroid tumors. Gene Chromosome Cancer 2011;50:735–745.

49 Corbetta S, Vaira V, Guarnieri V, Scillitani A, Eller-Vainicher C, Ferrero S, Vicentini L, Chiodini I, Bisceglia M, Beck-Peccoz P, Bosari S, Spada A: Differential expression of microRNAs in human parathyroid carcinomas compared with normal tissue. Endocr Relat Cancer 2010;17:135–146.

50 Haven CJ, Howell VM, Eilers PHC, Dunne R, Takahashi M, van Puijenbrock M, Furge K, Kievit J, Tan M-H, Fleuren GJ, Robinson BG, Delbridge LW, Philips J, Nelson AE, Krause U, Dralle H, Hoang-Vu C, Gimm O, Morreau H, Marsh DJ, Teh BT: Gene expression of parathyroid tumors: molecular subclassification and identification of the potential malignant phenotype. Cancer Res 2004;64:7405–7411.

51 Giusti L, Cetani F, Ciregia F, Da Valle V, Donadio E, Giannaccini G, Banti C, Pardi E, Saponaro F, Basolo F, Berti P, Miccoli P, Pinchera A, Marcocci C, Lucacchini A: A proteomic approach to study parathyroid glands. Mol Biosyst 2011;7:687–699.

52 Cromer MK, Starker LF, Choi M, Udelsman R, Nelson-Williams C, Lifton RP, Carling T: Identification of somatic mutations in parathyroid tumors using whole exome sequencing. J Clin Endocrinol Metab 2012;97:E1774–E1781.

Geoffrey N. Hendy
Departments of Medicine, Physiology, and Human Genetics, McGill University, and Calcium Research Laboratory, and Hormones and Cancer Research Unit, Rm. H4.67, Royal Victoria Hospital
687 Pine Avenue West, Montreal, QC H3A 1A1 (Canada)
E-Mail geoffrey.hendy@mcgill.ca

Stratakis CA (ed): Endocrine Tumor Syndromes and Their Genetics.
Front Horm Res. Basel, Karger, 2013, vol 41, pp 166–181 (DOI: 10.1159/000345676)

Endocrine Tumors Associated with Neurofibromatosis Type 1, Peutz-Jeghers Syndrome and Other Familial Neoplasia Syndromes

Esra Kalkan · Steven G. Waguespack

Department of Endocrine Neoplasia and Hormonal Disorders, University of Texas MD Anderson Cancer Center, Houston, Tex., USA

Abstract

Endocrine tumors are a less common but important component of the clinical spectrum of a number of hereditary tumor syndromes such as neurofibromatosis type 1, Peutz–Jeghers syndrome, Beckwith-Wiedemann syndrome, the tuberous sclerosis complex, Li-Fraumeni syndrome, *PTEN* hamartoma tumor syndrome, and *APC*-associated polyposis. It is important to recognize the often unique clinical presentations of these tumors and possible strategies for presymptomatic screening and early diagnosis.

Endocrine tumors can occur within any endocrine gland, and these neoplasms are typically sporadic events without an underlying germline genetic defect. In a minority of cases, an endocrine tumor occurs within the context of a broader tumor-predisposition syndrome such as the multiple endocrine neoplasia syndromes, von Hippel-Lindau disease, Carney complex, and the familial paraganglioma syndromes (reviewed elsewhere). Although not the predominant tumor type, endocrine tumors are also identified within the phenotypic spectrum of several other familial neoplasia syndromes such as neurofibromatosis type 1 (NF1), Peutz-Jeghers syndrome (PJS), Beckwith-Wiedemann syndrome (BWS), the tuberous sclerosis complex (TSC), Li-Fraumeni syndrome (LFS), *PTEN* hamartoma tumor syndrome (PHTS), and *APC*-associated polyposis (table 1). The intent of the current work is to provide an overview of the types of endocrine tumors identified in these genetic syndromes that are less frequently associated with endocrine neoplasia and to highlight the unique clinical aspects of these tumors as well as current recommendations for screening. Because

Table 1. Endocrine neoplasia in hereditary tumor syndromes

	Gene (chromosomal location)	Type(s) of endocrine neoplasia (percent of affected population) and other unique endocrine Issues	Screening guidelines
Beckwith-Wiedemann syndrome	Several genes on chromosome 11p15.5 (BWS critical region)	– ACT (up to 8% of BWS tumors)/ adrenocortical cytomegaly, adrenal hyperplasia – PHEO (case reports) – Thyroid carcinoma (case report) – Neonatal hypoglycemia	– Abdominal ultrasound examination every 3 months until the age of 8 years – Adrenal evaluation if evidence of adrenocortical hyperfunction (hypertension, Cushing's, virilization) or mass effect (back/ flank pain
PTEN hamartoma tumor syndrome (Cowden syndrome, Bannayan-Riley-Ruvalcaba syndrome, *PTEN*-related Proteus syndrome, and Proteus-like syndrome)	*PTEN* (10q23)	– Multiple adenomatous thyroid nodules/multinodular goiter – Thyroid follicular adenomas – DTC (up to 35%) • FTC over-represented	– Yearly thyroid ultrasound beginning at the age of diagnosis
APC-associated polyposis (FAP, attenuated FAP, Gardner syndrome, and Turcot syndrome)	*APC* (5q21–q22)	– ACT (~13%) – PTC (1–2%) • Cribriform-morular histological variant	– No universally accepted guidelines for ACT screening – Adrenal evaluation if evidence of adrenocortical hyperfunction (hypertension, Cushing's, virilization) or mass effect (back/ flank pain – Annual thyroid examination; thyroid US if abnormal physical examination – Consider prospective US screening in female patients starting at age 15, especially those with congenital hyperplasia of the retinal pigment epithelium
Li-Fraumeni syndrome	*TP53* (17p13.1)	– ACT (10%) – Thyroid carcinoma (case reports)	– No universally accepted guidelines for ACT screening – Consider prospective testing for adrenal hyperfunction and obtain serial abdominal ultrasounds in children with LFS – Parent education about the signs and symptoms of virilization and hypercortisolism – Adrenal evaluation if evidence of adrenocortical hyperfunction (hypertension, Cushing's, virilization) or mass effect (back/ flank pain
Neurofibromatosis type 1	*NF1* (17q11.2)	– PHEO/PGL (2-6%) • Composite PHEO (rare) – GEP-NET (<10%) • Primarily peri-ampullary duodenal somatostatinomas but also insulinomas, gastrinomas, and non-functioning tumors – Parathyroid tumors (case reports) – Adrenocortical tumors (case reports) – GH excess and/or central precocious puberty in children with optic glioma (case reports)	– Obtain plasma or urine metanephrines in any NF1 patient with: • Hypertension or other signs/symptoms of catecholamine excess • An incidental adrenal or para-aortic mass – Consider metanephrine testing in women of child-bearing potential who plan to become pregnant and in any patient prior to an elective surgical procedure – No standard recommendation for surveillance of GEP-NET

Table 1. Continued

	Gene (chromosomal location)	Type(s) of endocrine neoplasia (percent of affected population) and other unique endocrine Issues	Screening guidelines
Peutz-Jeghers syndrome	*STK11* (19p13.3)	– Sertoli cell tumors of the testis in males – Ovarian sex cord tumors with annular tubules (SCTAT) in females – DTC (case reports)	– Annual testicular palpation ages 0–12 years – Testicular ultrasound if an abnormal exam or the presence of gynecomastia – No universally accepted guidelines for SCTAT screening – No universally accepted guidelines for DTC screening
Tuberous sclerosis complex	*TSC1*(9q34) *TSC2* (16p13.3)	– GEP-NETs (rare) • Insulinomas predominant – Functional PA (case reports) – Parathyroid adenoma/hyperplasia (case reports) – PHEO (case report)	– No universally accepted guidelines for endocrine neoplasia screening – Low threshold for investigation in patients with *TSC2* mutations who have signs or symptoms of hypoglycemia, including those with worsening neurological symptoms

ACT = Adrenocortical tumor; DTC = differentiated thyroid carcinoma; FTC = follicular thyroid carcinoma; GEP-NET = gastroenteropancreatic neuroendocrine tumors; GH = growth hormone; PA = pituitary adenoma; PGL = paraganglioma; PHEO = pheochromocytoma; PTC = papillary thyroid carcinoma.

these tumors are diagnosed and treated similarly to sporadic endocrine neoplasms, the current review will not focus on those aspects of management.

Neurofibromatosis Type 1

NF1, also known as von Recklinghausen disease, is an autosomal-dominant disorder caused by mutations in the *NF1* gene, a tumor suppressor gene located on chromosome 17 [1]. Almost 50% of cases represent de novo mutations. The *NF1* gene is large with more than 500 mutations identified, and there is significant clinical variability with very poor genotype-phenotype correlations [1]. Therefore, the diagnosis of NF-1 is made on well-established clinical criteria rather than genetic testing [2–4]. Café-au-lait macules, neurofibromas, axillary and inguinal freckling, optic pathway gliomas, skeletal dysplasia, and Lisch nodules of the iris are the main clinical features.

NF-1 patients are at an increased risk of developing benign and malignant tumors [5, 6], and the primary endocrine neoplasias associated with NF1 are pheochromocytoma (PHEO)/paraganglioma (PGL) (fig. 1) and gastroenteropancreatic neuroendocrine tumors (GEP-NET). Several case reports of primary hyperparathyroidism due to benign and malignant parathyroid tumors and adrenocortical tumors have also been reported to occur in NF1 [7–9]. However, it is unclear if mutations in the *NF1* gene are directly involved in the pathogenesis of these tumors. Finally, a unique endocrinopathy associated with NF1 in children with infiltrating optic pathway gliomas is the clinical syndrome of gigantism due to unregulated growth hormone secretion [10].

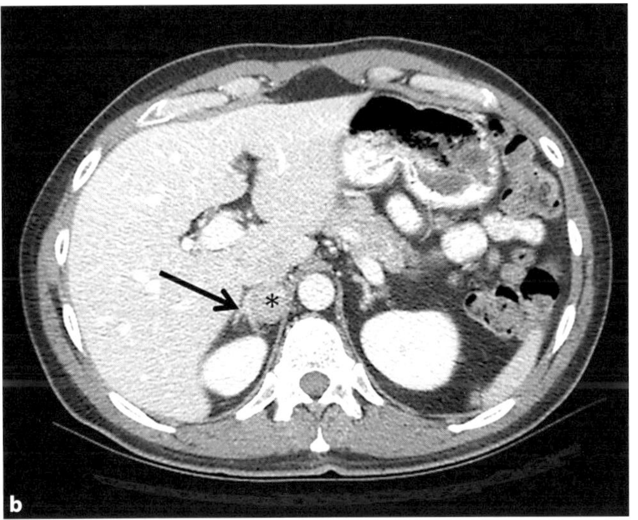

Fig. 1. A 40-year-old man with NF1 and borderline hypertension was found to have a right adrenal mass (white arrow) on a routine MRI (note classic signal hyperintensity on T2-weighted imaging). A 24-hour urine for metanephrines revealed elevated metanephrine levels over 8 times the upper limits of normal and minimally elevated normetanephrine levels. CT scan after contrast revealed a vascular mass (*) arising from the right adrenal gland (black arrow). The patient was prepared for surgery with alpha and beta blockade and a posterior retroperitoneoscopic resection of the right adrenal gland was performed. Pathology revealed a 3.2-cm pheochromocytoma.

Pheochromocytoma/Paraganglioma

PHEO and PGL are rare neuroendocrine neoplasms that arise from the adrenal medulla (PHEO) or extra-adrenal paraganglia (PGL). Functional tumors produce and metabolize catecholamines and can have primary noradrenergic or adrenergic biochemical phenotypes [11, 12]. The diagnosis of PHEO/PGL will be made in 2–6% of NF1 patients.[13, 14] PHEO (10% bilateral) represent the majority of NF1-associated cases but intraabdominal and pelvic PGL are diagnosed in up to 6% [13, 15]. Onset is usually in adulthood (mean age of presentation 41.6 years [15]) and NF1-associated PHEO are characterized by an adrenergic phenotype (elevated epinephrine, norepinephrine, and their metabolites) [12]. Malignancy is uncommon and occurs in about 10% of cases [15]. Rarely, a composite PHEO (a mixed tumor comprised of

PHEO and neuroblastoma, ganglioneuroma, or ganglioneuroblastoma) may occur in the setting of NF1 [16]. Such tumors may portend a more aggressive clinical course [13].

The diagnosis of a catecholamine-producing tumor should be considered in any NF1 patient with hypertension or any other signs or symptoms of catecholamine excess (e.g. palpitations, diaphoresis, headache) [13]. Prospective screening for PHEO/PGL is not recommended for the asymptomatic patient with NF1, unless an incidental adrenal or para-aortic mass is discovered. Screening can also be considered in women of child-bearing potential who plan to become pregnant and in any adult NF1 patient prior to an elective surgical procedure [13].

Gastroenteropancreatic Neuroendocrine Tumors

GEP-NET are an uncommon (<10%) occurrence in NF-1 and are almost exclusively duodenal somatostatinomas that occur in the peri-ampullary region [14, 17]. Age of diagnosis is during the 5th decade of life [17]. NF1-associated somatostatinomas rarely produce the clinical somatostatinoma syndrome and are less frequently associated with metastasis, compared with somatostatinomas of pancreatic origin [18]. These tumors are more likely to present clinically with signs and symptoms due to mass effect or bleeding [14, 17]. Other types of GEP-NETs that have been reported in NF1 patients include insulinomas, gastrinomas, and nonfunctioning pancreatic endocrine tumors [14, 19, 20]. There is no standard recommendation for surveillance of GEP-NET in NF1, although a low threshold for evaluation should exist for any patient with symptoms that would suggest an underlying GEP-NET.

Peutz-Jeghers Syndrome

PJS is an autosomal-dominant syndrome characterized by hamartomatous polyps in the gastrointestinal tract and mucocutaneous hyperpigmentation [21, 22]. The diagnosis of PJS is based on clinical findings and 50% of patients have no family history of the disease [21, 22]. PJS is caused by inactivating mutations in the *STK11 (LKB1)* gene, which encodes for a serine/threonine kinase, and it was the first cancer-susceptibility syndrome to be associated with mutations in a protein kinase [23, 24]. Although most cases of PJS are associated with *STK11* mutations, genetic heterogeneity may exist [25]. Individuals with PJS are at an increased risk for malignancies [26], chiefly luminal gastrointestinal cancers and breast cancer, followed by pancreatic cancer, cervical and ovarian malignancies, and lung cancer. Although there are several case reports of differentiated thyroid cancer occurring in PJS [27], it remains unclear if this is a random occurrence or a direct association with PJS. Outside of the physical examination, prospective screening for thyroid cancer has not been validated [21]. Finally, PJS patients are at risk for unique gonadal tumors that may clinically present with an endocrinopathy: Sertoli cell tumors of the testis in males and ovarian sex cord tumors with annular tubules in females.

Sertoli Cell Tumors of the Testis

Testicular Sertoli cell tumors in PJS are clinically benign lesions that typically occur in prepubertal boys (mean age 6.8 years) who present with gynecomastia and bilateral (rarely unilateral) testicular enlargement [28]. The microscopic findings are distinctive and the term 'intratubular large cell hyalinizing Sertoli cell neoplasia' has been proposed [28]. Calcifications are unusual and not extensive in these lesions, although large-cell calcifying Sertoli cell tumors (similar to those identified in the Carney complex) can also occur within the PJS spectrum [29]. Ultrasonographic evaluation can reveal bilateral echogenic foci and microcalcifications. The gynecomastia is due to estrogen overproduction secondary to high levels of aromatase activity [28], making the use of an aromatase inhibitor a rational approach to medically treating the gynecomastia in such cases [30]. Annual testicular palpation is recommended for male PJS patients starting at birth until 12 years of age, and testicular ultrasound should be obtained in any boy with an abnormal exam or the presence of gynecomastia [21].

Ovarian Sex Cord Tumors with Annular Tubules

Sex cord tumor with annular tubules (SCTATs) is a distinctive neoplasm that has morphologic features that lie between those of a Sertoli cell tumor and a granulosa cell tumor [31]. When occurring in the PJS, these tumors are typically small, calcified, multifocal and bilateral lesions, as compared with non-PJS SCTATs. SCTAT is almost always a benign neoplasm with a mean age of diagnosis of 27 years (range 4–57 years) [31]. Clinical presentation is often due to estrogen overproduction and manifested by menstrual irregularity in postmenarchal women and sexual precocity in prepubertal girls. Abdominal pain and a palpable adnexal mass can also be presenting features, and SCTAT can also be an incidental finding [31]. There are no formal surveillance guidelines for SCTAT or other ovarian tumors in PJS [21], although some groups do recommend prospective pelvic examination, transvaginal ultrasound, and measurement of CA-125 to screen for ovarian malignancy [26].

Beckwith-Wiedemann Syndrome

BWS is a congenital overgrowth disorder associated with abnormal regulation of gene transcription in an imprinted domain on chromosome 11p15.5 (also known as the BWS critical region) [32, 33]. Multiple molecular mechanisms are implicated in pathogenesis, and the majority of BWS cases are sporadic. When familial, the family history is consistent with autosomal dominant transmission and incomplete penetrance. The diagnosis of BWS is primarily based on clinical criteria [32, 33] and can be further confirmed by molecular genetic studies. Major findings include macrosomia and

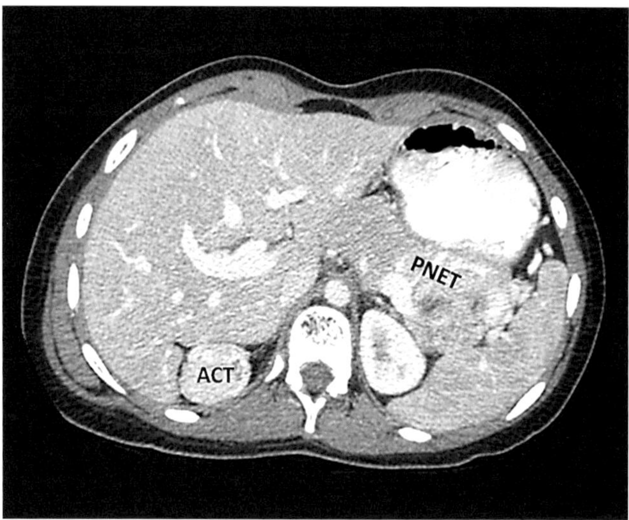

Fig. 2. A 12-year-old girl with Beckwith-Wiedemann syndrome diagnosed as an infant was found to have an adrenal and pancreatic mass on routine radiographic screening, in addition to a fibroadenoma of the breast. She had a history of hemihyperplasia, cleft lip/palate, and bilateral Wilms' tumor, in addition to neonatal hypoglycemia that recurred as a child and that was requiring ongoing treatment with diazoxide. The hormonal evaluation was normal and she was taken to surgery. Pathology confirmed an ACT of the right adrenal and the pancreatic mass was identified to be a multifocal well-differentiated neuroendocrine tumor (PNET). She has had no further hypoglycemia and no recurrence of the ACT or progression of residual PNET during almost 3 years of follow-up.

hemihyperplasia, macroglossia, visceromegaly, embryonal tumors (e.g. Wilms' tumor, hepatoblastoma, neuroblastoma, pancreatoblastoma, and rhabdomyosarcoma), omphalocele, neonatal hypoglycemia, ear creases/pits, adrenocortical tumors/cytomegaly, and renal abnormalities (e.g. medullary dysplasia, nephrocalcinosis, medullary sponge kidney, and nephromegaly). A variety of benign and malignant tumors that are typically restricted to childhood onset have been associated with BWS and occur in up to 7.5% of all cases [33]. Pheochromocytoma and thyroid carcinoma have also been reported [34], but given that there are only isolated cases, it remains unclear if they are truly associated with BWS.

Adrenocortical Tumors

Adrenocortical tumors, both benign and malignant, are among the more common neoplasia identified in BWS (fig. 2), representing up to 8% of benign and 7% of malignant tumors [34]. Fetal adrenocortical cytomegaly (a component of the underlying visceromegaly) and adrenal cystic lesions also occur [34, 35]. The *IGF2* gene is located within the BWS critical region, and overexpression of IGF2 (the effect of which is mediated via the IGF-1 receptor) is observed in the vast majority of sporadic adrenocortical carcinomas, thus suggesting an etiologic role between the IGF-1 receptor signaling pathway and adrenocortical neoplasia [35, 36].

Tumor surveillance in BWS includes quarterly abdominal ultrasound examination every 3 months until the age of 8 years [32]. If an adrenal lesion is suspected based upon screening ultrasound or (at any age) signs/symptoms suggestive of the same, a more comprehensive biochemical and imaging evaluation should be undertaken.

Tuberous Sclerosis Complex

The TSC is an autosomal-dominant, multiorgan hamartomatous disorder characterized by abnormalities of the skin (hypomelanotic macules, facial angiofibromas, shagreen patches, fibrous facial plaques, ungual fibromas); brain (cortical tubers, subependymal nodules and subependymal giant cell astrocytomas, seizures, intellectual disability/developmental delay); kidney (angiomyolipomas, cysts, renal cell carcinomas); heart (rhabdomyomas, arrhythmias), and lungs (lymphangioleiomyomatosis) [37]. Most patients represent de novo cases, and in those with who meet diagnostic criteria for TSC [37, 38], mutations can be identified in about 85%. The two known genes that cause the TSC include *TSC1* and *TSC2*, which encode for the proteins hamartin and tuberin, respectively [39, 40]. The hamartin-tuberin complex is an important negative regulator of the mammalian target of rapamycin (mTOR) signaling and cell growth [41].

Various endocrine neoplasms occurring within the context of the TSC have been reported (reviewed by Dworakowska and Grossman [42]), including functional pituitary adenomas, parathyroid hyperplasia and adenomas, GEP-NETs, and a single case report of a PHEO. The pancreatic NETs can be benign or malignant and functioning or nonfunctioning, with a large proportion of cases associated with *TSC2* gene mutations [43]. It remains unclear if all such tumors are a direct consequence of mutations in *TSC1* or *TSC2*, but evidence from the animal model of TSC [44], reports of very rare endocrine tumors (especially insulinomas) in TSC patients [42], knowledge that abnormalities in the mTOR pathway occur in sporadic GEP-NETs [45], and cases demonstrating loss of heterozygosity in the TSC2 gene [46] would support such an association.

Current recommendations for the care of TSC patients do not include standard screening for endocrine neoplasia. Nevertheless, some groups have suggested that there may be value in broadening the treatment algorithm to include investigation for such tumors, particularly in patients with any signs or symptoms of hypoglycemia, including those with worsening neurological symptoms [42]. It would also seem prudent to have a low threshold for screening for a GEP-NET in a patient with a *TSC2* mutation who has any signs or symptoms that might suggest an underlying pancreatic neuroendocrine tumor.

Li-Fraumeni Syndrome

Dominantly inherited germline mutations in the tumor suppressor gene *TP53* (tumor protein p53) cause the highly penetrant, cancer predisposition syndrome, LFS [47]. Soft tissue and bone sarcomas, premenopausal breast cancer, adrenocortical carcinoma, and brain tumors are considered the core tumors of LFS [48, 49]. Families with incomplete features of LFS are referred to as Li-Fraumeni-like syndrome [49]. Several cases of thyroid carcinoma have also been reported to occur in LFS patients [50].

Adrenocortical Tumors
The adrenal cortex is the third most common site of neoplasia development in LFS [48, 51], and adrenocortical carcinomas represented 10% (4/44) of cancers diagnosed in patients younger than 14 years in the initial report of 24 kindreds with LFS [52]. In one study, 80% (12/15) of patients with adrenocortical carcinoma <age 18 years had a germline *TP53* mutation, including 3 *de novo* cases diagnosed at age ≤2 years [48]. Adrenocortical tumors (ACT) have a very early onset, with diagnosis most common in young children but also seen in adults age <40 years [48, 53, 54]. A child diagnosed with adrenocortical carcinomas may also be the proband for a LFS kindred [55], thus supporting the notion that germline TP53 testing should be a standard of care in all children presenting with an ACT. In southern Brazilian families, the *TP53* mutation Arg337His is associated with a higher susceptibility to isolated ACT in children (median age of diagnosis 3 years; range 4 months to 13.5 years) [56], but recent studies have suggested that this mutation is also associated with other LFS features and is likely a *TP53* mutation with lower penetrance for the other major LFS cancers [57]. During childhood, ACTs typically present with virilization [53, 56], but at all ages, these tumors can present with other signs/symptoms of adrenocortical hyperfunction (such as Cushing syndrome) and/or with symptoms due to tumor mass effect, particularly in the case of nonfunctioning tumors.

Outside of an annual comprehensive physical examination and a high index of suspicion, there are currently no universally accepted screening recommendations for ACT in LFS [58]. However, screening protocols are being researched at several North American institutions [59]. Prospective testing of children with LFS has identified asymptomatic children with an ACT, and an active surveillance program may improve survival in *TP53* mutation carriers [59]. Therefore, it would seem reasonable to prospectively test for adrenal hyperfunction and obtain serial abdominal ultrasounds in a child with LFS. In all cases, parents should be educated about the signs and symptoms of virilization and hypercortisolism. The optimal timing and length of prospective surveillance remains undetermined. As a second primary ACT can occur years after the original ACT diagnosis (fig. 3), it appears important to undertake more diligent and perhaps life-long screening in any patient with a previous history of adrenocortical neoplasia. Patients with a strong family history of ACT may also want to consider more aggressive organ-targeted surveillance [49, 58].

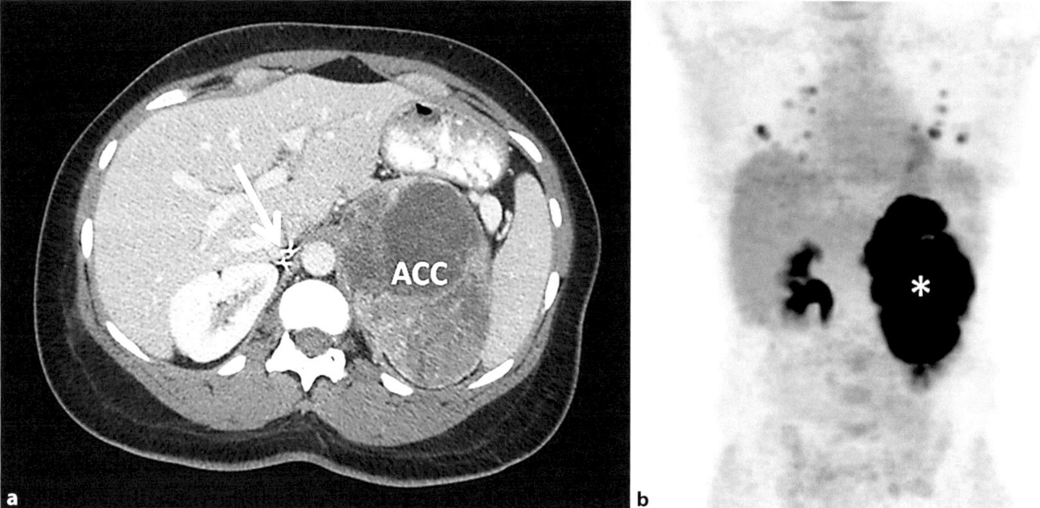

Fig. 3. A 28-year-old with LFS and a history of a functional adrenocortical tumor treated with surgery alone at age 2 years and a juvenile granulosa cell tumor of the ovary diagnosed at age 13 developed hypertension and was ultimately identified to have pulmonary metastases when chest imaging was done for a complaint of chest pain. The patient had clinical evidence of cortisol and androgen hypersecretion. **a** Computerized tomography of the abdomen revealed a large heterogeneous and partially necrotic left ACC and surgical clips related to prior right adrenalectomy (large arrow). **b** FDG-PET scan demonstrated significant uptake in the ACC (*) as well as multiple FDG-avid pulmonary metastases. Despite aggressive medical therapy, she died of disease 9 months after diagnosis.

PTEN Hamartoma Tumor Syndrome

The PHTS results from germline mutations in the *PTEN* (phosphatase and tensin homolog) tumor suppressor gene and is inherited in an autosomal-dominant manner, although the majority of cases are not associated with an obvious family history [60]. The PHTS encompasses the clinical phenotypes of Cowden syndrome (CS), Bannayan-Riley-Ruvalcaba syndrome, *PTEN*-related Proteus syndrome, and Proteus-like syndrome [60, 61]. CS, the most common PHTS phenotype, is a multiple hamartoma syndrome with an increased risk for both benign and malignant tumors arising from the thyroid follicular cell and, in women, the breast and endometrium. Macrocephaly is a consistent finding, occurring in 94% of patients with a PTEN mutation [62], and common skin manifestations include papillomatous papules, trichilemmomas, and acral keratoses. Clinical criteria have been established for the diagnosis of CS and other components of the PHTS [58, 60].

Thyroid Neoplasia

Thyroid neoplasia occurs in the majority of individuals with CS and primarily includes multiple adenomatous nodules (fig. 4), follicular adenomas, and differentiated

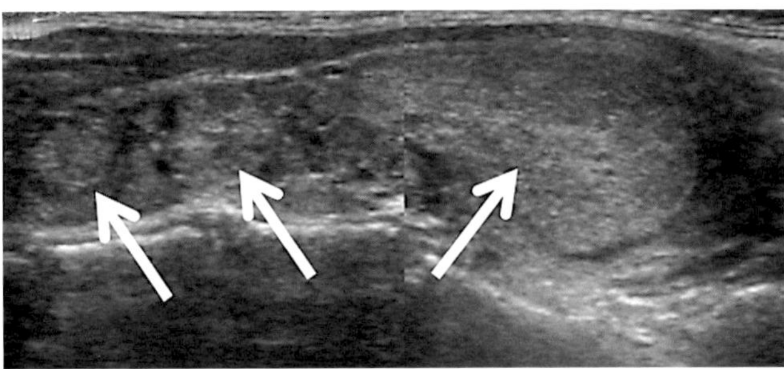

Fig. 4. A 12-year-old girl with CS and a known mutation in the *PTEN* gene was identified to have a multinodular goiter with multiple vascular nodules (arrows) scattered throughout a significantly enlarged thyroid gland. Total thyroidectomy was recommended and pathology demonstrated a multinodular adenomatous goiter without evidence for malignancy.

thyroid carcinoma (papillary and follicular thyroid carcinomas) [63–65]. The risk for thyroid malignancy in patients with deleterious *PTEN* mutations is significantly greater than expected and the lifetime risk may be as high as 35% [66]. Follicular thyroid carcinoma appears to be overrepresented in *PTEN* mutation positive patients [67], but papillary carcinomas are also common [64, 65, 67]. The risk of thyroid neoplasia begins during early childhood, with a reported case of follicular thyroid carcinoma as young as age 7 years [64]. Because of the early onset of thyroid neoplasia, a yearly thyroid ultrasound beginning at the age of diagnosis has been recommended [64, 66].

APC-Associated Polyposis

The *APC*-associated polyposis disorders result from dominantly inherited germline mutations in the *APC* (adenomatous polyposis coli) tumor suppressor gene and include the clinical syndromes of familial adenomatous polyposis (FAP), attenuated FAP, Gardner syndrome, and Turcot syndrome [68]. FAP is the predominant clinical syndrome whereas Gardner syndrome and Turcot syndrome are phenotypic variants associated with osteomas/soft tissue tumors and CNS tumors (namely medulloblastoma), respectively. Patients with an APC mutation are at greatest risk for colon cancer, but 30% or more can develop an extraintestinal manifestation [69], including adrenocortical and thyroid tumors.

Adrenocortical Tumors

Tumors arising from the adrenal cortex are 2–4 times as high in the *APC*-associated polyposis syndromes compared with the general population [69, 70]. In one prospective study, 13% of patients with FAP had an adrenal mass ≥1 cm identified on abdominal CT scan [71]. In patients with an *APC* mutation, adrenocortical tumorigenesis appears to be mediated by biallelic *APC* inactivation, leading to activation of the Wnt/

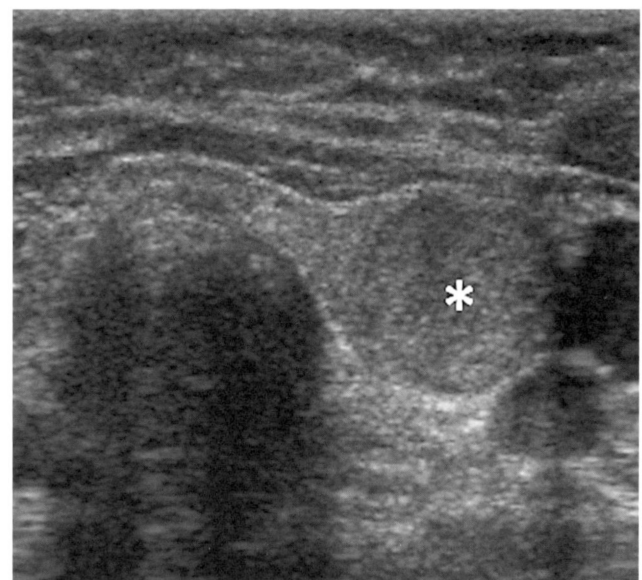

Fig. 5. A 27-year-old woman with a diagnosis of Turcot syndrome (medulloblastoma and diffuse colonic polyposis/colon cancer) and a known *APC* mutation was found to have a thyroid nodule on routine screening ultrasound. Ultrasound revealed an isoechoic to hypoechoic left thyroid lobe nodule (*) without increased vascularity. Fine-needle aspiration biopsy was positive for papillary thyroid cancer, and subsequent surgery was performed, with pathology documenting a unifocal 1.7 cm cribriform-morular variant of PTC.

β-catenin pathway [72]. Similar to sporadic adrenal neoplasia, *APC*-associated ACTs may be hormonally active or non-functioning and may rarely be malignant [9]. Although there are currently no universally accepted guidelines for screening, there should be a low threshold for clinical evaluation in any patient with signs or symptoms of adrenal hyperfunction (e.g. hypertension, weight gain, new diabetes, hirsutism, etc.) or mass effect (unexplained back or flank pain). Incidentally discovered adrenal masses should be managed similar to patients without an *APC* mutation [70, 73].

Papillary Thyroid Carcinoma

Patients with an *APC* mutation have a 1–2% lifetime risk for thyroid malignancy [69], with some studies suggesting a prevalence in FAP patients as high as 12% [74]. The primary subtype is papillary thyroid carcinoma, and it is a diagnosis almost exclusively made in young women during the third decade of life [74–77]. Unique to *APC*-associated PTC is the more common identification of the cribriform-morular histological variant [74, 78] (fig. 5). FAP-associated cribriform-morular PTC is more likely to be a multifocal tumor with a low likelihood of extrathyroidal extension and lymph node metastases, and hence, an excellent prognosis [74, 78, 79].

Prospective screening for thyroid neoplasia is not well established [69], and, at a minimum, should include an annual physical examination of the thyroid, with consideration for prospective screening ultrasound starting at age 15 in females. Screening ultrasound may identify presymptomatic PTC in up to 7% of patients [74]. However, it should be recognized that the cribriform-morular variant of PTC may not have the classic ultrasonographic findings of malignancy [74, 79], and biopsy will still be required for definitive diagnosis. Genotype and a concomitant diagnosis of congenital hyperplasia of the retinal pigment epithelium may predict the risk for thyroid cancer and also help to guide the age at which to initiate ultrasound screening [69, 76].

Conclusion

Endocrine tumors are a less common but important component of the clinical spectrum of a number of hereditary tumor syndromes such as NF1, PJS, BWS, the TSC, LFS, PHTS, and *APC*-associated polyposis. It is important to recognize the often unique clinical presentations of these tumors and possible strategies for presymptomatic screening and early diagnosis.

Acknowledgement

We thank Thereasa A. Rich, MS, CGC, for her thoughtful review of this manuscript.

References

1 Friedman JM: Neurofibromatosis 1; in Pagon RA BT, Dolan CR, et al (ed): GeneReviews™ [Internet]. Seattle, University of Washington, 1998.

2 National Institutes of Health consensus development conference statement: Neurofibromatosis. Bethesda, 1987. Neurofibromatosis 1988;1:172–178.

3 Ferner RE: Neurofibromatosis 1. Eur J Hum Genet 2007;15:131–138.

4 Williams VC, Lucas J, Babcock MA, Gutmann DH, Korf B, Maria BL: Neurofibromatosis type 1 revisited. Pediatrics 2009;123:124–133.

5 Walker L, Thompson D, Easton D, Ponder B, Ponder M, Frayling I, Baralle D: A prospective study of neurofibromatosis type 1 cancer incidence in the UK. Br J Cancer 2006;95:233–238.

6 Brems H, Beert E, de Ravel T, Legius E: Mechanisms in the pathogenesis of malignant tumours in neurofibromatosis type 1. Lancet Oncol 2009;10:508–515.

7 Kodama H, Iihara M, Okamoto T, Obara T: Water-clear cell parathyroid adenoma causing primary hyperparathyroidism in a patient with neurofibromatosis type 1: report of a case. Surg Today 2007;37: 884–887.

8 Demirjian AN, Grossman JM, Chan JL, Parangi S: Parathyroid carcinoma and neurofibromatosis. Surgery 2008;144:827–829.

9 Else T: Association of adrenocortical carcinoma with familial cancer susceptibility syndromes. Mol Cell Endocrinol 2012;351:66–70.

10 Josefson J, Listernick R, Fangusaro JR, Charrow J, Habiby R: Growth hormone excess in children with neurofibromatosis type 1-associated and sporadic optic pathway tumors. J Pediatr 2011;158:433–436.

11 Waguespack SG, Rich T, Grubbs E, Ying AK, Perrier ND, Ayala-Ramirez M, Jimenez C: A current review of the etiology, diagnosis, and treatment of pediatric pheochromocytoma and paraganglioma. J Clin Endocrinol Metab 2010;95:2023–2037.

12 Eisenhofer G, Pacak K, Huynh TT, Qin N, Bratslavsky G, Linehan WM, Mannelli M, Friberg P, Grebe SK, Timmers HJ, Bornstein SR, Lenders JW: Catecholamine metabolomic and secretory phenotypes in phaeochromocytoma. Endocr Relat Cancer 2011;18:97–111.

13 Walther MM, Herring J, Enquist E, Keiser HR, Linehan WM: Von Recklinghausen's disease and pheochromocytomas. J Urol 1999;162:1582–1586.

14 Jensen RT, Berna MJ, Bingham DB, Norton JA: Inherited pancreatic endocrine tumor syndromes: advances in molecular pathogenesis, diagnosis, management, and controversies. Cancer 2008;113: 1807–1843.

15 Welander J, Soderkvist P, Gimm O: Genetics and clinical characteristics of hereditary pheochromocytomas and paragangliomas. Endocr Relat Cancer 2011;18:R253–R276.

16 Kimura N, Watanabe T, Fukase M, Wakita A, Noshiro T, Kimura I: Neurofibromin and nf1 gene analysis in composite pheochromocytoma and tumors associated with von Recklinghausen's disease. Mod Pathol 2002;15:183–188.

17 Relles D, Baek J, Witkiewicz A, Yeo CJ: Periampullary and duodenal neoplasms in neurofibromatosis type 1: two cases and an updated 20-year review of the literature yielding 76 cases. J Gastrointest Surg 2010;14:1052–1061.

18 Mao C, Shah A, Hanson DJ, Howard JM: Von Recklinghausen's disease associated with duodenal somatostatinoma: contrast of duodenal versus pancreatic somatostatinomas. J Surg Oncol 1995;59: 67–73.

19 Perren A, Wiesli P, Schmid S, Montani M, Schmitt A, Schmid C, Moch H, Komminoth P: Pancreatic endocrine tumors are a rare manifestation of the neurofibromatosis type 1 phenotype: molecular analysis of a malignant insulinoma in a NF-1 patient. Am J Surg Pathol 2006;30:1047–1051.

20 Lee WS, Koh YS, Kim JC, Park CH, Joo YE, Kim HS, Cho CK, Choi SK, Rew JS, Kim SJ: Zollinger-Ellison syndrome associated with neurofibromatosis type 1: a case report. BMC Cancer 2005;5:85.

21 Beggs AD, Latchford AR, Vasen HF, et al: Peutz-Jeghers syndrome: a systematic review and recommendations for management. Gut 2010;59:975–986.

22 Amos CI, Frazier ML, Wei C, McGarrity TJ: Peutz-jeghers syndrome; in Pagon RA BT, Dolan CR, et al (eds): GeneReviews™ [Internet]. Seattle, University of Washington, 2001.

23 Jenne DE, Reimann H, Nezu J, Friedel W, Loff S, Jeschke R, Muller O, Back W, Zimmer M: Peutz-Jeghers syndrome is caused by mutations in a novel serine threonine kinase. Nat Genet 1998;18:38–43.

24 Hemminki A, Markie D, Tomlinson I, et al: A serine/threonine kinase gene defective in Peutz-Jeghers syndrome. Nature 1998;391:184–187.

25 Olschwang S, Boisson C, Thomas G: Peutz-jeghers families unlinked to stk11/lkb1 gene mutations are highly predisposed to primitive biliary adenocarcinoma. J Med Genet 2001;38:356–360.

26 van Lier MG, Wagner A, Mathus-Vliegen EM, Kuipers EJ, Steyerberg EW, van Leerdam ME: High cancer risk in Peutz-Jeghers syndrome: a systematic review and surveillance recommendations. Am J Gastroenterol 2010;105:1258–1264; author reply 1265.

27 Triggiani V, Guastamacchia E, Renzulli G, Giagulli VA, Tafaro E, Licchelli B, Resta F, Sabba C, Bagnulo R, Lastella P, Stella A, Resta N: Papillary thyroid carcinoma in Peutz-Jeghers syndrome. Thyroid 2011;21:1273–1277.

28 Ulbright TM, Amin MB, Young RH: Intratubular large cell hyalinizing sertoli cell neoplasia of the testis: a report of 8 cases of a distinctive lesion of the peutz-jeghers syndrome. Am J Surg Pathol 2007;31: 827–835.

29 Dreyer L, Jacyk WK, du Plessis DJ: Bilateral large-cell calcifying sertoli cell tumor of the testes with Peutz-Jeghers syndrome: a case report. Pediatr Dermatol 1994;11:335–337.

30 Lefevre H, Bouvattier C, Lahlou N, Adamsbaum C, Bougneres P, Carel JC: Prepubertal gynecomastia in Peutz-Jeghers syndrome: incomplete penetrance in a familial case and management with an aromatase inhibitor. Eur J Endocrinol 2006;154:221–227.

31 Young RH, Welch WR, Dickersin GR, Scully RE: Ovarian sex cord tumor with annular tubules: review of 74 cases including 27 with Peutz-Jeghers syndrome and four with adenoma malignum of the cervix. Cancer 1982;50:1384–1402.

32 Shuman C, Beckwith JB, Smith AC, Weksberg R: Beckwith-Wiedemann syndrome; in Pagon RA BT, Dolan CR, et al (eds): GeneReviews™ [Internet]. Seattle, University of Washington, 2000.

33 Cohen MM Jr: Beckwith-Wiedemann syndrome: historical, clinicopathological, and etiopathogenetic perspectives. Pediatr Dev Pathol 2005;8:287–304.

34 Lapunzina P: Risk of tumorigenesis in overgrowth syndromes: a comprehensive review. Am J Med Genet C Semin Med Genet 2005;137C:53–71.

35 Ribeiro RC, Pinto EM, Zambetti GP: Familial predisposition to adrenocortical tumors: clinical and biological features and management strategies. Best Pract Res Clin Endocrinol Metab 2010;24:477–490.

36 Fassnacht M, Libe R, Kroiss M, Allolio B: Adrenocortical carcinoma: a clinician's update. Nat Rev Endocrinol 2011;7:323–335.

37 Northrup H, Koenig MK, Au KS: Tuberous sclerosis complex; in Pagon RA BT, Dolan CR, et al (eds): GeneReviews™ [Internet]. Seattle, University of Washington, 1999.

38 Roach ES, Sparagana SP: Diagnosis of tuberous sclerosis complex. J Child Neurol 2004;19:643–649.

39 European Chromosome 16 Tuberous Sclerosis Consortium: Identification and characterization of the tuberous sclerosis gene on chromosome 16. Cell 1993;75:1305–1315.

40 van Slegtenhorst M, de Hoogt R, Hermans C, et al: Identification of the tuberous sclerosis gene tsc1 on chromosome 9q34. Science 1997;277:805–808.

41 Huang J, Wu S, Wu CL, Manning BD: Signaling events downstream of mammalian target of rapamycin complex 2 are attenuated in cells and tumors deficient for the tuberous sclerosis complex tumor suppressors. Cancer Res 2009;69:6107–6114.

42 Dworakowska D, Grossman AB: Are neuroendocrine tumours a feature of tuberous sclerosis? A systematic review. Endocr Relat Cancer 2009;16:45–58.

43 Arva NC, Pappas JG, Bhatla T, Raetz EA, Macari M, Ginsburg HB, Hajdu CH: Well-differentiated pancreatic neuroendocrine carcinoma in tuberous sclerosis – case report and review of the literature. Am J Surg Pathol 2012;36:149–153.

44 Fukuda T, Kobayashi T, Yasui H, Tsutsumi M, Konishi Y, Hino O: Distribution of tsc2 protein in various normal rat tissues and renal tumours of tsc2 mutant (eker) rat detected by immunohistochemistry. Virchows Arch 1999;434:341–350.

45 Kasajima A, Pavel M, Darb-Esfahani S, Noske A, Stenzinger A, Sasano H, Dietel M, Denkert C, Rocken C, Wiedenmann B, Weichert W: Mtor expression and activity patterns in gastroenteropancreatic neuroendocrine tumours. Endocr Relat Cancer 2011;18:181–192.

46 Francalanci P, Diomedi-Camassei F, Purificato C, Santorelli FM, Giannotti A, Dominici C, Inserra A, Boldrini R: Malignant pancreatic endocrine tumor in a child with tuberous sclerosis. Am J Surg Pathol 2003;27:1386–1389.

47 Malkin D, Li FP, Strong LC, Fraumeni JF Jr, Nelson CE, Kim DH, Kassel J, Gryka MA, Bischoff FZ, Tainsky MA, et al: Germ line p53 mutations in a familial syndrome of breast cancer, sarcomas, and other neoplasms. Science 1990;250:1233–1238.

48 Gonzalez KD, Noltner KA, Buzin CH, Gu D, Wen-Fong CY, Nguyen VQ, Han JH, Lowstuter K, Longmate J, Sommer SS, Weitzel JN: Beyond Li Fraumeni syndrome: clinical characteristics of families with p53 germline mutations. J Clin Oncol 2009;27:1250–1256.

49 Schneider K, Garber J: Li-Fraumeni syndrome; in Pagon RA BT, Dolan CR, et al (eds): GeneReviews™ [Internet]. Seattle, University of Washington, 1999.

50 Masciari S, Van den Abbeele AD, Diller LR, Rastarhuyeva I, Yap J, Schneider K, Digianni L, Li FP, Fraumeni JF Jr, Syngal S, Garber JE: F18-fluorodeoxyglucose-positron emission tomography/computed tomography screening in Li-Fraumeni syndrome. JAMA 2008;299:1315–1319.

51 Olivier M, Hollstein M, Hainaut P: Tp53 mutations in human cancers: origins, consequences, and clinical use. Cold Spring Harb Perspect Biol 2010;2:a001008.

52 Li FP, Fraumeni JF Jr, Mulvihill JJ, Blattner WA, Dreyfus MG, Tucker MA, Miller RW: A cancer family syndrome in twenty-four kindreds. Cancer Res 1988;48:5358–5362.

53 Ribeiro RC, Pinto EM, Zambetti GP, Rodriguez-Galindo C: The international pediatric adrenocortical tumor registry initiative: contributions to clinical, biological, and treatment advances in pediatric adrenocortical tumors. Mol Cell Endocrinol 2012;351:37–43.

54 Herrmann LJ, Heinze B, Fassnacht M, Willenberg HS, Quinkler M, Reisch N, Zink M, Allolio B, Hahner S: Tp53 germline mutations in adult patients with adrenocortical carcinoma. J Clin Endocrinol Metab 2012;97:E476–E485.

55 Choong S, Latiff Z, Mohamed M, Lim L, Chen K, Vengidasan L, Razali H, Abdul Rahman E, Ariffin H: Childhood adrenocortical carcinoma as a sentinel cancer for detecting families with germline tp53 mutations. Clin Genet 2012;82:564–568.

56 Ribeiro RC, Sandrini F, Figueiredo B, Zambetti GP, Michalkiewicz E, Lafferty AR, DeLacerda L, Rabin M, Cadwell C, Sampaio G, Cat I, Stratakis CA, Sandrini R: An inherited p53 mutation that contributes in a tissue-specific manner to pediatric adrenal cortical carcinoma. Proc Natl Acad Sci USA 2001;98:9330–9335.

57 Achatz MI, Olivier M, Le Calvez F, Martel-Planche G, Lopes A, Rossi BM, Ashton-Prolla P, Giugliani R, Palmero EI, Vargas FR, Da Rocha JC, Vettore AL, Hainaut P: The tp53 mutation, r337h, is associated with Li-Fraumeni and Li-Fraumeni-like syndromes in Brazilian families. Cancer Lett 2007;245:96–102.

58 National Comprehensive Cancer Network: Genetic/familial high-risk assessment: Breast and ovarian: NCCN Clinical Practice Guidelines in Oncology (NCCN Guidelines) 2012, Version 1.2012.

59 Villani A, Tabori U, Schiffman J, Shlien A, Beyene J, Druker H, Novokmet A, Finlay J, Malkin D: Biochemical and imaging surveillance in germline tp53 mutation carriers with Li-Fraumeni syndrome: a prospective observational study. Lancet Oncol 2011;12:559–567.

60 Eng C: PTEN hamartoma tumor syndrome (PHTS); in Pagon RA BT, Dolan CR, et al (ed): GeneReviews™ [Internet]. Seattle, University of Washington, 2001.

61 Liaw D, Marsh DJ, Li J, Dahia PL, Wang SI, Zheng Z, Bose S, Call KM, Tsou HC, Peacocke M, Eng C, Parsons R: Germline mutations of the pten gene in Cowden disease, an inherited breast and thyroid cancer syndrome. Nat Genet 1997;16:64–67.

62 Mester JL, Tilot AK, Rybicki LA, Frazier TW 2nd, Eng C: Analysis of prevalence and degree of macrocephaly in patients with germline PTEN mutations and of brain weight in PTEN knock-in murine model. Eur J Hum Genet 2011;19:763–768.

63 Harach HR, Soubeyran I, Brown A, Bonneau D, Longy M: Thyroid pathologic findings in patients with Cowden disease. Ann Diagn Pathol 1999;3:331–340.

64 Smith JR, Marqusee E, Webb S, Nose V, Fishman SJ, Shamberger RC, Frates MC, Huang SA: Thyroid nodules and cancer in children with PTEN hamartoma tumor syndrome. J Clin Endocrinol Metab 2011;96:34–37.
65 Laury AR, Bongiovanni M, Tille JC, Kozakewich H, Nose V: Thyroid pathology in PTEN-hamartoma tumor syndrome: characteristic findings of a distinct entity. Thyroid 2011;21:135–144.
66 Tan MH, Mester JL, Ngeow J, Rybicki LA, Orloff MS, Eng C: Lifetime cancer risks in individuals with germline PTEN mutations. Clin Cancer Res 2012;18:400–407.
67 Ngeow J, Mester J, Rybicki LA, Ni Y, Milas M, Eng C: Incidence and clinical characteristics of thyroid cancer in prospective series of individuals with Cowden and Cowden-like syndrome characterized by germline PTEN, SDH, or KLLN alterations. J Clin Endocrinol Metab 2011;96:E2063–E2071.
68 Jasperson KW, Burt RW: Apc-associated polyposis conditions; in Pagon RA BT, Dolan CR, et al (eds): GeneReviews™ [Internet]. Seattle, University of Washington, 1998.
69 Groen EJ, Roos A, Muntinghe FL, Enting RH, de Vries J, Kleibeuker JH, Witjes MJ, Links TP, van Beek AP: Extra-intestinal manifestations of familial adenomatous polyposis. Ann Surg Oncol 2008; 15:2439–2450.
70 Marchesa P, Fazio VW, Church JM, McGannon E: Adrenal masses in patients with familial adenomatous polyposis. Dis Colon Rectum 1997;40:1023–1028.
71 Smith TG, Clark SK, Katz DE, Reznek RH, Phillips RK: Adrenal masses are associated with familial adenomatous polyposis. Dis Colon Rectum 2000; 43:1739–1742.
72 Gaujoux S, Pinson S, Gimenez-Roqueplo AP, Amar L, Ragazzon B, Launay P, Meatchi T, Libe R, Bertagna X, Audebourg A, Zucman-Rossi J, Tissier F, Bertherat J: Inactivation of the *APC* gene is constant in adrenocortical tumors from patients with familial adenomatous polyposis but not frequent in sporadic adrenocortical cancers. Clin Cancer Res 2010; 16:5133–5141.
73 Will OC, Hansmann A, Phillips RK, Palazzo FF, Meeran K, Marshall M, Clark SK: Adrenal incidentaloma in familial adenomatous polyposis: a long-term follow-up study and schema for management. Dis Colon Rectum 2009;52:1637–1644.
74 Herraiz M, Barbesino G, Faquin W, Chan-Smutko G, Patel D, Shannon KM, Daniels GH, Chung DC: Prevalence of thyroid cancer in familial adenomatous polyposis syndrome and the role of screening ultrasound examinations. Clin Gastroenterol Hepatol 2007;5:367–373.
75 Plail RO, Bussey HJ, Glazer G, Thomson JP: Adenomatous polyposis: An association with carcinoma of the thyroid. Br J Surg 1987;74:377–380.
76 Cetta F, Montalto G, Gori M, Curia MC, Cama A, Olschwang S: Germline mutations of the *APC* gene in patients with familial adenomatous polyposis-associated thyroid carcinoma: results from a European cooperative study. J Clin Endocrinol Metab 2000;85:286–292.
77 Truta B, Allen BA, Conrad PG, Kim YS, Berk T, Gallinger S, Bapat B, Terdiman JP, Sleisenger MH: Genotype and phenotype of patients with both familial adenomatous polyposis and thyroid carcinoma. Fam Cancer 2003;2:95–99.
78 Ito Y, Miyauchi A, Ishikawa H, Hirokawa M, Kudo T, Tomoda C, Miya A: Our experience of treatment of cribriform morular variant of papillary thyroid carcinoma: difference in clinicopathological features of FAP-associated and sporadic patients. Endocr J 2011;58:685–689.
79 Chong Y, Shin JH, Oh YL, Han BK, Ko EY: Cribriform-morular variant of papillary thyroid carcinoma: US and clinical characteristics. Thyroid 2012;Epub

Steven G. Waguespack, MD, Associate Professor
Department of Endocrine Neoplasia and Hormonal Disorders, University of Texas MD Anderson Cancer Center, PO Box 301402, Unit 1461
Houston TX 77230–1402 (USA)
E-Mail swagues@mdanderson.org

Author Index

Subject Index